Elsevier's Integrated
Pharmacology

Elsevier's Integrated
Pharmacology

Mark Kester PhD
Distinguished Professor of Pharmacology
Professor of Cellular and Molecular Physiology
Penn State College of Medicine

Kent E. Vrana PhD
Elliot S. Vesell Professor
Chair, Department of Pharmacology
Penn State College of Medicine

Sadeq A. Quraishi MD, MHA
Instructor, World Campus Graduate School Program
on Homeland Security in Public Health Preparedness
Pennsylvania State University
Resident, Department of Anesthesiology
Milton S. Hershey Medical Center
Penn State College of Medicine

Kelly Dowhower Karpa PhD, RPh
Assistant Professor, Department of Pharmacology
Penn State College of Medicine

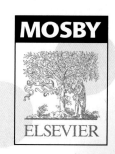

MOSBY

ELSEVIER

1600 John F. Kennedy Blvd
Suite 1800
Philadelphia, PA 19103-2899

ELSEVIER'S INTEGRATED PHARMACOLOGY   ISBN-13: 978-0-323-03408-1

Notice

Knowledge and best practice in this field are constantly changing. As new research and experience broaden our knowledge, changes in practice, treatment and drug therapy may become necessary or appropriate. Readers are advised to check the most current information provided (i) on procedures featured or (ii) by the manufacturer of each product to be administered, to verify the recommended dose or formula, the method and duration of administration, and contraindications. It is the responsibility of the practitioner, relying on their own experience and knowledge of the patient, to make diagnoses, to determine dosages and the best treatment for each individual patient, and to take all appropriate safety precautions. To the fullest extent of the law, neither the Publisher nor the Authors assume any liability for any injury and/or damage to persons or property arising out or related to any use of the material contained in this book.

The Publisher

Library of Congress Cataloging-in-Publication Data

Kester, Mark.
  Elsevier's integrated pharmacology / Mark Kester, Kent E. Vrana, Sadeq A. Quraishi, and Kelly D. Karpa.—1st ed.
    p. ; cm.
  ISBN 978-0-323-03408-1
  1. Drugs—Administration. 2. Pharmacology. 3. Therapeutics. I. Vrana, Kent E. II. Quraishi, Sadeq A. III. Karpa, Kelly D. IV. Title. V. Title: Integrated pharmacology.
  [DNLM: 1. Pharmacology Preparations. 2. Drug Therapy. 3. Pharmacologic Actions.
4. Pharmacology—methods. QV 55 K42e 2007]
RM125.K47 2007
615'.1—dc22

                                                                              2006044859

Acquisitions Editor: Kate Dimock
Developmental Editor: Andrew Hall

Printed in China

Last digit is the print number: 9 8 7 6 5 4 3 2 1

To my past, present, and future: Lee and Allen Kester,
Karen Kester, and Johanna and Saul Kester.
MK

To my best friend, confidant, and wife, Sheila,
and the two reasons I do what I do—Caroline and Erin.
KEV

I wish to thank the individuals who have aided and
encouraged me through the years, making this book a reality,
including the Dowhower and Karpa parents, Barry, Patricia,
Karl, and Linda Lee. I would especially like to recognize my
husband, Karl, and my children, Kyle and Kieri, for their
unconditional love and unwavering support.
KDK

Finally, to Professor Elliott Saul Vesell
(founding Chair of Penn State Pharmacology),
for putting the "art" in Pharmacology.

Preface

It's all about integration. In fact, integration is essential for the study of pharmacology. Practitioners must consider mechanisms of action, adverse effects, and contraindications for any given drug to ensure proper and safe use by patients. Crucial to these considerations is a thorough understanding of the biochemistry, physiology, and anatomy of the targets affected by the drug. Thus, the overarching concept of the Elsevier series of integrated review texts is to consider each basic science discipline within the overall context of all the other basic sciences. The foundation of clinical medicine requires that all basic sciences be integrated across disciplines. To facilitate this important learning paradigm, we have created Integration Boxes that highlight an essential pharmacologic principal that can be dramatically reinforced with information from another basic or clinical science discipline. This mode of learning facilitates deeper understanding and more complete memory of the concept.

It's also all about forging a team. Frequently, pharmacology is taught by basic research-based scientists only. We have taken a different and more dynamic approach. The authors of *Elsevier's Integrated Pharmacology* comprise basic science researchers and educators, as well as a pharmacist and a clinician. It is our concept that integration must occur not only between "-ologies" but also between practitioners who prescribe, dispense, and create drugs. In this way, in one voice, basic research scientists can effectively describe mechanisms of action for a drug, the clinician can highlight adverse effects, and the pharmacist can discuss potential drug interactions with other drugs or complementary alternative medicines. It is these coordinated interactions between Ph.D.s., M.D.s and PharmDs that are now the core of Penn State College of Medicine's clinically relevant and organ-based pharmacology curriculum.

It is also about voice—one consistent voice. Each chapter reflects the input of each of the four authors, reflecting an integration of basic, clinical, and pharmaceutical sciences. Each chapter includes Top 5 Lists of important concepts and case-based learning questions that reinforce the Integration Boxes.

In the end, it's all about the students. *Elsevier's Integrated Pharmacology* provides students with a rich tapestry from which to draw conclusions about specific drug classes. Detailed information is provided for major drugs in each of the classes. More importantly, this book provides students with the tools necessary to deal with the myriad new drugs that are presently moving through pharmaceutical drug evaluation "pipelines" or are first being contemplated or discovered by academic or industrial scientists. For the student, it should be more than just memorization of every minor adverse side effect for each and every drug. It's really about applying the principles of pharmacology to evaluate and assess the usefulness and effectiveness of new drugs as they come to market. Indeed, a core competency for the health care professional of the 21st century is to become a life-long learner. We hope that we have provided the pharmacologic foundation for such an educational journey.

Mark Kester, PhD
Kent E. Vrana, PhD
Sadeq A. Quraishi, MD, MHA
Kelly Dowhower Karpa, PhD, RPh

Acknowledgments

To our editors at Elsevier:

To Alex Stibbe, whose "integrative" vision is now an educational reality.

To Andrew Hall, who had to be constantly reminded that there is no such thing as a "hard and fast" deadline. Andy, more than anyone else, ensured that this labor-of-love came to fruition.

And to Kate Dimock, who joined the team as we finished this project.

To Eileen Mitchell and the team at Electronic Publishing Services, Inc. (EPS), who masterfully changed our stick figures into elegant illustrations.

To our many basic and clinical science resources: Dr. Robert Zelis, Penn State College of Medicine; Dr. Cheston Berlin, Penn State College of Medicine; Dr. Michael White, Drexel University; Dr. Kevin Mulieri, Hershey Medical Center; and Dr. Dominic Solimando, Jr., Oncology Pharmacy Services, Inc.

To the hard-working Penn State College of Medicine medical students of the classes of 2007 and 2008, who provided valuable feedback concerning selected chapters and subject materials (especifically Ms. Nina Manni).

For administrative and secretarial assistance, Ms. Elaine Neidigh, Ms. Kristi Bracale, Ms. Maxine Gerberich, and Ms. Vicki Condran.

To all of the above, we offer our heartfelt gratitude and appreciation of the fact that you can all work so well with such difficult personalities as ours.

Editorial Review Board

Contents

Series Preface

How to Use This Book

The idea for Elsevier's Integrated Series came about at a seminar on the USMLE Step 1 exam at an American Medical Student Association (AMSA) meeting. We noticed that the discussion between faculty and students focused on how the exams were becoming increasingly integrated—with case scenarios and questions often combining two or three science disciplines. The students were clearly concerned about how they could best integrate their basic science knowledge.

One faculty member gave some interesting advice: "read through your textbook in, say, biochemistry, and every time you come across a section that mentions a concept or piece of information relating to another basic science—for example, immunology—highlight that section in the book. Then go to your immunology textbook and look up this information, and make sure you have a good understanding of it. When you have, go back to your biochemistry textbook and carry on reading."

This was a great suggestion—if only students had the time, and all of the books necessary at hand, to do it! At Elsevier we thought long and hard about a way of simplifying this process, and eventually the idea for Elsevier's Integrated Series was born.

The series centers on the concept of the *integration box*. These boxes occur throughout the text whenever a link to another basic science is relevant. They're easy to spot in the text—with their color-coded headings and logos. Each box contains a title for the integration topic and then a brief summary of the topic. The information is complete in itself—you probably won't have to go to any other sources—and you have the basic knowledge to use as a foundation if you want to expand your knowledge of the topic.

You can use this book in two ways. First, as a review book . . . When you are using the book for review, the integration boxes will jog your memory on topics you have already covered. You'll be able to reassure yourself that you can identify the link, and you can quickly compare your knowledge of the topic with the summary in the box. The integration boxes might highlight gaps in your knowledge, and then you can use them to determine what topics you need to cover in more detail.

Second, the book can be used as a short text to have at hand while you are taking your course . . . You may come across an integration box that deals with a topic you haven't covered yet, and this will ensure that you're one step ahead in identifying the links to other subjects (especially useful if you're working on a PBL exercise). On a simpler level, the links in the boxes to other sciences and to clinical medicine will help you see clearly the relevance of the basic science topic you are studying. You may already be confident in the subject matter of many of the integration boxes, so they will serve as helpful reminders.

At the back of the book we have included case study questions relating to each chapter so that you can test yourself as you work your way through the book.

Online Version

An online version of the book is available on our Student Consult site. Use of this site is free to anyone who has bought the printed book. Please see the inside front cover for full details on the Student Consult and how to access the electronic version of this book.

In addition to containing USMLE test questions, fully searchable text, and an image bank, the Student Consult site offers additional integration links, both to the other books in Elsevier's Integrated Series and to other key Elsevier textbooks.

Books in Elsevier's Integrated Series

The nine books in the series cover all of the basic sciences. The more books you buy in the series, the more links that are made accessible across the series, both in print and online.

 Anatomy and Embryology

 Histology

 Neuroscience

 Biochemistry

 Physiology

 Pathology

 Immunology and Microbiology

 Pharmacology

 Genetics

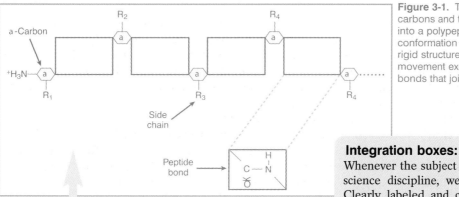

Figure 3-1. The peptide bond linking α-carbons and their side chains together into a polypeptide. The *trans* conformation is favored, producing a rigid structure that restricts freedom of movement except for rotation around bonds that join to the α-carbons.

Artwork:
The books are packed with 4-color illustrations and photographs. When a concept can be better explained with a picture, we've drawn one. Where possible, the pictures tell a dynamic story that will help you remember the information far more effectively than a paragraph of text.

Integration boxes:
Whenever the subject matter can be related to another science discipline, we've put in an Integration Box. Clearly labeled and color-coded, these boxes include nuggets of information on topics that require an integrated knowledge of the sciences to be fully understood. The material in these boxes is complete in itself, and you can use them as a way of reminding yourself of information you already know and reinforcing key links between the sciences. Or the boxes may contain information you have not come across before, in which case you can use them as a springboard for further research or simply to appreciate the relevance of the subject matter of the book to the study of medicine.

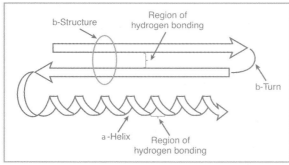

Figure 3-3. Secondary structure includes α-helix and β-pleated sheet (β-sheet).

MICROBIOLOGY

Prion Diseases

Prions (PrP^{Sc}) are formed from otherwise normal neurologic proteins (PrP) and are responsible for encephalopathies in humans (Creutzfeldt-Jakob disease, kuru), scrapie in sheep, and bovine spongiform encephalopathy. Contact between the normal PrP and PrP^{Sc} results in conversion of the secondary structure of PrP from predominantly α-helical to predominantly β-pleated sheet. The altered structure of the protein forms long, filamentous aggregates that gradually damage neuronal tissue. The harmful PrP^{Sc} form is highly resistant to heat, UV irradiation, and protease enzymes.

Since proline has no free hydrogen to contribute to helix stability, it is referred to as a "helix breaker." The α-helix is found in most globular proteins and in some fibrous proteins (e.g., α-keratin).

Text:
Succinct, clearly written text, focusing on the core information you need to know and no more. It's the same level as a carefully prepared course syllabus or lecture notes.

rmation

-structure) consists of

tabilized by hydrogen f adjacent sequences.

The orientation of the adjacent chains can be the same (parallel) or opposite (antiparallel) direction. β-Structures are found in 80% of all globular proteins and in silk fibroin.

Supersecondary Structure and Domains

Supersecondary structures, or *motifs*, are characteristic combinations of secondary structure 10–40 residues in length that recur in different proteins. They bridge the gap between the less specific regularity of secondary structure and the highly specific folding of tertiary structure. The same motif can perform similar functions in different proteins.

- The four-helix bundle motif provides a cavity for enzymes to bind prosthetic groups or cofactors.
- The β-barrel motif can bind hydrophobic molecules such as retinol in the interior of the barrel.
- Motifs may also be mixtures of both α and β conformations.

Pharmacokinetics

1

It's all about delivery—drug delivery, that is—ensuring that an optimal concentration of drug reaches its specific target. Obstacles to drug delivery include absorption, metabolism, elimination, and distribution of drug to other body compartments. In the end, it all boils down to a dynamic equilibrium —balancing a drug's absorption and distribution with its metabolism and elimination.

A complete understanding of any drug must take into account the mechanism of action, potential side effects, and interactions with other drugs. To fully understand "how drugs work," practitioners (this includes physicians, pharmacists, nurses, and physician assistants) must know the general pharmacokinetic and pharmacodynamic characteristics of the prescribed drug to maximize therapeutic benefits and avoid toxicity. Pharmacokinetic principles covering the integrated processes of drug absorption, distribution, metabolism

(biotransformation), and excretion cooperatively determine the drug concentration at the receptor site. Pharmacodynamic mechanisms determine how drug/receptor molecular interactions produce pharmacologic effects by altering intracellular signaling mechanisms (see Chapter 2).

Simply put, pharmacology is the science that studies the effects of drugs on the body (Table 1-1). A drug is any substance that alters the structure or function of living organisms. A poison is any substance that irritates, damages, or impairs the body's tissues. It is worth noting that *all* drugs, if given in large enough doses, have the potential to be toxic, since all drugs are associated with some adverse effects. Thus, the practitioner is responsible for hitting the bull's eye or, in "pharmacology language," the therapeutic window—a concentration of drug at the active site that exerts a biological response without exerting a toxic effect. The underlying principles of drug therapy can be reduced to four key statements:

TABLE 1-1. Pharmacology Terminology

Term	Definition
Pharmacology	The study of drugs and their effects on the body
Drug	Any substance that alters the structure or function of a living organism
Poison	Any substance that irritates, damages, or harms tissues
Pharmacokinetics	The study of the rates and movements of drugs through the body
Absorption	The process of getting a drug from its site of delivery into the bloodstream
Distribution	The process of getting a drug from the bloodstream to the tissue where its actions are needed
Biotransformation	Conversion of a drug molecule to a more water-soluble form
Elimination	The process of removing a drug from the body

- The intensity and duration of drug action depend on the time course of drug concentration at the receptor.
- Optimal steady state drug concentration must be maintained at receptor sites to sustain the pharmacologic effect.
- Practitioners control these drug concentrations through selection of appropriate dose, dosage interval, and route of drug administration.
- The physical properties and mathematical models that determine drug absorption, distribution, metabolism, and excretion ultimately are responsible for drug/drug interactions and potential toxic side effects.

Pharmacokinetics can be reduced to mathematical equations, which determine the transit of the drug throughout the body, a net balance sheet from absorption and distribution (in) to metabolism and excretion (out). By understanding these mathematical equations, practitioners are able to determine optimal dosing for patients with impaired or altered mechanisms of absorption, metabolism, or excretion resulting from diet, genetics, environment, disease, allergy, behavior, and other drugs (prescription, nonprescription, and complementary or alternative medicines). Together, these complicating issues are known as host factors and represent the interface of environment, genetics, and pharmacology.

●●● ABSORPTION

Absorption is the process of delivering a drug into the bloodstream. Drugs can be administered by a variety of routes: orally (PO), intravenously (IV), intramuscularly (IM), rectally (PR), topically, and via inhalation. Ultimately, in order to exert systemic effects, drugs must reach the vasculature. Unexpected alterations in absorption can significantly impact therapeutic goals, and certainly there are pros and cons associated with each route of administration, which will be discussed. The general physical principles that govern the rate of absorption, regardless of the route by which the drug was administered, are passive diffusion, concentration gradients, lipid solubility, drug ionization, size of the drug, and dosage form of the drug.

PHYSIOLOGY

Fick's Law of Diffusion

Fick's law of diffusion states that in a steady state of diffusion the flux of a substance is proportional to the concentration gradient in the system. To be precise,

$$J = -DA \frac{\Delta c}{\Delta x}$$

where J is the net flux (rate of diffusion), D is the diffusion coefficient, A is the area available for diffusion, and $\frac{\Delta c}{\Delta x}$ is the concentration gradient. It's all about moving from areas of high drug concentration to areas of lower drug concentration.

For a drug to be absorbed—to enter the bloodstream—the drug must cross biologic barriers. For orally administered drugs, barriers include the epithelial cells lining the gut and the endothelial cells of the vasculature. Most drugs move down their concentration gradients from an area of high concentration to an area with a lower drug concentration. This movement, called *passive diffusion,* requires no energy expenditure but does depend on the size (molecular weight) of the drug and the lipid solubility of the drug. Most drugs cross biologic barriers by passive diffusion.

On the other hand, a few drugs cross biologic barriers using active transport mechanisms. In this case, the drug moves "uphill" against its concentration gradient—from an area of low concentration to an area with higher concentration. This type of transport requires energy expenditure, typically ATP. Some ions, vitamins, and amino acids are absorbed in this way.

For drugs that are absorbed by passive diffusion, the lipid solubility of the drug is a key determinant for predicting how well the drug will be absorbed. Drugs that are lipid soluble easily pass through the lipid bilayer of cell walls. As a general rule of thumb, the more carbon atoms and the fewer oxygen atoms a drug has, the more lipid soluble the drug is. However, the problem with lipid solubility is that a drug must be *lipid soluble* (hydrophobic) enough to pass through cell membranes but *water soluble* (hydrophilic) enough to dissolve in aqueous fluids (gastric juice, bloodstream). If a drug is too water soluble, it won't penetrate cell membranes. An example of an extremely water-soluble class of drugs is the aminoglycoside antibiotics. When used to treat systemic infections, aminoglycosides must be given IV because the drugs are not absorbed when administered PO. On the other hand, drugs like phenytoin and griseofulvin are so lipid soluble that it is difficult for these agents to dissolve in aqueous media. Because of the need to be both lipid soluble and water soluble simultaneously, most drugs are administered as either weak acids or weak bases, i.e., a molecule that fluctuates between charged and uncharged states at physiologic pH.

Ionization

Weak acids and weak bases exist in solution as a mixture of ionized and un-ionized forms. Ionized drugs are poorly lipid soluble and don't readily cross lipid membranes, but they dissolve well in aqueous media. Un-ionized drugs, on the other hand, are highly lipid soluble and readily cross biologic membranes. Hence, the transfer of drug across a biologic barrier is proportional to the concentration gradient of the un-ionized form across the membrane; this is known as the *degree of ionization.* The ratio of ionized versus un-ionized fraction of drug depends on the pK_a (ionization constant) of the drug and the pH of the surrounding tissues or fluids. See Box 1-1 for an example.

When the pH of the solution is below the pK_a, acids are preferentially un-ionized and bases are mostly ionized. On the other hand, when the pH of a solution is above the pK_a, acids are mostly ionized and bases are mostly un-ionized.

Box 1-1. EFFECT OF pH ON THE IONIZATION OF SALICYLIC ACID (pKa = 3)

When pH = 1   99% of salicylic acid is un-ionized
When pH = 2   90.9% of salicylic acid is un-ionized
When pH = 3   50% of salicylic acid is un-ionized. (Note: By definition, the pKa of a drug is the pH at which 50% of the drug is ionized and 50% is un-ionized.)
When pH = 4   9.09% of salicylic acid is un-ionized
When pH = 5   0.99% of salicylic acid is un-ionized
When pH = 6   0.10% of salicylic acid is un-ionized

BIOCHEMISTRY

The Henderson-Hasselbach Equation

The Henderson-Hasselbach equation states that there is a relationship between the pH of a solution and the relative concentrations of an acid and its conjugate base in that solution. Recall that the pKa (or ionization constant) is numerically equivalent to the pH of the solution when the molar concentrations of an acid and its conjugate base are equal.

Biochemists express this as the log ratio of protonated over unprotonated. In pharmacologic terms, this translates to:

$$\text{For acids (A): } \log \frac{A^-}{HA} \left(\frac{unprotonated}{protonated} \right) = pH - pKa$$

$$\text{For bases (B): } \log \frac{B}{BH^+} \left(\frac{unprotonated}{protonated} \right) = pH - pKa$$

You will notice that for acids the protonated form is unchanged and is the denominator. This is the more permeable chemical form. In contrast, for bases the protonated form is charged and is the denominator. However, this is the less permeable chemical form. In practical terms, this means that acids are preferentially absorbed under acidic conditions (pH below the pKa), while bases are preferentially absorbed at alkaline pHs (above their pKa).

The above principles may be illustrated in a different manner: in biochemistry, the following notation is often used to indicate the ionization status of weak acids:

$$HA \rightleftharpoons H^+ + A^-$$

In an acidic environment, such as the stomach, the weak acid, A^-, accepts a proton and becomes un-ionized. Therefore, in an acidic environment, an acidic drug is likely to be uncharged and thus preferentially absorbed. Alternatively, in an alkaline environment, acidic drugs are more likely to remain ionized and relative absorption is reduced. However, it should be realized that even though the generalization suggests that weak acids are preferentially absorbed at low pH, there is still relatively little, if any, absorption in the acidic environment of the stomach, an organ not suited for absorption. The stomach is mostly a storage depot for drugs rather than an organ for drug absorption. Thus, the rate of gastric emptying into the intestines greatly impacts the overall rate of absorption. Most drugs are absorbed in the intestines. The small intestines have the greatest capacity for absorption, because villi and microvilli markedly increase the absorptive surface area. The proximal areas of the small intestines (duodenum) primarily absorb drugs that are weak acids because of the acidic pH of stomach secretions. See Box 1-2 for examples of drugs that are best absorbed in an acidic environment.

Ammonia, NH_3, is an example of a weak base.

$$NH_3 + H^+ \rightleftharpoons NH_4^+$$

In contrast to weak acids, when a weak base is in an acidic environment and picks up a proton, the compound becomes ionized and, in our example, ammonium ion is preferentially formed. An alkaline drug is un-ionized in a high pH environment (like the small intestines) and thus more likely to be absorbed in this alkaline environment. The distal portions of the small intestines predominately absorb drugs that are weak bases, due to the alkalinity of bile secretions. The key point to remember is that even though weak acids are preferentially absorbed in acidic environments, they will still be absorbed in the intestines because of the large intestinal surface area designed for absorption.

Box 1-2. EXAMPLES OF DRUGS BEST ABSORBED IN AN ACIDIC ENVIRONMENT

Ketoconazole
Itraconazole
Iron
Digoxin
Vitamin B_{12}
Aspirin

Molecular Weight

Absorption is slow for drugs that are large in size or that possess "bulky" or oxygenated side chain groups. Most drugs are less than 100 to 200 Da in size and can readily cross membranes.

Dosage Form

Many drugs are available in multiple dosage forms. The formulation of a drug affects the drug's absorption and onset of action. Consider, for example, an orally administered drug that is available as a tablet, a capsule, a liquid suspension, and a liquid solution. To be absorbed, the solid tablet must disintegrate into small particles, which must then dissolve into aqueous gastrointestinal fluids. On the other hand, drugs that are formulated into capsules can skip the "disintegration step" because capsules contain drugs that are already in "small particle" form. A drug suspension contains even

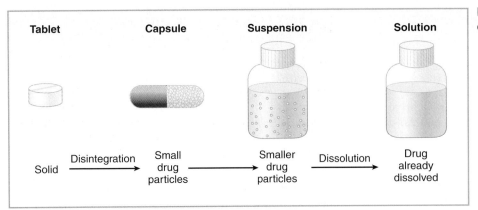

Figure 1-1. Disintegration and dissolution characteristics of various dosage forms.

smaller particles than capsules. With liquid formulations, the drug has already been dissolved. Hence, drugs that are available as liquid formulations are absorbed faster than drugs that are suspensions, suspensions are absorbed more rapidly than capsules, and capsules are absorbed more rapidly than tablets (Fig. 1-1).

Routes of Administration

The enteral (relating to the alimentary canal) route of administration is the safest, most economical, and most convenient way of administering drugs. Orally, sublingually, and rectally administered medications are in this category.

Sublingual and Oral

Medications that are administered sublingually dissolve under the tongue, without chewing or swallowing. Absorption is very quick, and higher drug levels are achieved in the bloodstream by sublingual routes than by oral routes because (1) the sublingual route avoids "first-pass metabolism" by the liver (Fig. 1-2), and (2) the drug avoids destruction by gastric

juices or complexation with foods. Remember that drugs absorbed from the gut travel first to the liver via the portal vein. Drugs absorbed through the intestine may, thus, reach systemic circulation at a concentration significantly below the initial dose. The keys to understanding drug absorption are highlighted in Box 1-3.

Box 1-3. KEYS TO DRUG ABSORPTION

- The biochemical properties of a drug determine the optimal route of administration.
- Optimal absorption of weak acids/bases depends on the pH of the gastrointestinal tract or surrounding environment.
- Gastrointestinal disease can affect the absorption of drugs.

ANATOMY

Drug Absorption

The first-pass effect is a major mechanism that determines the ultimate concentration of a drug in the plasma. Based solely on the anatomy of the body, drugs absorbed beyond the oral cavity are transported to the liver via the portal vein, where most drugs are metabolized to less active metabolites. After metabolism in the liver, drug metabolites are transported to the systemic circulation by the hepatic vein.

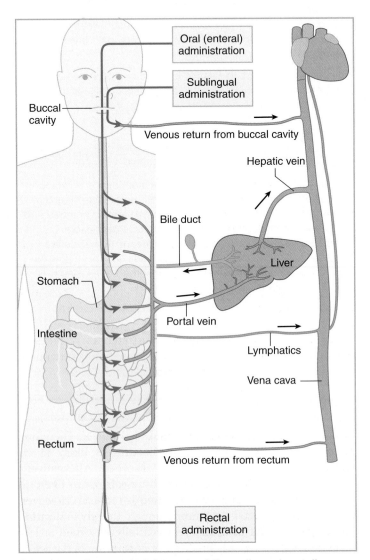

Figure 1-2. Drugs administered sublingually and rectally avoid "first-pass metabolism" in the liver.

TABLE 1-2. Drugs Commonly Prescribed Sublingually

Drug	Use
Loratadine	Allergies
Mirtazapine	Anxiety
Nitroglycerin	Angina
Rizatriptan	Migraine headache

TABLE 1-3. Effect of Intestinal Disease on Drug Absorption

Disease	Absorption Increased	Absorption Decreased
Celiac sprue	Aspirin Cephalexin Clindamycin Erythromycin Propranolol Sulfamethoxazole Trimethoprim	Acetaminophen Amoxicillin Penicillin V
Crohn's disease	Clindamycin Propranolol Sulfamethoxazole Trimethoprim	Acetaminophen Cephalexin Methyldopa Metronidazole

TABLE 1-4. Drug Effects That Alter Absorption

Effect	Drug
Changes in gastric or intestinal pH	H_2 blockers, antacids, proton pump inhibitors
Changes in gastrointestinal motility	Laxatives, anticholinergics, metoclopramide
Changes in gastrointestinal perfusion	Vasodilators
Interference with mucosal function	Neomycin, colchicine
Chelation	Tetracycline, calcium, magnesium, aluminum
Resin binding	Cholestyramine
Absorption	Charcoal

TABLE 1-5. Effect of Food on Absorption of Selected Drugs

Reduced Absorption	Delayed Absorption	Increased Absorption
Ampicillin	Acetaminophen	Carbamazepine
Aspirin	Aspirin	Diazepam
Atenolol	Cephalosporins	Griseofulvin
Captopril	Sulfonamides	Labetalol
Hydrochlorothiazide	Diclofenac	Metoprolol
Tetracyclines	Digoxin	Propranolol
Iron	Furosemide	Nitrofurantoin
Levodopa	Valproate	
Penicillamine		
Sotalol		
Warfarin		

Box 1-4. WHEN TO AVOID GIVING DRUGS ORALLY

- If the drug causes nausea and vomiting
- If the patient is currently vomiting
- If the patient is unwilling or unable to swallow (child, mentally retarded, unconscious)
- If the drug is destroyed by digestive enzymes (insulin)
- If the drug is not absorbed through the gastric mucosa (aminoglycosides)
- If the drug is rapidly degraded (lidocaine)

Ideally, for a drug to be delivered sublingually, the drug should dissolve rapidly, produce desired therapeutic effects with small amounts of drug, and be tasteless. Examples of commonly prescribed sublingual tablets include nitroglycerin, loratadine, mirtazapine, and rizatriptan (Table 1-2).

Some diseases alter rates of drug absorption. For example if gastrointestinal motility is dramatically increased, as in inflammatory bowel diseases (Crohn's disease, ulcerative colitis) or malabsorptive syndromes (celiac sprue), absorption of some drugs may be reduced (Table 1-3). On the other hand, absorption of other drugs may be increased in patients with these inflammatory gut disorders, since gastrointestinal membranes often do not remain intact as a consequence of these autoimmune diseases. Alternatively, consider situations in which gastrointestinal motility is slowed (i.e., diabetic gastroparesis). Here, drug absorption could be enhanced as a result of prolonged contact time with the absorptive areas of the intestine. Likewise, there are drugs that alter the rate of absorption for other orally administered medications (Table 1-4).

Food can also affect absorption of drugs by either increasing, decreasing, or delaying the rate at which absorption occurs (Table 1-5). As a generalization, food tends to slow the rate of gastric emptying. This results in slower absorption of many drugs. For this reason, drugs are often administered on an empty stomach—to increase absorption. However, if drugs are irritating to the gastrointestinal tract, a light, nonfatty meal may be recommended. There are other reasons to consider giving drugs with or without food. For example, penicillin V should be administered on an empty stomach (1 hour before meals or 2 to 3 hours after meals) because it is unstable in gastric acids. On the other hand, metoprolol and propranolol (β-blockers) should be taken with meals because food enhances their bioavailability. Although the oral route of administration is the most common, there are a few instances when the oral route of administration should not be used (Box 1-4).

Rectal

Sometimes drugs are administered rectally via suppository or enema. Absorption from the rectum is erratic and unpredictable, since the rectum contains no microvilli. Additionally, most drugs irritate the rectum. However, rectal administration can be useful in patients who are unconscious or vomiting or in those with severe inflammatory bowel disease. An additional benefit of this route of administration is that the "first-pass effect" of the liver is avoided, since a portion of the rectal blood supply (inferior and middle hemorrhoidal veins) bypasses hepatic portal circulation.

Parenteral

The parenteral routes of administration include any routes that bypass the gastrointestinal tract entirely. The intravenous route of administration is the quickest way to get a drug to its site of action, so intravenous drugs are of the greatest value during emergencies when speed is vital. Advantages and disadvantages of intravenous drug administration are found in Boxes 1-5 and 1-6.

Intramuscular and subcutaneous administrations are not affected by "first-pass" hepatic metabolism, but both routes of administration are directly affected by blood flow at the site of injection. Exercise, activity, and massage at the injection site increase blood flow, which speeds drug absorption by allowing drug contact with vasodilated capillaries.

Relatively large volumes of solution can be administered intramuscularly with less pain or irritation than subcutaneous injections. This route is particularly useful for lipophilic substances. Aqueous solutions administered intramuscularly are typically absorbed within 10 to 30 minutes, although depot formulations have been designed for some drugs that promote gradual absorption over a prolonged period of time. Subcutaneously administered drugs are absorbed slightly more slowly than intramuscularly administered drugs. Patients are more likely to be able to give themselves subcutaneous injections (e.g., insulin) than to self-administer medications by any other parenteral route.

In the event of an overdose following intramuscular or subcutaneous injections, absorption may be reduced by immobilizing the limb, applying ice, administering a vasoconstrictive agent (e.g., epinephrine), or applying a tourniquet.

Other examples of parenteral administration options are listed in Table 1-6.

Inhalation

Anesthetic gases, metered-dose inhalers, and dry-powder inhalers all deliver drugs to the lungs. The smaller the particle size of the drug, the more likely the drug will reach the alveoli. Inhaled glucocorticoids and β-adrenergic agonists are often given to *directly* target inflamed bronchial and alveolar targets, thus achieving efficacy with minimal systemic effects. However, it should be remembered that a proportion of inhaled drugs still reaches the systemic circulation.

Mucous Membranes

A variety of drugs are administered topically to mucous membranes of the eye, nose, throat, and vagina. Although typically only local effects are desired, some level of systemic drug absorption does occur through mucous membranes. In fact, some vaginal estrogen products are specifically formulated to provide systemic effects. Likewise, undesired systemic side effects can occur from drug administration to mucous membranes, such as when ocular β-blockers aggra-

---

Box 1-5. ADVANTAGES OF INTRAVENOUS ADMINISTRATION

- Drug immediately enters circulation
- Drug is rapidly distributed to tissues
- Rapid response
- Permits instant dosage titration
- Useful if drug is destroyed by gastric contents or heavily metabolized by the first pass effect
- Allows maintenance of constant blood levels
- Large quantities can be administered for a long time
- Reduced irritation due to diluting/buffering by blood
- Always available (unconscious patients)

Box 1-6. DISADVANTAGES OF INTRAVENOUS ADMINISTRATION

- Once injected, the drug cannot be removed
- Injections given too rapidly can cause serious reactions if too much drug arrives at organs as a concentrated solution (respiratory, circulatory failure)
- Not suited for easy self-administration
- Must use sterile technique
- Discomfort with drug administration
- Irritation, allergy, overdoses difficult to manage

TABLE 1-6. Additional Parenteral Routes of Administration and Rationale for Use

Site of Administration	Rationale (Example)
Intra-arterial	Local perfusion of an organ (cancer chemotherapy, radiocontrast agent)
Bone marrow	Other sites inaccessible (burn patients)
Intradermal	Allergy testing
Intracardiac	Emergency treatment of cardiac arrest
Intraperitoneal	Home dialysis

vate asthma or when nasally delivered corticosteroids contribute to osteoporosis, cataracts, or elevated intraocular pressure.

Topical

In general, absorption through the skin is extremely slow. Absorption can be increased by incorporating drugs into fatty, lipid-soluble vehicles such as lanolin, by rubbing the application site to increase blood flow, or by applying a keratolytic (e.g., salicylic acid) to reduce the keratin layer. Drugs applied topically may be used either for their local effects (e.g., hydrocortisone) or for systemic effects (e.g., nitroglycerin, scopolamine, estrogen, nicotine). The latter examples are available as *transdermal* formulations and are time-released.

●●● DISTRIBUTION

The process of translocating drugs from the bloodstream into the tissues is referred to as distribution. The apparent *volume of distribution* (Vd) describes the area of the body to which drugs are distributed and may be defined as the fluid volume required to contain all the drug in the body at the same concentration observed in the blood. The Vd may be calculated by dividing the total amount of drug in the body by the concentration of drug in the plasma. Remember, Vd assumes that the concentration of drug is the same in all locations throughout the body (which isn't always true). Mathematically, Vd (in liters) is equivalent to

$$\frac{\text{Dose (mg)}}{\text{Concentration (mg/L)}}$$

Another way to think about Vd is that it is equal to the amount of space in the body that a drug needs to fill up. It should in no way be confused or associated with any particular physiologic compartment. In many cases, the volume of distribution is normalized to body weight and will then have units of liters per kilogram (L/kg).

Vascularity is the most important determinant of distribution. After all, very little drug can be distributed to an area of the body that gets minute amounts of blood flow. Frankly, most drugs are not uniformly distributed. Drugs are typically distributed in several phases. In the first phase, drugs are distributed to "high flow" areas like the heart, liver, kidneys, and brain. In later phases, drugs are distributed to "low flow" areas such as bones, fat, and skin.

There are many body compartments in which drugs can be distributed, and the Vd varies for each drug, depending on how widely distributed the drug is. Some hydrophilic drugs remain primarily in the vasculature, a compartment with a Vd of about 5 L, the volume of plasma. Other drugs distribute to both the vasculature and extracellular fluid compartments, with a Vd of about 15 L. Still other agents distribute throughout all body fluids, including cellular fluids, and possess a Vd of about 40 L. With respect to Vd, some key points to understand are (1) when a drug has a large Vd, it means that a larger dose of drug will be needed to achieve a target drug concentration in the plasma; and (2) lipid-soluble drugs have a larger Vd than water-soluble drugs. In fact, lipophilic drugs can dissolve in fat and can accumulate in adipose tissues, yielding Vd > 100 L. Note that a drug may have a high Vd and distribute to peripheral compartments, but those compartments are not necessarily the sites of drug action. However, the real "value" of Vd is that it allows determination of steady-state dosing regimens.

Plasma Protein Binding

Numerous drugs bind nonspecifically to serum proteins, especially albumin, as well as other cell constituents in the skeletal system (bones, teeth), through a process known as nonspecific protein binding. Protein-bound drugs are not bioactive, i.e., protein-bound drugs have no therapeutic efficacy while bound nonspecifically to plasma proteins. Bound drugs cannot be filtered by the glomerulus nor are they subject to metabolism by microsomal P-450 enzymes. Protein-bound drug can be thought of as a *reservoir*—with drug gradually released from nonspecific binding sites when plasma concentrations of the drug decline. For sports enthusiasts, think of plasma proteins as the hockey penalty box; when bound to plasma proteins, drugs (i.e., hockey players) can no longer participate in excretion, metabolism, and distribution. Unbound (or "free") drugs are able to distribute and bind to their specific receptor targets and exert biologic effects.

When a drug is nonspecifically protein bound, the disappearance of the drug from the blood is slowed, since only free drug (1) distributes to tissues, interacts with receptors, and exerts biological effects, and (2) is filtered by renal glomeruli and eliminated. Since albumin is the primary plasma protein to which drugs bind nonspecifically, alterations in albumin levels can affect free drug concentrations (Table 1-7). Other plasma proteins that nonspecifically bind drugs include α_1-acid glycoproteins and lipoproteins.

There is a theoretical risk of drug-drug interactions any time a drug is greater than 80% protein bound. Drugs compete with one another for binding to plasma proteins, and drugs frequently displace each other. Consider the anticoagulant drug warfarin, which is greater than 99% protein bound. This means that less than 1% of warfarin is circulating freely, and it is this small amount of free drug that is therapeutically active. If a patient has been stabilized on a dosage of warfarin and another highly protein-bound drug is

TABLE 1-7. "Free" Drug Levels with Albumin Alterations

Albumin Level	Illness	Free Drug Levels
Hyperalbuminemia	Dehydration	Decreased
Hypoalbuminemia	Burns	Increased
	Renal disease	Increased
	Hepatic disease	Increased
	Malnutrition	Increased

Box 1-7. EXAMPLES OF HIGHLY PROTEIN BOUND DRUGS

Warfarin
Sulfonamides
Valproate
NSAIDs
Sulfonylureas
Nifedipine

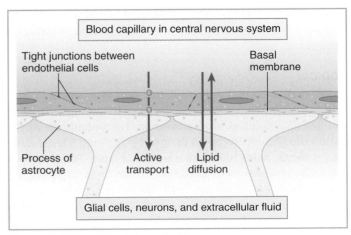

Figure 1-3. The blood-brain barrier.

Box 1-8. CHARACTERISTICS OF DRUGS THAT READILY PENETRATE THE CNS

- Low ionization at plasma pH
- Low binding to plasma proteins
- Highly lipophilic
- Small molecular size

Box 1-9. KEYS TO DRUG DISTRIBUTION

- Drugs are distributed into interstitial or cellular fluids after absorption or injection into the bloodstream.
- Drug distribution may be limited by drug binding to plasma proteins.
- Lipid solubility, pH gradients, and binding characteristics to intracellular or membrane components are determinants that can lead to accumulation of drug in some tissues at higher concentrations than would be expected from diffusion equilibrium alone.

administered (e.g., a sulfonylurea; see Box 1-7), the second drug may compete with warfarin for binding sites and may displace some warfarin from albumin. Even if this displacement results in only 2% of warfarin circulating freely, the amount of free drug has doubled, and this may lead to toxic, potentially life-threatening consequences.

There is a growing feeling that plasma protein binding is not as important as originally thought, since drugs displaced from plasma proteins would then be subject to distribution, excretion, and metabolism. As such, concentrations of free drug in plasma may only be transiently and minimally increased. However, clear cases of toxicity have been observed following administration of highly protein-bound drugs. For example, sulfonamide antibiotics are never used in infants less than 2 months of age. Sulfonamides are highly protein-bound drugs, and in neonates, these drugs have displaced bilirubin from plasma protein-binding sites. This has resulted in hyperbilirubinemia and kernicterus (brain damage caused by bilirubin). Additionally, numerous examples of drug-drug interactions involving warfarin and other highly protein-bound drugs exist in the literature.

Selective Distribution

Some molecules are preferentially taken up by specific cell membranes (e.g., iodide by thyroid). As a result, it is important to remember that tissues with the highest drug concentrations are not always the sites of drug action.

Just as there are reservoirs for drugs, there are also barriers. The term *blood-brain barrier* is a bit of a misnomer. There is not a true barrier that keeps all drugs from entering the central nervous system. The blood-brain barrier refers to decreased permeability of brain capillaries due to endothelial cells fitting tightly together. To enter the central nervous system, drugs must first transverse the capillary endothelium and then cross astrocyte membranes (Fig. 1-3). The so-called blood-brain barrier is impermeable to water-soluble drugs, but Box 1-8 lists criteria for drugs that readily permeate the central nervous system.

The placental barrier protects the fetus from maternal drugs and metabolites. However, the placental barrier is also not a true barrier. In fact, the barrier becomes thinner during pregnancy, decreasing from the beginning of gestation through term. Drugs are distributed to a developing fetus if they are (1) highly lipid soluble, (2) un-ionized, and (3) small in size. Key points about drug distribution are highlighted in Box 1-9.

METABOLISM

Biotransformation is "pharmacology language" for metabolism and is the first step toward metabolizing a drug. The end result of metabolism is that the original drug molecule is altered in ways that make the drug more polar, hydrophilic, and water soluble (and hence excretable). Remember that "free" metabolites are readily filtered in the glomerulus (in contrast to those that are protein bound) and that these polar hydrophilic metabolites are preferentially excreted rather than reabsorbed across the lipid barrier of the peritubular capillary network of the nephron. While metabolism can occur in any tissue, the liver is typically thought of as being the primary metabolic site. Without metabolism, 99.9% of all drugs filtered at the glomerulus would be reabsorbed into systemic circulation by the peritubular capillaries of the kidney.

Rates of Metabolism

In the liver, drugs are metabolized at various rates, either by zero-order kinetics or first-order kinetics. Only a few drugs, (e.g., alcohol and phenytoin, an anticonvulsant drug) follow zero-order kinetics for metabolism. With zero-order kinetics, the rate of metabolism is constant and does not vary with the amount of drug present. With drugs eliminated in this manner, there is a *fixed amount* of drug that can be handled at any one time. That is because the enzymes involved with metabolism are saturable. Consider alcohol as an example. Only 10 to 14 grams of alcohol can be eliminated per hour, because alcohol dehydrogenase gets saturated with drug at these doses and simply cannot handle any more drug. When an amount greater than this is ingested, an individual suffers from side effects (i.e., "gets drunk"). The amount of time necessary for alcohol to be metabolized increases with the amount of alcohol ingested. If 100 g of alcohol is initially ingested but only 10 g can be metabolized per hour, it will take 10 hours for that alcohol to be metabolized and eliminated. Zero-order reactions are shown graphically in Figure 1-4.

Figure 1-4. Zero-order reactions are linear.

Most drugs, however, are metabolized by first-order kinetics. In other words, a *constant fraction* of the drug is metabolized per unit of time. Another way to think about first-order kinetics is that metabolism increases proportionately as the concentration of drug in the body increases. The more drug in the body, the faster metabolism will occur. The enzymes involved with metabolizing most drugs are not saturable at normal drug concentrations. Graphically, first-order reactions are shown as illustrated in Figure 1-5. When plotted on linear paper, the resulting graph is curvilinear. However, if the log of drug concentration versus time is plotted, the result is a straight line. In fact, this line can provide very useful information. Since a constant fraction of drug is metabolized per unit time and metabolism increases proportionately as the concentration of drug in the body increases, the time to clear the body of 50% of drug will always be constant. This is, in fact, the definition of half-life ($t_{1/2}$). The $t_{1/2}$ of a drug is defined as the time necessary to remove 50% of drug from the body. With first-order reactions, the $t_{1/2}$ of a drug is constant and independent of the dosage given. For example, if 100 mg of a drug is administered and it takes 4 hours to eliminate 50 mg, the $t_{1/2}$ is 4 hours. Knowing that information, it will take 4 more hours to eliminate 25 mg, 4 additional hours to eliminate 12.5 mg,

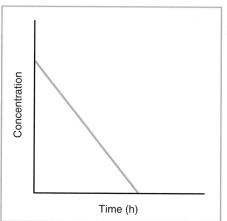

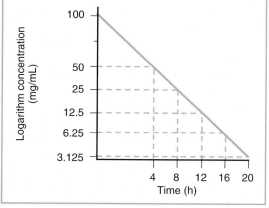

Figure 1-5. First-order reactions are curvilinear (**A**) unless the concentration is plotted on a logarithmic scale (**B**).

A   B

and another 4 hours to eliminate 6.25 mg. Another way to say this is that the peak plasma concentration is reduced in half every $t_{1/2}$. As a general rule of thumb, it takes five $t_{1/2}$ to effectively eliminate (>97%) a drug from the body.

Microsomal P-450 Isoenzymes

In the liver, the microsomal (endoplasmic reticulum) P-450 mixed-function oxidases play a major role in drug metabolism. P-450 enzymes have modest specificity for substrates and catalyze the metabolism of widely differing chemical structures. The ability of a drug to be metabolized by various enzymatic reactions depends on the drug's side chain groups and chemical structure. There are 17 families of cytochrome (CYP) P-450 genes and 39 subfamilies. Three of these families preferentially metabolize drugs—CYP 1, 2, and 3. Genetic polymorphisms exist for these genes. For example, 7% to 10% of whites are deficient in CYP2D6, and CYP2C19 is completely absent in 3% of whites and 20% of Asians. Since these two genes largely determine how people break down drugs, genetic variations in these "metabolism genes" can have important consequences for patients. "Poor metabolizers" have a greater risk than the general population of experiencing adverse drug reactions. These P-450 polymorphisms (genetic variants) are the basis for the emerging field of pharmacogenomics. That is, genetic information provides guidance on the best choice of drug and dose for a specific patient.

Phase I Reactions

Also known as nonsynthetic reactions, phase I reactions include oxidation, hydrolysis, and reduction reactions. Cytochrome P-450s are the enzymes that catalyze phase I reactions. Addition of oxygen groups or removal of methyl groups causes drugs to be more polar than the parent compounds, but even after phase I reactions, the drugs often lack the water solubility necessary for elimination. One aspect of phase I reactions is to prepare drugs for subsequent phase II conjugation reactions.

In addition to serving as a first step in normal metabolism, phase I reactions can have beneficial or negative consequences (Box 1-10). In some cases, phase I reactions activate pro-drugs. For example, the inactive enalapril is activated to enalaprilat (an angiotensin-converting enzyme [ACE] inhibitor). Conversely, phase I metabolism of benzo[a]pyrene (a tobacco pyrolysis product) produces genotoxic diol epoxide metabolites.

BOX 1-10. RESULTS OF BIOTRANSFORMATION

Active drug → Active metabolite
Active drug → Inactive metabolite
Pro-drug → Active drug
Active drug → Toxic metabolite

Phase II Reactions

Phase II, or "synthetic," reactions are energy-dependent reactions in which chemical structures are added to the drug to increase polarity and enhance water solubility. Such chemical modifications include glycine conjugation, glutathione conjugation, sulfate formation, acetylation, methylation and glucuronidation (the addition of the polar sugar glucuronic acid, $C_6H_9O_6$). Phase II reactions typically cause drugs to be inactivated. In additon, phase II reactions often enhance polarity so that the molecules can be readily excreted.

Enzyme Induction and Inhibition

Frequent administration of certain drugs leads to increased synthesis (transcription or translation), or induction, of P-450 enzymes. Enzyme induction increases metabolism of all drugs that are metabolized by that particular P-450 isoenzyme. Therefore, when multiple drugs are given, drug interactions are likely at the level of P-450 metabolism. *This is the major mechanism for drug-drug interactions!* For example, the antiepileptic drug phenytoin induces the CYP1A2 P-450 isoenzyme. The antipsychotic drug haloperidol is metabolized by the same isoenzyme. If haloperidol is given concurrently with phenytoin, the metabolism of haloperidol will occur faster than normal as a result of enzyme induction, and the drug will be less effective. In this situation, practitioners may need to prescribe larger doses of haloperidol to achieve desired therapeutic effects. Other chronic inducers of CYP-450 enzymes include the anticonvulsant drug phenobarbital and the antimycobacterial drug rifampin. As a potent P-450 enzyme inducer, rifampin is associated with drug interactions of substantial clinical significance. Rifampin induces the P-450 enzymes responsible for metabolizing oral contraceptives and immunosuppressant drugs. The end result of these drug interactions could be an unplanned pregnancy or immune rejection in a transplant patient. The antiseizure medication carbamazepine is a unique example of an "auto-inducer." Carbamazepine induces its own metabolism via CYP3A4, meaning that the longer the drug is given, the more rapidly it is metabolized.

In contrast to enzyme induction, some drugs block, or inhibit, the CYP enzymes that metabolize other drugs. The H_2 (histamine) blocker cimetidine (used to treat acid reflux) is an example of a CYP2C9 P-450 enzyme inhibitor. Since diazepam (an anxiolytic) is metabolized by the same CYP-450 enzyme, when cimetidine (available as an over-the-counter medication) is administered concurrently, diazepam will not be metabolized as rapidly as normal and may accumulate in the body. This can lead to a longer $t_{1/2}$ for diazepam and associated toxic effects. Box 1-11 lists major drugs whose metabolism may be altered if they are given concurrently with P-450 enzyme inhibitors or inducers. Remember, the plasma level of substrates increases with coadministration of a P-450 enzyme inhibitor and decreases with coadministration of a P-450 enzyme inducer, with varying degrees of clinical significance. Natural and herbal products can also alter the activities of the microsomal P-450

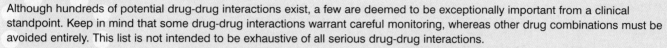

CLINICAL MEDICINE

Drug Interactions

Although hundreds of potential drug-drug interactions exist, a few are deemed to be exceptionally important from a clinical standpoint. Keep in mind that some drug-drug interactions warrant careful monitoring, whereas other drug combinations must be avoided entirely. This list is not intended to be exhaustive of all serious drug-drug interactions.

Drug-Drug Interactions of Significant Clinical Importance

Object Drug (or Drug Class)	Precipitant Drug (or Drug Class)	Potential Adverse Clinical Outcome
Benzodiazepines	Azole antifungal	Increased benzodiazepine toxicities
Carbamazepine	Propoxyphene	Increased carbamazepine toxicities
Cyclosporine	Rifampin	Decreased cyclosporine efficacy
Dextromethorphan	MAO inhibitors	Serotonin syndrome; avoid combination
Digoxin	Clarithromycin	Increased digoxin toxicities
Ergot alkaloids	Macrolide antibiotics	Increased ergotamine toxicities
Estrogen-progestin products (oral contraceptives)	Rifampin	Decreased oral contraceptive efficacy
MAO inhibitors	Anorexiants; sympathomimetics	Hypertensive crisis; avoid combination
Meperidine	MAO inhibitors	Serotonin syndrome; avoid combination
Methotrexate	Trimethoprim	Increased methotrexate toxicities
Nitrates	Phosphodiesterase-5 inhibitors	Enhanced vasodilatory effects; avoid combination
Pimozide	Macrolide antibiotics; azole antifungal agents	QT prolongation, life-threatening arrhythmias; avoid combination
Selective serotonin reuptake inhibitors	MAO inhibitors	Serotonin syndrome; avoid combination
Theophylline	Ciprofloxacin, enoxacin; fluvoxamine	Increased theophylline toxicities, especially seizure risk
Thiopurines (azathioprine, mercaptopurine)	Allopurinol	Increased thiopurine toxicities
Warfarin	Sulfinpyrazone, NSAIDs, cimetidine, fibric acid derivatives, barbiturates thyroid hormone	Increased bleeding risk
Zidovudine	Ganciclovir	Increased zidovudine toxicities

Data from Malone DC, Abarca J, Hansten PD, et al. Identification of serious drug-drug interactions: results of the partnership to prevent drug-drug interactions. *J Am Pharm Assoc (Wash DC)* 2004;44:142–151.

isoenzymes and alter drug metabolism (Table 1-8). To prevent adverse drug-drug interactions that occur as a result of altered metabolism, remember the key points highlighted in Box 1-12.

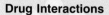 ELIMINATION

Elimination is the process of excreting drugs or their metabolites from the body. The kidneys play a large role in drug removal. When glomerular filtration rates are decreased in disease, as evidenced by decreased creatinine clearance (see Chapter 9), the dose of drugs that are eliminated by the kidney must be reduced to avoid toxicity. In other words, renal disease leads to reduced drug excretion, drug accumulation, and increases the risk of drug toxicities. Physicians often need to lower drug dosages for patients with renal disease.

As blood enters the renal glomeruli, plasma is filtered of all substances that (1) are less than 60 Da in size and (2) are not protein bound. Drugs that are un-ionized and lipid soluble are readily reabsorbed into the peritubular capillaries from the renal tubules, whereas drugs that are ionized or polar tend to be retained in the renal tubule and excreted in the urine (Fig. 1-6). Changes in urine pH can alter (increase or decrease) drug elimination, just as discussed in the section on absorption. Briefly, acidifying the urine (with vitamin C or NH_4Cl) promotes reabsorption of drugs that are weakly acidic (acidic environments render weak acids un-ionized, $H^+ + A^- \rightarrow HA$). On the other hand, alkalinizing the urine ($NaHCO_3$) causes a weak acid to be ionized and thus accelerates its excretion. This is a great way to detoxify weak acids (i.e., salicylate). Equally, toxins that are weak bases can be preferentially excreted by acidifying the urine.

Additionally, some drugs are actively secreted out of the bloodstream and into the proximal renal tubule via energy-dependent cationic and anionic transport pumps (Table 1-9). Drugs can compete with one another for binding sites on these transport pumps; as a result, one drug can inhibit the elimination of another. Probenecid (used for chronic gout) competes with penicillins and cephalosporins for binding to the anionic transporter, hence extending the actions of the antibiotics. Likewise, cimetidine competes with metformin (an antihyperglycemic) for the cationic transporter, causing

BOX 1-11. P-450 ENZYME INHIBITORS AND INDUCERS*

P-450 Substrates

Benzodiazepines
β-Blockers
Ca++ channel blockers
Carbamazepine
Cyclosporine
Haloperidol
Oral contraceptives

Phenytoin
Theophylline
Tricyclic antidepressants
Warfarin

P-450 Inducers

Carbamazepine
Phenobarbital
Phenytoin

Rifampin

P-450 Inhibitors

Cimetidine
Erythromycin
Fluoxetine
Isoniazid

Ketoconazole
Ritonavir

*This list is not exhaustive. It is merely a representation of selected drugs that have been associated with clinically significant drug interactions resulting from altered P-450 metabolism.

TABLE 1-8. Examples of Natural Products That Alter P-450 Isoenzyme Metabolism*

P-450 Inducers	P-450 Inhibitors
Cabbage	Dandelion
Broccoli	Milk thistle
Brussels sprouts	St. John's wort†
Cauliflower	Black tea
Charbroiled meats	Chamomile
Cigarette smoking	Clove
Oregano	Ginger
Chasteberry	Gotu kola
Bloodroot	Kava kava
	Grapefruit juice
	Licorice

*This list is not exhaustive. More than 40 foods and natural products are known to alter P-450 metabolism.
†Although St. John's wort appears to inhibit CYP3A4 acutely, it also seems to induce the enzyme with repeated administration.

Box 1-12. KEYS TO DRUG METABOLISM

- Most drugs undergo metabolism before being eliminated from the body.
- Drug metabolites are generally more polar than their parent compound.
- The cytochrome P-450 enzymes are selective but not specific.
- Concurrent ingestion of two or more drugs can affect the rate of metabolism of one or more of them.

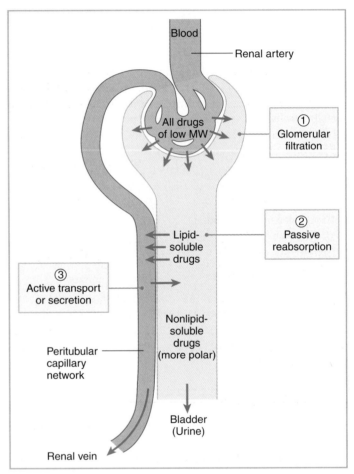

Figure 1-6. Elimination of drugs in the renal tubule.

metformin levels to increase substantially. These types of competitive interactions are another classical example of how drug-drug interactions may lead to toxicity.

Other organs also play roles in drug elimination. The mammary glands typically secrete drugs, such that drug concentrations found in breast milk approximate 1% of the total maternal dose. As breast milk is slightly acidic, some weak bases may be preferentially concentrated (trapped) and eliminated through this "excretory" organ. Some drugs are eliminated via sweat glands, saliva, or tears. Although these are minor routes of drug elimination, they may account for skin rashes associated with use of some drugs. Substances such as alcohol and volatile anesthetics are eliminated by the lungs. The liver also plays a role in elimination, since some drugs are eliminated via the bile and pass out of the body with fecal matter. This latter route of elimination is also associated with *enterohepatic recirculation* for some lipid-soluble drugs. For example, polar estrogen metabolites are excreted by the liver into the bile and are then returned to the intestines by the bile duct. Once in the intestines, normal gut flora can cleave the estrogen glucuronide, thus recycling the estrogenic parent compound. Because of the lipophilic nature of steroids, estrogen can then be reabsorbed and

TABLE 1-9. Drugs That Are Actively Secreted

Anionic Transporter	Cationic Transporter
Furosemide	Amiloride
Thiazides	Digoxin
Penicillins	Morphine
Cephalosporins	Procainamide
Probenecid	Quinidine
NSAIDs	Ranitidine
	Triamterene
	Trimethoprim
	Vancomycin

Box 1-13. KEYS TO DRUG ELIMINATION

- Renal and fecal excretion are the most important routes of drug elimination.
- Urine pH can be manipulated to enhance renal clearance of drugs.
- Some drug conjugates are hydrolyzed in the lower gastrointestinal tract back to the parent compound and reabsorbed in a process called enterohepatic recirculation. This process extends the duration of drug action.

Box 1-14. THERAPEUTIC CONSIDERATIONS WHEN SELECTING DRUG DOSAGES

- Dose
- Bioavailability (F)
- Route of administration (PO, IV, etc.)
- Drug interactions
- Interval between doses (τ)
- Plasma level of drug initially (Co)
- Plasma concentration of drug reported by laboratory (Cp)
- Desired steady-state plasma concentration of drug (Cpss)
- Volume of distribution (Vd)
- Clearance (Cl)
- Half-life ($t_{1/2}$)

recycled. The end result for a drug that is recycled in this manner is a prolonged $t_{1/2}$. Note that when antibiotics are administered and the gut flora has been reduced, estrogen is less likely to be recycled and hence excreted in feces. Whenever antibiotics are administered to women using hormonal contraception, there is a possible risk of reduced efficacy of the contraceptive and a back-up barrier method of contraception should be utilized. The key points to remember about drug elimination are highlighted in Box 1-13.

●●● APPLYING THE BASIC PRINCIPLES TO CLINICAL PRACTICE (DOING THE MATH)

When health care professionals administer medication to patients, numerous factors need to be considered (Box 1-14). In the final sections of this chapter, basic pharmacokinetic principles and equations will be applied to determine dosing regimens for patients.

Desired Drug Level

Any time a drug is given, there is a "target" level of drug in the plasma that the physician is trying to achieve. Typically, the drug concentrations should become relatively constant and stable when the amount of drug administered during each $t_{1/2}$ is equal to the amount of drug metabolized and eliminated from the body during the same time interval. Thus, it is said that the physician is trying to reach *steady state* (drug concentration in plasma at steady state, or Cpss).

If a drug is given once every $t_{1/2}$, it takes 4 to 5 $t_{1/2}$ for that drug to reach Cpss. Likewise, it takes 4 to 5 $t_{1/2}$ for the drug to be eliminated from the body. When the dosage "in" equals the dosage "out" at any time after 4 to 5 $t_{1/2}$, the Cpss has been reached.

Steady-state concentrations can be achieved either by administering a continuous IV infusion or by giving a series of intermittent doses (either as IV bolus injections or orally) (Fig. 1-7). Note several key points illustrated in Figure 1-7: (1)

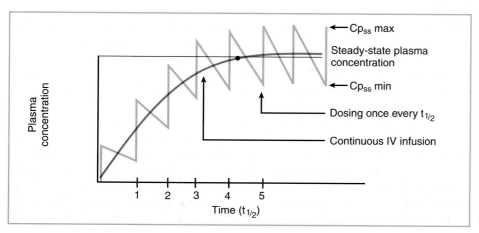

Figure 1-7. Multiple dosing regimens attain steady-state plasma concentrations.

a new dose is administered once every $t_{1/2}$, (2) 50% of the preceding peak plasma concentration is eliminated each $t_{1/2}$, and (3) Cpss is attained after 4 to 5 $t_{1/2}$, regardless of whether the drug was given by constant IV infusion or by repeated intermittent doses. It is important to realize that the steady state presented in Figure 1-7 can be achieved more quickly by administering a large "loading dose" early in therapy.

It is worth noting, too, that controlled-release dosage formulations have been created whose plasma levels mimic continuous IV infusions. A few advantages of controlled-release formulations include (1) reduced dosing frequency, (2) reduced fluctuations in drug levels, and (3) a more uniform pharmacologic response.

Drug Factors Affecting Pharmacokinetics

The bioavailability (F) of a drug refers to the fraction of a drug that reaches the systemic circulation. For drugs given IV, F = 1.0. Two major factors that alter oral bioavailability are (1) the amount of drug *absorbed* from the gastrointestinal tract and (2) the amount of drug *metabolized* by the liver during the first-past effect. Note that bioavailability does not take into account metabolism subsequent to first-pass metabolism or excretion. Often, pharmacologists refer to a term known as area under the curve (AUC). This is a reference to the graphical representation of the systemic concentration of a drug versus time. This analysis encompasses the factors that elevate concentration (absorption, bioavailability) versus those factors that decrease concentration (metabolism, excretion). This is illustrated in Figure 1-8. Although generic drugs must contain the same active ingredients as their trade name counterparts, inactive ingredients are permitted to vary. Sometimes, this change in

inert ingredients may alter the dissolution rate of a drug, and thus, the shape of the curve may vary. Clinically, this can be important if two different products (albeit containing the same active ingredient) produce differential pharmacologic responses. Similarly, different dosage forms (tablets, gelcaps, liquid) of the same drug may not always be bioequivalent with each other.

For drugs eliminated by first-order kinetics, the $t_{1/2}$ is constant. That is to say, the time to remove 50% of drug from the body is always the same. Doubling the dosage of a drug will not alter its $t_{1/2}$.

When a drug's $t_{1/2}$ is known (or looked up), it provides the information that helps determine or predict (1) how often a drug should be readministered, (2) the time necessary to reach Cpss, (3) how long it will take to completely eliminate the drug, and (4) plasma levels of the drug (Cp) at various time points.

Patient-Specific Variables—Determination of Loading Dose

Briefly, Vd is the apparent volume in which a drug is at equilibrium in the body:

$$Vd = \frac{Dose}{Cp}$$

Importantly, the term *Vd* assumes that the body is a single compartment in which drugs are equally distributed. This apparent Vd allows us to calculate a loading dose (a higher initial dose to quickly achieve the desired Cpss) for a desired Cpss:

$$Loading\ dose = \frac{(Vd)\ (Cpss)}{F}$$

Reduced to its simplest form, this calculation takes into account the size of the patient (Vd) multiplied by the plasma concentration desired (Cpss).

Sometimes, the desired Cpss is not being attained (e.g., impaired bioavailability due to gastrointestinal disease, enhanced metabolism due to CYP-450 enzyme induction, unusual body composition, etc.), and the loading dose may need to be boosted. If a patient has already been receiving a drug but is below the desired Cpss, the loading dose can be recalculated according to

$$Loading\ dose = \frac{(Vd)\ (Cpss\ desired - Cp\ initial)}{F}$$

Patient-Specific Variables—Determination of Maintenance Dose

Knowing a person's rate of clearance (Cl) is especially important for calculating maintenance doses. Clearance is defined as the volume of plasma from which a drug is completely removed by the processes of excretion or metabolism per unit time. Clearance has the units of flow (L/h, mL/min). When the physician wants to achieve Cpss, it is important

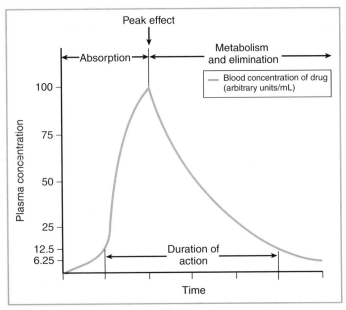

Figure 1-8. Plasma levels of drug during absorption and elimination phases. The integral of this curve represents the area under the curve.

that the amount of drug cleared from the body in a given time interval is equivalent to the next dose given (e.g., what goes "in" must come "out"). Clearance is the "out" component for the drug. The 0.693 term is a mathematical constant that reflects first-order clearance (metabolism and excretion).

$$Cl = \frac{0.693 \ (Vd)}{t_{1/2}}$$

Using this information, maintenance doses can be calculated:

$$Maintenance \ dose = \frac{(Cl) \ (Cpss) \ (\tau)}{F}$$

where τ stands for the interval of time between doses of the drug.

Additionally, for some drugs (e.g., aminoglycosides) it is useful to predict "peak" and "trough" levels. This can be estimated using the following equation, where Cp max stands for maximal plasma concentration (i.e., the peak) and Cp min represents the minimal plasma concentration (i.e., the trough).

$$Cp \ max = Cp \ min + \frac{(F) \ (Dose)}{Vd}$$

●●●● TOP FIVE LIST

1. Pharmacokinetics is a collection of equations that determine drug concentrations at the target site over time.
2. Pharmacokinetic principles integrate drug *a*bsorption, *d*istribution, *m*etabolism, and *e*xcretion (ADME).
3. Practitioners often need to know mathematical terms specific for a drug ($t_{1/2}$, bioavailability) as well as for a patient (volume of distribution, clearance) to determine the steady-state concentration of drug in plasma (Cpss).
4. Since clearance and volume of distribution change in patients as a function of disease or age, practitioners often need to quantify plasma concentrations of drug directly (via laboratory measurements) to ensure that drugs reach therapeutically effective concentrations without causing toxic effects.
5. Frequently, practitioners must determine volume of distribution and clearance in selected groups of patients (i.e., in renal, gastrointestinal, or hepatic disease). This is necessary to achieve appropriate therapeutic responses.

Pharmacodynamics and Signal Transduction

2

CONTENTS

It's all about the targets. The targets may be membrane or cytosolic receptors, ion channels, transporters, signal transduction kinases, enzymes, or specific sequences of RNA or DNA, but the pharmacodynamic principles that govern these interactions remain the same (Table 2-1). Drugs bind to specific targets, activating (stimulating) or inactivating (blocking) their functions and altering their biological responses.

●●● DOSE-RESPONSE RELATIONSHIPS

Often, the lock-and-key concept is useful to understand the way drugs work. In this analogy, the target is the lock and the drug is the key. If the key fits the lock and is able to open it (i.e., activate it), the drug is called an *agonist*. If the key fits the lock but can't get the lock to open (i.e., just blocks the lock), the drug is called an *antagonist*.

The pharmacodynamic properties of drugs define their interactions with selective targets. Pharmaceutical companies identify and then validate, optimize, and test drugs for specific targets via rational drug design or high-throughput drug screening. Table 2-2 identifies some pharmacodynamic concepts that determine the properties of drugs.

Terms such as *affinity* and *potency* (see Table 2-2) are most appreciated in graphical form. Figure 2-1A illustrates a graded (quantitative) dose-response curve. Often, this type of curve is graphed as a semi-log plot (see Fig. 2-1B). Notice that the y-axis is depicted as a percentage of the maximal effect of the drug, and the x-axis is the dose or concentration of the drug. Several important relationships can be appreciated through graded dose-response curves:

1. *Affinity* is a measure of binding strength that a drug has for its target.
2. Affinity can be defined in terms of the K_D (the dissociation constant of the drug for the target). In this instance, affinity is the inverse of the K_D ($1/K_D$). The smaller the K_D, the greater affinity a drug has for its receptor.
3. The dose of a drug that produces 50% of the maximal effect is known as the ED_{50} (effective dose to achieve 50% response). If concentrations are used, then the concentration to achieve 50% of the maximal effect is known as the EC_{50}.
4. When plotted on *linear* graph paper, the dose-response relationship for most drugs is exponential, often assuming the shape of a rectangular hyperbola.
5. By plotting response vs *log* dose, we can transform a graded dose-response curve into more linear (sigmoidal) relationships. This facilitates comparison of the dose-response curves for drugs that work by similar mechanisms of action. Without knowing anything about the mechanisms of opioids or aspirin, a glance at Figure 2-1C tells you that hydromorphone, morphine, and codeine work by the same mechanism, but aspirin works by a different mechanism. Often, the slope of the curves and the maximal effects are identical for drugs that work via the same

TABLE 2-1. Examples of Drug Targets

General Target Class	Specfic Target	Drug Example
Plasma membrane receptor	β-Adrenergic receptor	Isoproterenol
Cytosolic receptor	Corticosteroid receptor	Prednisone
Enzyme	Cyclooxygenase	Aspirin
Ion channel	GABA receptor	Barbiturates
Transporter	Serotonin transporter	Fluoxetine
Nucleic acid	Alkylating chemotherapeutics	Chlorambucil
Signal transduction kinases	Bcr-Abl mTOR	Imatinib Sirolimus

TABLE 2-2. Pharmacodynamic Concepts for Determining Properties of Drugs

Term	Definition
Affinity	The attraction (ability) of a drug to interact (bind) with its target. The greater the affinity, the greater the binding
Efficacy	The ability of a drug to interact with its target and elicit a biological response
Agonist	A drug that has both affinity and efficacy
Antagonist	A drug that has affinity but *not* efficacy
Selectivity	Interaction of drug with receptor elicits primarily one effect or response (preferably a therapeutic response)
Specificity	Interaction of a drug with preferentially one receptor class or a single receptor subtype
Potency	Term for comparing efficacies of two or more drugs that work via the same receptor or through the same mechanism of action*

*In the comparison potency of two drugs, the drug that can achieve the same biologic effect at the lower concentration/dosage is considered more potent.

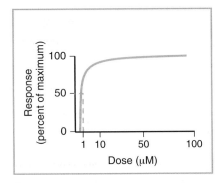

A

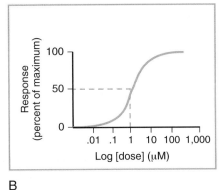

B

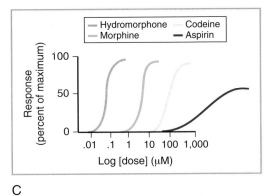

C

Figure 2-1. Graded dose-response curves, where the K_D value is 1 µm.

mechanism. These curves also tell you that of the three opioids, hydromorphone is the most potent. *Potency* is a comparative term that is used to compare two or more drugs that have different affinities for binding to the same target.

6. Below the *threshold* dose, there is no measurable response.
7. E_{max} is a measure of maximal response or *efficacy*, not a dose or concentration. Once the maximal response is achieved, increasing the concentration/dose of the drug beyond the E_{max} will not produce a further therapeutic effect but can lead to toxic effects.

Doesn't the curve depicted in Figure 2-1B look familiar? The same mathematical relationships that define how a drug (ligand) interacts with a receptor to elicit or diminish a biological response also governs the ways in which substrates (ligands) interact with enzymes to generate metabolic end products. In fact, the terms K_D and E_{max} (ceiling effect) can easily be redefined as K_m and V_{max}, which you recall from Michaelis-Menten enzyme kinetics.

Another useful mathematical concept is quantal ("all-or-none") dose-response curves. These population-based dose-response curves include data from multiple patients, often plotting percentages of patients who meet a predefined criterion (e.g., a 10 mm Hg reduction in systolic blood pressure, going to sleep after taking a sleep aid) on the y-axis versus the dose of drug that produced the biological response

BIOCHEMISTRY

Gene Targeting

The future of pharmacology may well be to target signaling elements at transcriptional or translational levels. Strategies being investigated to selectively silence genes include:
Antisense oligonucleotides
siRNAs (small interfering RNAs)
RNAzymes (enzymes that degrade RNA)
DNAzymes (enzymes that degrade DNA)
These strategies are presently limited by the technology needed to selectively and efficiently deliver these nucleic acids to specific tissues without inducing toxicity.

on the x-axis (Fig. 2-2A). These curves often take the shape of a normal frequency distribution (i.e., bell shape). These all-or-none responses can easily be thought of in terms of drugs that are sleep aids. The drug either puts people to sleep or it doesn't. There is no in-between. However, the dosage that induced sleep may vary among various people. Most folks will fall asleep with a medium-range dose, but there will be outliers—some will be very sensitive to the drug at low doses, whereas others will be relatively resistant to hypnotic effects until higher drug levels are achieved.

These data can be transformed into a cumulative frequency distribution (see Fig. 2-2B), where cumulative percent

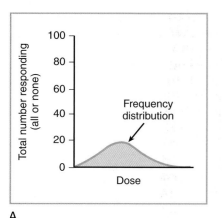
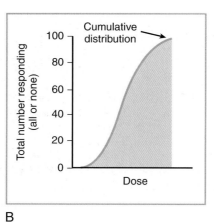
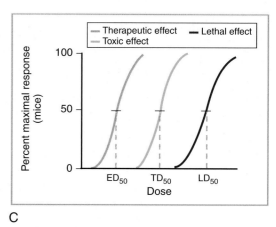

A   B   C

Figure 2-2. Quantal dose-response curves.

Box 2-1. DRUGS WITH NARROW THERAPEUTIC WINDOWS	
Theophylline	Digoxin
Warfarin	Carbamazepine
Valproate	Phenytoin
Lithium	Gentamicin

maximal patient responses are plotted versus dose. This type of sigmoidal curve yields useful safety information when the all-or-nothing responses are defined as therapeutic maximal responses, toxic responses, or lethal responses. In this way, for a single drug, cumulative frequency distributions can be compared for therapeutic efficacy, toxicity, and lethality (see Fig. 2-2C). This type of analysis can be used to compute the therapeutic index for any drug. The therapeutic index is defined as the TD_{50} (the dose that results in toxicity in 50% of the population) divided by the ED_{50} (the dose at which 50% of the patients meet the predefined criteria). As a rule of thumb, when a drug's therapeutic index is less than 10 (meaning that less than a tenfold increase in the therapeutic dose will lead to 50% toxicity), then the drug is defined as having a narrow therapeutic window. Examples of drugs with narrow therapeutic windows are listed in Box 2-1. Plasma concentrations are routinely assessed for drugs with narrow therapeutic windows. This is especially critical for patients whose pharmacokinetic parameters are compromised by renal or hepatic diseases.

TIME-RESPONSE RELATIONSHIPS

For some analyses, it is often advantageous to graph time to drug action versus defined response. This time-response curve (Fig. 2-3) depicts the latent period (time to onset of action), the time to peak effect, as well as the duration of action. Often the y-axis for this type of relationship is given as the plasma concentration of the drug (since plasma concentration is directly related to response). The maximal peak response

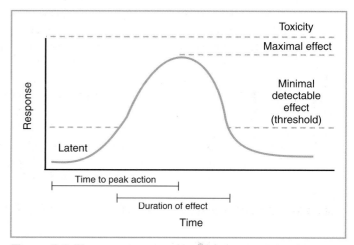

Figure 2-3. Time-response curve.

should be below the toxic dose and above the minimal effective dose. If it isn't obvious why the processes of absorption, distribution, metabolism, and excretion determine the shape of this curve, please refer back to Chapter 1.

DRUGS AS AGONISTS

How does a practitioner interpret two drugs that have equal affinities (binding) for a specific target but have different efficacies (degree of response) (Fig. 2-4)? In this example, even though all these drugs are agonists for the target, the drugs that elicit a maximal response are full agonists (drugs C and D), while those that do not elicit a maximal response are often referred to as *partial agonists* (drugs A and B in Fig. 2-4). In other words, despite occupying all of the receptors for the drug at the target site, the biological response for partial agonists is muted or lower than that of full agonists. Often the reasons for this muted or weak biological response at full receptor occupancy (saturation) is unknown. However, the key point is that partial agonists are often used clinically to competitively inhibit the responses of full agonists, and thus they can be thought of as competitive pharmacologic antagonists. Buspirone is an example of a partial agonist; buspirone exhibits full agonist properties at presynaptic

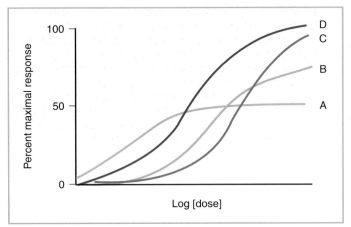

Figure 2-4. Graded dose-response curves for four drugs of the same class. Drugs C and D are full agonists, while drugs A and B are partial agonists. Drug A is the most potent agent, despite being a partial agonist. Drug D is more potent than C, even though both are full agonists.

$5HT_{1A}$ serotonin receptors but very weak agonist activity at postsynaptic $5HT_{1A}$ receptors. The net result of these disparate biological responses leads to classification of this drug as a partial agonist.

Continuing with Figure 2-4, there can be cases when partial agonists (drug A) display greater potency (greater effect at a lower concentration) than full agonists (drug D). Understanding these dose-response curves requires an appreciation of the two-state model for receptor activation. Receptors can be thought to undergo a dynamic conformational or structural transition between inactive and active states in the presence of ligands. This model can be useful to explain why partial agonists exhibit weak biological responses at full saturation of receptors. In this model, full agonists preferentially bind to the active form of the target with high affinity, whereas partial agonists have affinities to both the active and the inactive conformations of the target. By extending this model, drugs can be designed to stabilize the inactive form of targets. These drugs theoretically would exhibit negative efficacy, and they are called *inverse agonists*. For inverse agonism to be observed, there must be some level of constitutive activity in the absence of agonist. Although these issues are frequently incorporated into test questions, there are few, if any, demonstrated examples of inverse agonism in vivo.

●●● DRUGS AS ANTAGONISTS

Often physicians prescribe a drug that blocks or competes with an endogenous metabolite or pathway or exogenous *xenobiotic* (foreign substance) or drug. These agents are antagonists in that they block (or antagonize) the natural signal. These antagonists change the shape of dose-response curves. For example, a competitive, reversible antagonist shifts the dose-response curve to the right, indicating that the agonist must now be given at a higher dose to elicit a similar response in the presence of the antagonist (Fig. 2-5A). In contrast, an irreversible antagonist shifts the dose response

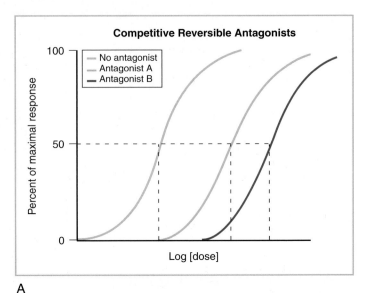

A

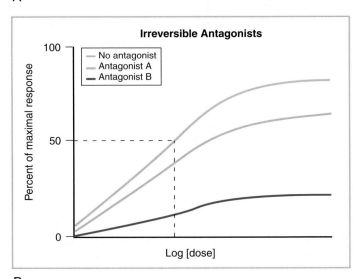

B

Figure 2-5. Antagonists shift dose-response curves of agonists. **A**, Competitive reversible antagonists. **B**, Irreversible antagonists.

curve downward, indicating that the agonist can no longer exert maximal effects at any therapeutic dose (see Fig. 2-5B). There are also allosteric interactions (binding at an alternative or "distant" site), where different drugs bind to distinct sites on one target in a reversible but not competitive manner. In these cases, the action of one drug positively or negatively impacts the binding of a second drug to the target, a phenomenon known as *cooperativity*.

Antagonists, such as β-adrenergic receptor antagonists, ("β-blockers") have affinity, but no efficacy, for β-adrenergic receptors. These drugs compete for and block endogenous norepinephrine or epinephrine from stimulating adrenergic receptors. Because membrane receptors may be recycled after drug binding (desensitization), may be newly transcribed, or may have amplified responses through actions at multiple effectors, the actual magnitude of antagonism corresponding to a reduced biological response may not

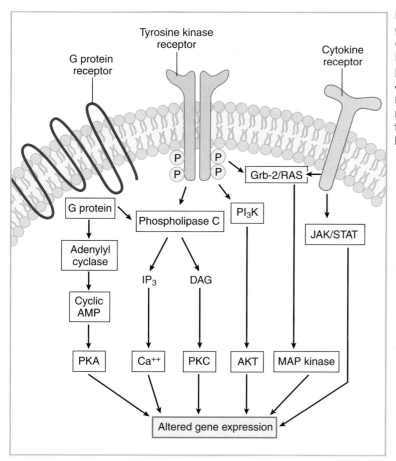

Figure 2-6. Signal transduction: it all leads to altered gene expression. IP$_3$, inositol-trisphosphate; DAG, diacylglycerol; cAMP, cyclic adenosine monophosphate; PKA, protein kinase A; PKC, protein kinase C; PI$_3$K, phosphatidylinositol-3-kinase; AKT, a cell-survival kinase; JAK/STAT, dimerized proteins that couple cytokine receptors to downstream targets; Grb-2/Ras, scaffold network of proteins that couple tyrosine kinase receptors to downstream targets such as the MAP kinases; MAP kinases, mitogen-activated protein kinases.

always be linear and, in fact, may be less than expected. The term *spare receptor* is often used to describe this phenomenon.

●●● SIGNALING AND RECEPTORS

The critical concepts of signal transduction pathways are amplification, redundancy, cross-talk, and integration of biological signals. From a pharmacological perspective, identification of individual signal transduction elements often uncovers potential targets for drugs to selectively disrupt the integrated circuits that control cell growth, survival, and differentiation. To fully appreciate the complexity of signaling networks requires an understanding of a "New York City subway map" of interconnected receptors, effectors, targets, and scaffold proteins. The physician should understand the critical concepts of cell signaling, as well as some of the therapeutic targets that can now be modified with drugs.

Figure 2-6 depicts several intracellular signals that are regulated via receptor activation. A major family of membrane receptors is the 7 transmembrane-spanning domain G protein–coupled receptors. These receptors couple to heterotrimeric GTP-binding proteins, which regulate downstream effectors, including adenylate cyclase. This is a critical element in the discussion of the autonomic (see Chapter 6) and central nervous systems (see Chapter 13).

As depicted in Figure 2-7, amplification of the signal occurs as one receptor interacts with multiple G proteins that remain activated even after the receptors dissociate. In a cyclical fashion, activated receptors couple to the $\alpha/\beta/\gamma$ subunits of the inactivated G protein (bound to GDP). This interaction induces GDP dissociation, followed by GTP binding, and activation of the G protein. The activated G protein dissociates into distinct α and β/γ subunits. The α subunit interacts with adenylyl cyclase, the enzyme that produces cyclic AMP, the biological cofactor for protein kinase A (PKA). Hydrolysis of GTP to GDP dissociates the α subunit from adenylyl cyclase and permits reassociation with the β/γ subunits, resetting the cycle for subsequent activation by another receptor. Leading to further complexity is that fact that distinct α subunits couple to different and specific effectors (Fig. 2-8) as well as the fact that β/γ subunits themselves can interact with other downstream effectors including phospholipases.

Examples of a receptor class that couples to G$_s$ ("s" stands for "stimulatory" as opposed to G$_i$, in which the "i" stands for "inhibitory") to activate adenylate cyclase and generate cAMP are the β-adrenergic receptors. Pharmacologic intervention with a β-agonist like isoproterenol activates β-adrenergic receptors, whereas antagonists such as propranolol, a β-blocker, prevent endogenous activation of these receptors.

Understanding the mechanisms by which these receptors undergo desensitization or internalization helps explain

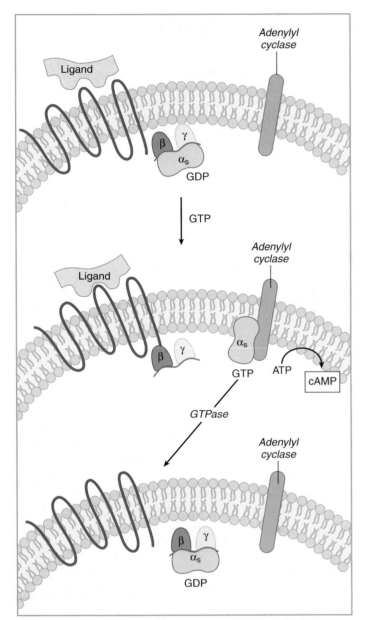

Figure 2-7. A G protein–centric view of signaling. GTP, guanosine triphosphate; GDP, guanosine diphosphate.

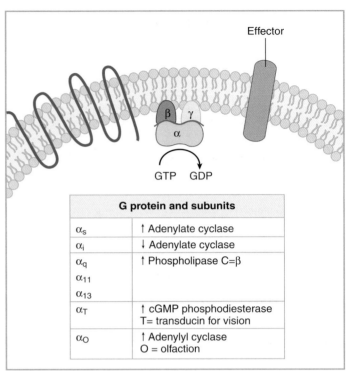

G protein and subunits	
α_S	↑ Adenylate cyclase
α_i	↓ Adenylate cyclase
α_q	↑ Phospholipase C=β
α_{11}	
α_{13}	
α_T	↑ cGMP phosphodiesterase T= transducin for vision
α_O	↑ Adenylyl cyclase O = olfaction

Figure 2-8. G proteins come in different flavors. The G-protein complex is composed of α-, β-, and γ-subunits. The α-subunits are distinct proteins that subserve different functions by coupling to different effectors.

why receptor responses dissipate over prolonged activation (Fig. 2-9). Interaction of β-adrenergic receptors with epinephrine promotes phosphorylation of the receptor by β-adrenergic receptor kinases (BARKs). The hyperphosphorylated receptors interact with arrestin, a molecule that either prevents activation of G proteins by the receptor and/or induces receptor internalization. One of the critical concepts in signal transduction is that posttranslational modifications of targets by phosphorylation alter receptor function.

Besides coupling to adenylate cyclase, G protein–linked receptors can regulate lipid turnover in membranes. Another critical concept in signaling is that altered lipid metabolism generates lipid-derived second messengers that amplify primary signals. Simply put, it's all about metabolism of a phosphorylated lipid that makes up less than 0.01% of the total lipid content of the membrane. G protein–coupled receptors, like the angiotensin II receptor, activate phospholipase C via Gq, which preferentially hydrolyzes phosphatidylinositol 4,5-bisphosphate (PIP_2) to form two distinct lipid-derived second messengers (Fig. 2-10A): inositol 1,4,5-trisphosphate (IP_3) and diacylglycerol (DAG). IP_3, being hydrophilic, leaves the membrane and interacts with calcium channels on the endoplasmic reticulum, producing an increase in intracellular free calcium. Calcium-regulated kinases impact multiple systems responsible for blood clotting, neuronal function, and proton secretion in the stomach. In contrast, DAG, being hydrophobic, remains at the plasma membrane, where it is a lipid cofactor that activates protein kinase C.

To complicate matters, growth factor receptors, such as platelet-derived growth factor, which are tyrosine kinases, also couple to phospholipases to form lipid-derived second messengers (see Fig. 2-6). Another critical concept in signaling is that dimerization and resultant autophosphorylation of tyrosine kinase receptors often leads to propagation of the signal. Many of the latest therapeutic approaches work through inhibiting these tyrosine kinase receptor activation mechanisms. In addition, these tyrosine kinase receptors also activate phosphatidylinositol-3-kinase (PI_3K; Fig. 2-10B), which can form a third messenger from phosphatidylinositol 4,5-bisphosphate. The generated phosphatidylinositol 3,4,5-triphosphate can interact with proteins containing pleckstrin homology domains, such as AKT, which are critical kinases for cell survival. Growth factor receptors are overexpressed in

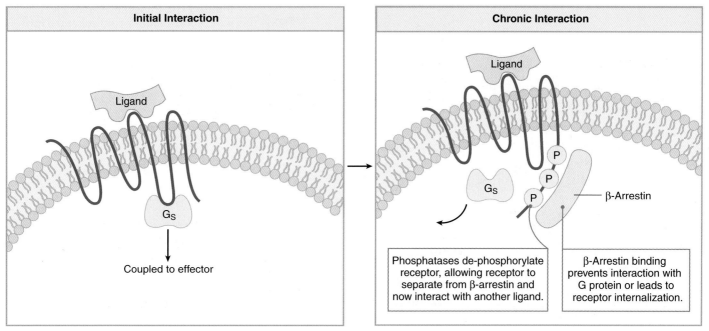

Figure 2-9. Hyperphosphorylation of G protein receptors leads to desensitization.

cancerous lesions. Figure 2-11 depicts several of the pro-mitogenic cascades activated by this class of receptors, as well as designated targets for therapeutic intervention.

Figure 2-12 illustrates another lipid metabolite formed from hydrolysis of phosphatidylinositol 4,5-bisphosphate (PIP_2). Phospholipase A_2 hydrolyzes fatty acids from lipids, such as PIP_2 or phosphatidylcholine. These fatty acids are often highly unsaturated, containing multiple double bonds. Fatty acids containing 20 carbons with 4 double bonds that occur starting 6 carbons from the carboxyl terminus are known as *arachidonic acid*. These fatty acids can be oxidized by multiple enzymes to form prostaglandins, leukotrienes, and epoxides (HETEs) by cyclooxygenase, lipoxygenase, and epoxygenases, respectively.

The onslaught of lipid-derived messengers is referred to as "arachidonophobia." Multiple drugs, either irreversibly (aspirin) or reversibly (nonsteroidal anti-inflammatory agents [NSAIDs]) inhibit cyclooxygenase and are reviewed in Chapter 10. Inhibitors of leukotriene synthesis, such as montelukast, are effective in asthmatic patients.

Another signaling concept is that lipid-derived second messengers such as prostaglandins can themselves activate G protein–coupled receptors, again amplifying responses (Fig. 2-13). It should be noted that lipid-derived messengers can signal by creating structured membrane microdomains (also called lipid rafts), directly interacting with lipid-binding domains on proteins, or by posttranslationally modifying proteins. Examples of posttranslational modifications include proteins made hydrophobic by covalent modifications with 14-carbon (myristoylate) or 16-carbon (palmitoylate) fatty acids. A critical example of a myristoylated target protein is Ras, which is over-expressed or mutated in multiple cancers.

CLINICAL MEDICINE

Why do physicians need to know Signaling 101?

More and more drugs that alter signal transduction cascades are being validated, tested, approved, and marketed. These drugs offer the promise of specificity, selectivity, and reduced toxicity, since signaling elements are often mutated or overexpressed in disease states, including cancer and inflammation. In this way, normal tissues may not be dramatically affected by the drug, resulting in reduced side effects. Examples of some approved designer drug targets are:

Target Signal	Approved Pathology
Erb-B_2 receptor	Breast cancer
Erb-B_2 receptor	Non–small cell lung cancer
Erb-B_2 receptor	Colorectal cancer
BCR-ABL	Chronic myelogenous leukemia
mTOR	Re-stenosis after coronary stenting
Peroxisome proliferator activator receptors (PPAR)	Diabetes

The Her2/neu gene product, the Erb-B_2 receptor, a member of the human epidermal growth factor family of tyrosine kinases, is overexpressed in multiple cancers and is associated with a poor prognosis. Erb-B_2 forms a heterodimer with other Erb receptors that exhibit enhanced mitogenic signaling potential. Several different strategies have been used to target this receptor. Monoclonal antibodies (trastuzumab) as well as low-molecular-weight inhibitors (gefitinib) have been designed to block these actions. Additional strategies, including coupling a specific antibody to cytotoxins or ligands that activate immune cells, are being investigated.

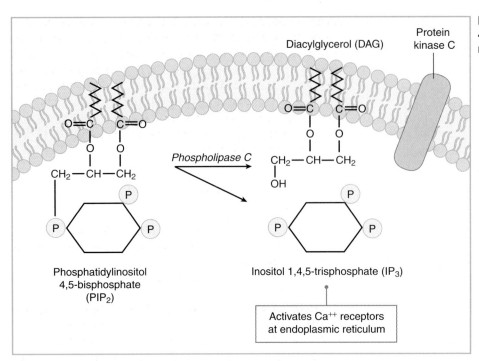

Figure 2-10. Phosphatidylinositol 4,5-bisphosphate, a lipid substrate for multiple enzymes.

A

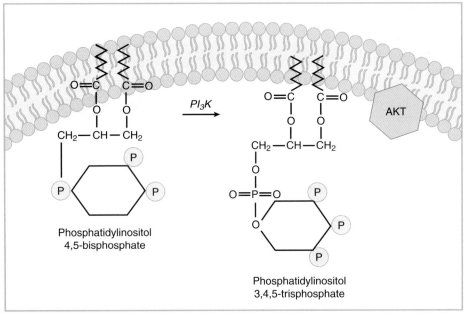

B

Signal transduction cascades can interact with and dramatically impact ion channels. In fact, ligand-gated ion channels themselves serve as targets for both intracellular signal transduction cascades as well as therapeutic drugs. Pharmacologic regulation of ion channels serves as one approach to controlling cardiac (verapamil, a Ca^{++} channel blocker), renal (furosemide, an $Na^+/K^+/Cl^-$ cotransporter antagonist), and neuronal (benzodiazepines, a Cl^- channel allosteric modulator) function. Modifying pathologic ion channel activity with therapeutics can be affected by direct interaction with the channel itself or upstream/downstream

signal transduction targets of that ion channel. Ligand-gated ion channels can be regulated by Ca^{++}, cAMP, lipid mediators, and tyrosine phosphorylation signal transduction mechanisms.

A detailed example of ion channel modulation with therapeutics is γ-aminobutyric acid (GABA)–activated neuronal chloride channels. Benzodiazepines are examples of drugs that work via modulation of GABA-activated chloride channels. GABA serves as the endogenous ligand for this ligand-gated ion channel (Fig. 2-14). Benzodiazepines cannot activate GABA receptors in the absence of GABA, but

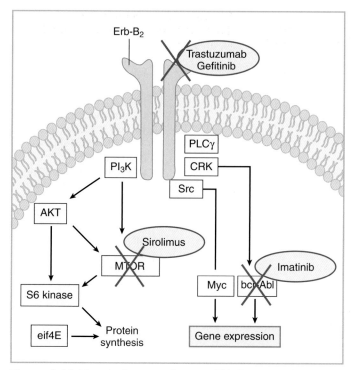

Figure 2-11. Targeted cancer therapy. Erb-B$_2$, a tyrosine kinase receptor; PLCγ, phospholipase C subtype that couples to tyrosine kinases; CRK/Src, another group of scaffold proteins that couple tyrosine kinases to downstream effectors; cABL, Myc, mTOR, S6 Kinase, various downstream kinases and transcriptional factors that can serve as selective "targets" for drugs.

benzodiazepines do facilitate the actions of GABA to alter the conformation of the receptor-ion channel, allowing the chloride channel to remain open longer than it would be otherwise. The enhanced chloride flux hyperpolarizes the membrane, diminishing neuronal transmission and inducing sedation or cessation of anxiety (anxiolytic). The target of benzodiazepines, then, is a ligand-gated ion channel. This is also an example of positive cooperativity between the GABA neurotransmitter and a drug.

●●● TOP FIVE LIST

1. Drugs bind to targets.
2. Targets themselves can be receptors, ion channels, transporters, signaling molecules, enzymes, or specific nucleic acid sequences.
3. Interactions between drugs and targets can be agonistic or antagonistic.
4. Pharmacodynamic terms used to define drug-target interactions include affinity, potency, and efficacy.
5. Drugs with a narrow therapeutic window (therapeutic index equals toxic dose [TD$_{50}$] divided by effective dose [ED$_{50}$]) must be closely monitored by the practitioner.

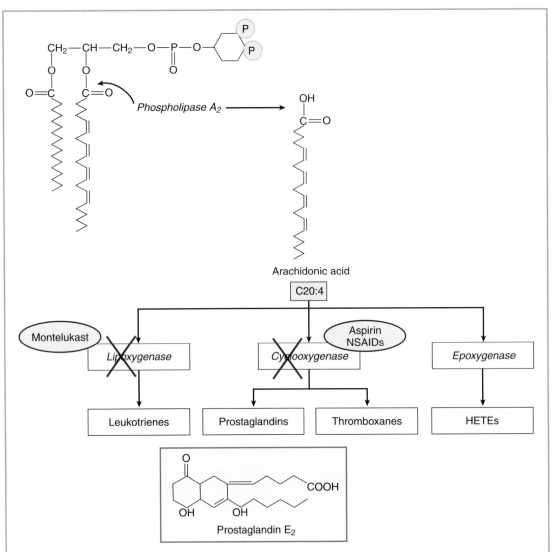

Figure 2-12. Arachidonophobia: 20 carbons, 4 double bonds, and the precursor to multiple lipid-derived second messengers (leukotrienes, prostaglandins, thromboxanes, and HETEs [hydroxyeicosatrienoic acids]) that regulate myriad physiologic responses from vasoreactivity, to bronchial constriction, to labor, to protection of the gastrointestinal tract, to inflammation, and so on. The inset prostaglandin E_2 is an example of the kinds of structures that are created.

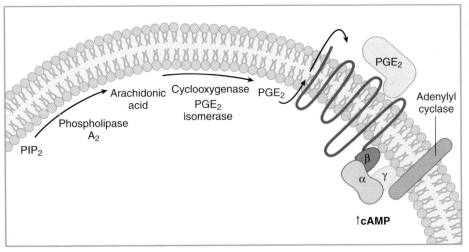

Figure 2-13. Lipid-derived second messengers can interact with their own G protein–coupled receptors. PGE$_2$, prostaglandin E$_2$; cAMP, cyclic adenosine monophosphate.

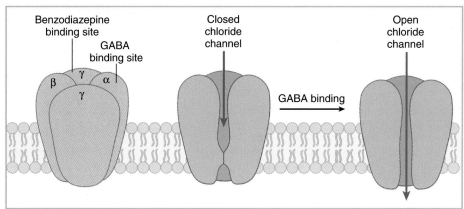

Benzodiazepine binding site

GABA binding site

β   γ   α
γ

Closed chloride channel

GABA binding →

Open chloride channel

Figure 2-14. Ligand-gated channels regulate the flow of ions through plasma membrane channels. This example depicts the GABA$_A$ receptor, which modulates chloride conductance.

Toxicology

3

CONTENTS

It's all about excess—too much of a good thing can be bad. In fact, according to the ancient pharmacology proverb, "If one is good, two is not necessarily better." More than just the memorization of acronyms or mnemonics, toxicology involves the practice of life-saving modalities and therapeutic interventions that reduce levels of hazardous substances within the body. Almost any substance, if taken in large enough doses, can produce harmful effects. It is therefore critical to be able to identify common toxins and to be able to initiate appropriate measures in a timely fashion.

●●● APPROACHES TO THE POISONED PATIENT

When managing the adverse effects associated with drugs or poisons, always begin with ABC (*a*irway, *b*reathing, and *c*irculation) and initiate cardiopulmonary resuscitation if necessary. That is, make sure the patient is stable before worrying about the specific treatments or antidotes.

Activated Charcoal

Activated charcoal is often utilized in emergency rooms for suspected overdose situations when antidotes with higher specificity are not available. Activated charcoal is a highly purified adsorbent form of charcoal that binds (adsorbs) drugs in the gastrointestinal tract, preventing their absorption. However, charcoal is ineffective for treating hydrocarbon (e.g., ethanol) or metal (e.g., iron, lead, lithium) overdoses. Risks associated with activated charcoal include emesis

(vomiting) following administration, pulmonary aspiration leading to pneumonitis, and constipation or bowel obstruction.

Gastric Lavage

Another common technique used in emergency rooms is gastric lavage ("pumping the stomach"), which is helpful only if a patient comes to the hospital within 1 hour of a toxic ingestion. Lavage decreases absorption of toxins by approximately 50% at 5 minutes, 25% at 30 minutes, and 15% at 60 minutes. Lavage may be used to speed removal of many drugs ingested orally, but it is contraindicated for ingestion of caustic substances or hydrocarbons. Complications associated with gastric lavage include aspiration pneumonitis, laryngospasm, mechanical injury to the esophagus or gastrointestinal tract, hypothermia, and fluid and electrolyte imbalances.

Ionized Diuresis

Ionized diuresis may be used to facilitate excretion of poisons that are eliminated by the kidneys. Ionized diuresis refers to the process in which excretion of weak acids or weak bases is enhanced by trapping the ionized portion of drug in the renal tubules. Let's use ammonia, $NH_3 + H^+ \rightleftharpoons NH_4^+$, as an example. Ammonia, NH_3, is a weak base that readily crosses biologic membranes because it is uncharged. If filtered from the plasma by the glomeruli, ammonia would be prone to reabsorption in the bloodstream since it is un-ionized and not particularly polar. However, the situation changes if the urine is acidified. In an acidic environment, the positively charged ammonium ion cannot easily penetrate biologic membranes and thus is not readily reabsorbed (i.e., a higher percentage of metabolite would be excreted). Historically, the ion-trapping principle was applied to hasten removal of drugs that are weak bases (amphetamines, phencyclidine). However, this practice is no longer recommended, since rhabdomyolysis (muscle breakdown) is common following these overdoses and acidification of urine may increase the risk of renal failure. On rare occasions, ammonium chloride can be used to acidify urine and facilitate secretion of weak bases.

The same principle applies to weak acids. We'll use

$$salicylic\ acid \rightleftharpoons salicylate + H^+ (HA \rightleftharpoons A^- + H^+)$$

PHYSIOLOGY

Anion Gap—Acids and Bases

The term anion gap refers to the concentration of all the unmeasured anions (negatively charged molecules) present in the plasma. It is estimated by subtracting measurable anions (chloride and bicarbonate) from the measurable cations (Na^+ and K^+). A normal anion gap is between 8–16 mEq/L. The resulting anion gap is then assessed as normal, high, or low. A high gap is deemed a sign of acidosis and is used in the emergency department as an indication of conditions such as ketoacidosis, lactic acidosis, or renal failure.

PHYSIOLOGY

Aspirin Toxicity Is an Acid-Base Problem

Aspirin is a commonly used drug that can potentially lead to fatalities in overdose situations. Acute intoxication causes an initial respiratory alkalosis via hyperventilation resulting from direct stimulation of the respiratory centers. High-dose salicylates also cause uncoupling of oxidative phosphorylation. Catabolism occurs secondary to the inhibition of ATP-dependent reactions, which leads to hyperpyrexia (markedly elevated body temperature) and metabolic acidosis from the accumulation of endogenous acids.

as an example. In other words, to excrete toxic weak acids, alkalinize the urine. In an alkalinized urine, drugs that are weak acids are ionized and excreted—not reabsorbed. To treat poisonings associated with weak acids (salicylates, phenobarbital), the urine can be alkalinized with intravenous sodium bicarbonate while the patient is monitored for alkalosis and fluid and electrolyte disturbances (Table 3-1).

●●● SPECIFIC ANTIDOTES

Specific antidotes are available for only a few drugs and poisonous substances. Be aware that (1) the duration of action of most antidotes is shorter than that of the toxic

agent, so antidotes may need to be given repeatedly until the effects of the poison are eliminated; and (2) antidotes should never replace good supportive care.

Neurally Active Drugs/Poisons

Organophosphates

Toxic exposure to irreversible acetylcholinesterase inhibitors like the organophosphates usually stems from occupational hazards, given that the chemicals are used as insecticides and pesticides in the agricultural industry (parathion, malathion) and as biologic warfare agents (soman). As a result, farmers are at risk of developing life-threatening complications if crop-dusting airplanes inadvertently spray them. Military personnel are also at risk in the event that they are attacked with weapons containing "nerve agents."

Organophosphates are very lipophilic and can permeate the body via inhalation or absorption through the skin. These agents covalently bind to and inhibit acetylcholinesterases, the enzymes that usually terminate the actions of acetylcholine. The most important thing for health care providers to remember when organophosphate poisoning is suspected is to protect themselves. Owing to the lipophilic nature of the drugs, health care professionals can become cross-contaminated simply from skin contact with the affected individual (Table 3-2).

Exposure to organophosphates results in widespread toxicity, since acetylcholine plays key roles within the sympathetic nervous system, the parasympathetic nervous system, and the neuromuscular junction. Signs and symptoms of organophosphate overdose include salivation, lacrimation, urination, defecation (known as the *SLUD syndrome*), miosis, bronchospasm, bradycardia, sweating, paralysis of respiratory muscles, convulsions, and coma. Another popular mnemonic is DUMBELS (*d*iarrhea, *u*rination, *m*iosis, *b*ronchoconstriction, *e*xcitation, *l*acrimation, *s*alivation). The most common cause of death is respiratory failure, so mechanical ventilation may be necessary.

Pharmacologic management of organophosphate poisoning includes atropine and pralidoxime. Atropine competitively blocks the actions of acetylcholine at muscarinic receptors.

TABLE 3-1. Presentation and Management of Salicylate Poisoning

Agent	Signs/Symptoms	Interventions	Antidotes

Salicylates (e.g., aspirin)	Acidosis
	Coma
	Confusion and lethargy
	Dehydration
	Hyperthermia
	Hyperventilation
	Hypokalemia
	Seizures
	Tinnitus
		Manage acidosis
		  and electrolytes
		IV hydration
		Intubation and mechanical
		  ventilation (severe cases)
			Urinary alkalinization
			Hemodialysis (severe cases)

TABLE 3-2. Presentation and Management of Acetylcholinesterase (AChE) Inhibitor Poisoning

Agent	Signs/Symptoms	Interventions	Antidotes
AChE inhibitors (e.g., physostigmine, insecticides [organophosphates, carbamates])	Diarrhea Urination Miosis Bronchoconstriction Excitation (muscle twitches) Lacrimation Salivation, sweating, seizures GI cramps	Respiratory support IV hydration	Atropine Pralidoxime

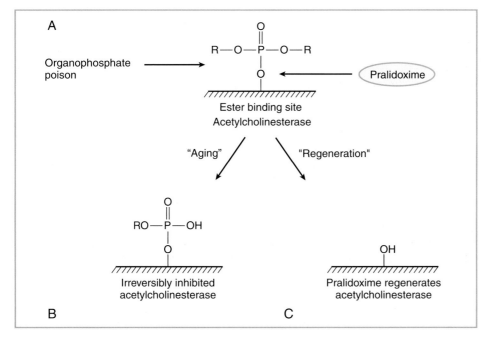

Figure 3-1. A, Organophosphate-inactivated acetylcholinesterase enzyme. **B**, With time, one of the R-groups leaves and this generates an irreversible complex and an inactive enzyme (the aging process). **C**, Pralidoxime attacks organophosphate-enzyme complex and causes organophosphate to release from enzyme, thereby regenerating active acetylcholinesterase. This drug does not work against the "aged" complex depicted in part B.

Thus, it is palliative in nature, since it does not reverse the inhibition of acetylcholinesterases caused by the organophosphates. Atropine will reverse bronchorrhea but not pupil size. Pralidoxime is truly an antidote for organophosphate poisoning. Pralidoxime breaks the covalent bond between organophosphates and acetylcholinesterases to regenerate the active enzyme. Pralidoxime is an effective antidote for organophosphate poisoning only if the antidote is administered prior to the "aging" process (i.e., within 24 hours of exposure), which stabilizes the organophosphate-enzyme complex (Fig. 3-1).

Anticholinergics

In contrast to organophosphates, numerous medications including muscarinic receptor antagonists, such as benztropine, possess anticholinergic properties. In addition, some antihistamines and phenothiazines possess anticholinergic properties, as do natural products like Jimson weed and some mushrooms (*Amanita muscaria*).

Signs and symptoms of anticholinergic syndrome are opposite those of the SLUD syndrome and include hypertension, tachycardia, fever, dry eyes/mouth, urinary retention, and ileus (intestinal obstruction). Central nervous system side effects, including visual hallucinations, disorientation and confusion, seizures, and coma also occur. Thus, a patient with anticholinergic syndrome may generally be described as being dry as a bone, red as a beet, hot as a pistol, blind as a bat, and mad as a hatter. To alleviate excessive anticholinergic side effects, acetylcholinesterase inhibitors like physostigmine may be administered. Physostigmine inhibits the degradation of acetylcholine in the synaptic cleft, thus enhancing the action of acetylcholine. Physostigmine is indicated if anticholinergic side effects of agitated psychosis, seizures, or supraventricular arrhythmias are occurring (Table 3-3).

Benzodiazepines

Benzodiazepines have largely replaced barbiturates as sedative-hypnotic agents because of their superior safety

TABLE 3-3. Presentation and Management of Anticholinergic Syndrome

Agent	Signs/Symptoms	Interventions	Antidotes
Muscarinic antagonists (e.g., atropine), mushrooms	Dry mouth, eyes Tachycardia Hypertension Hyperthermia Delirium and hallucinations Sedation Urinary retention Constipation Agitation, disorientaton, confusion Seizures Coma	Manage cardiovascular symptoms and hyperthermia	Physostigmine or neostigmine

TABLE 3-4. Presentation and Management of Sedative Hypnotic Syndrome

Agent	Signs/Symptoms	Interventions	Antidotes
Sedative-hypnotics (e.g., benzodiazepines, barbiturates, alcohol)	Lethargy Disinhibition Ataxia Nystagmus Miosis Stupor Coma Hypothermia Hypotension Bradycardia Respiratory failure	Ventilatory support	Flumazenil for benzodiazepines only

profile. However, in benzodiazepine overdose situations, respiratory depression is still a major concern. Other signs and symptoms accompanying sedative hypnotic syndrome include hypothermia, miosis, ileus, and bradycardia (Table 3-4).

Flumazenil competitively antagonizes the benzodiazepine binding site of the $GABA_A$ receptor. If benzodiazepine toxicity is suspected, flumazenil treatment may prevent the need for subsequent intubation of the patient. Flumazenil has a relatively short half-life ($t_{1/2}$) compared with many benzodiazepines, often necessitating readministration. Like benzodiazepines, flumazenil may cause sedation. Patients should avoid engaging in activities that require mental alertness for at least 18 to 24 hours following flumazenil administration. Caution is also necessary when using flumazenil during detoxification in patients who may be physically dependent upon benzodiazepines, since the antidote can induce seizures as a result of sudden benzodiazepine withdrawal.

Opioids: Heroin

The opioid analgesics and heroin possess a variety of depressant effects, the most dangerous of which is decreased respiratory drive. Naloxone was the first opioid receptor antagonist made available to reverse toxicities associated with

opioid overdoses. Use of this specific antidote may prevent both intubation and aspiration. Naloxone should be used if the patient has both respiratory depression and miosis. Since naloxone has a relatively short half-life compared with the depressant effects of most opioid receptor agonists, the antidote may need to be readministered numerous times to reverse respiratory depression (Table 3-5).

Serotonin Syndrome

Serotonin syndrome is a hyperserotonergic state that is dangerous and potentially fatal. It is a condition that has been on the rise since the 1960s, when drugs that affect serotonergic neurotransmission (e.g., LSD, SSRIs, MAOIs) came into use. In addition, toxicity due to excess serotonin is also observed in the case of carcinoid tumors.

Signs and symptoms of serotonin syndrome include euphoria, sustained rapid eye movements, overreaction of reflexes, clumsiness, rapid muscle contractions and relaxations in ankles and jaw, dizziness, feelings of intoxication, sweating, shivering, diarrhea, loss of consciousness, and death. Treatment of serotonin syndrome first involves discontinuing any offending drugs. Second, benzodiazepines may be administered, followed by drugs that possess

Carcinoid Syndrome

Toxicologic syndromes, such as the symptoms associated with serotonin syndrome, may not always be a result of improper uses of medication. As an example, carcinoid syndrome is a constellation of symptoms that arise as a result of a carcinoid tumor. Carcinoid tumors arise from peripheral neuroendocrine cells (especially of the gut) and are generally defined by their ability to synthesize and release large amounts of serotonin. Because of the inappropriate release of this bioactive amine neurotransmitter and neurohormone (see Chapter 13), patients have a wide range of symptoms, including flushing of the neck and face, diarrhea, wheezing, and palpitations. In some patients, right-sided heart problems arise as a result of tricuspid valve stenosis.

Serotonin Syndrome and Neuroleptic Malignant Syndrome

Physicians are required to make differential diagnoses based on a combination of symptoms and patient history. Many different clinical problems may present with similar symptoms. As an example, neuroleptic malignant syndrome (idiosyncratic toxicologic reaction to antipsychotic neuroleptic drugs; see Chapter 13) often presents with the same symptoms as serotonin syndrome. This latter condition is more predictably associated with excess serotonin activity as a result of treatments with serotonergic drugs such as the SSRI antidepressants (selective serotonin reuptake inhibitors; see Chapter 13). In this case, serotonin syndrome can be distinguished from neuroleptic syndrome on the basis of a detailed medical history with particular attention devoted to recent changes in drug administration.

TABLE 3-5. Presentation and Management of Opioid Overdose

Agent	Signs/Symptoms	Interventions	Antidotes
Opioid analgesics (e.g., morphine, heroin, oxycodone)	Lethargy and sedation Bradycardia Hypotension Hypoventilation Miosis Constipation Coma Respiratory failure	Ventilatory support	Naloxone

serotonin antagonist activity such as cyproheptadine or metoclopramide (Table 3-6).

Serotonin syndrome may occur as a consequence of inadvertent combinations of drugs that affect serotonin levels in the central nervous system. Combining drugs that act as selective serotonin reuptake inhibitors (SSRIs), serotonin receptor agonists, serotonin release agents, or serotonin catabolism inhibitors could result in a patient exhibiting the serotonin syndrome. Examples of agents that in combination elicit serotonin syndrome are monoamine oxidase inhibitors (MAOIs), clomipramine, trazodone, lithium, amphetamines, cocaine, dextromethorphan, meperidine, venlafaxine, tricyclic antidepressants, buspirone, the "triptans" (serotonin $5HT_{1D}$ agonists), and reserpine (Table 3-7; see Chapter 13 for details). The natural supplements L-tryptophan and St. John's wort have also been implicated in serotonin syndrome, as has electroconvulsive therapy.

Methanol

Methanol is found in fuel antifreeze, windshield washer fluids, and "moonshine." Its ingestion leads to optic nerve damage and associated blindness as well as severe metabolic acidosis.

Causes of a High Anion Gap

Numerous toxins, metabolic syndromes, and drugs produce a high anion gap acidosis. A simple mnemonic for these conditions and poisonings is MUDPILES.

M—methanol
U—uremia
D—diabetic acidosis
P—paraldehyde or phenformin
I—isoniazid or iron
L—lactic acid (carbon monoxide, cyanide—inhibition of aerobic metabolism)
E—ethylene glycol
S—salicylates

Metabolized by the same hepatic enzymes that biotransform ethanol, methanol is first converted by the enzyme alcohol dehydrogenase to formaldehyde, which is then converted to formic acid by aldehyde dehydrogenase (Fig. 3-2).

The formaldehyde and formic acid metabolites are responsible for the visual damage and acidosis. Ethanol is an

TABLE 3-6. Presentation and Management of Psychotropic Drug Overdoses

Agents	Interventions	Antidotes
Selective serotonin reuptake inhibitors (SSRIs; e.g., sertraline); serotonin receptor agonists (e.g., buspirone, sumatriptan)	Manage hyperthermia and seizures	Cyproheptadine Antipsychotics Benzodiazepines Dantrolene Metoclopramide
Tricyclic antidepressants (e.g., imipramine)	Manage seizures, hyperthermia, and acidosis	Antiarrhythmics
CNS stimulants (e.g., cocaine, amphetamines)	Manage cardiovascular symptoms, hyperthermia, and seizures	Benzodiazepines Antipsychotics Antiarrhythmics
Antipsychotics (e.g., haloperidol)	Dose reduction Switch to different agent Manage seizures	Botulinum toxin for acute dystonia Bromocriptine and/or Dantrolene for neuroleptic malignant syndrome Antimuscarinics and antihistamines for extrapyramidal reactions

TABLE 3-7. Drugs That Can Cause Serotonin Syndrome When Used in Combination

Selective Serotonin Reuptake Inhibitors	Nonselective Serotonin Reuptake Inhibitors	Serotonin Agonists
Fluoxetine Fluvoxamine Sertraline Paroxetine Citalopram Escitalopram	Trazodone Nefazodone Clomipramine Imipramine Desipramine Amitriptyline Nortriptyline	Buspirone LSD Mescaline "Triptans"

Drugs That Promote Serotonin Release	Drugs That Inhibit Serotonin Breakdown
Cocaine Amphetamines Codeine Dextromethorphan Reserpine	Pargyline Phenelzine Selegiline

effective antidote for methanol ingestion, since it successfully competes with methanol for alcohol dehydrogenase and saturates the enzyme. This slows the metabolism of methanol and provides time to remove methanol by dialysis, if needed (Table 3-8). Alternatively, fomepizole, an inhibitor of alcohol dehydrogenase, can also be used for methanol and ethylene glycol poisoning.

Cardiovascular Drugs/Poisons

Carbon Monoxide

Carbon monoxide (CO) is an odorless, colorless gas that binds to hemoglobin with a more than 200-fold greater affinity than O_2, resulting in tissue hypoxia. Most CO poisonings occur as a result of furnace or space heater malfunctions or automobile exhausts. Following hurricanes, CO poisoning incidence increases owing to the use of generators for power. Headache often is the first symptom, followed by confusion, malaise, tachycardia, syncope, coma, convulsions, and death. Administering either 100% O_2 or hyperbaric O_2 (available at selected facilities) reverses CO poisoning (Table 3-9). Hyperbaric O_2 treatment is the most rapid means of reducing CO content.

Hematologic and Cardiovascular Toxidromes

Overdoses of many cardiovascular medications result in toxic syndromes, or toxidromes, for which appropriate interventions must be employed (Table 3-10). As one example, bleed-

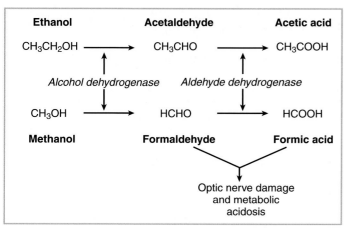

Figure 3-2. Ethanol can be used to treat methanol poisoning. Since ethanol has greater affinity for alcohol dehydrogenase than methanol, the conversion of methanol to active metabolites is slowed.

ing complications as a result of heparin or warfarin overdoses are particularly life-threatening. Protamine sulfate is a basic polypeptide that binds to and neutralizes the anticoagulant properties of heparin (see Chapter 7). As warfarin reduces vitamin K–dependent coagulation factors, the antidote for warfarin toxicity is slow intravenous infusion of vitamin K with transfusion of fresh-frozen plasma, if necessary. Both protamine and vitamin K therapies have a slight risk of anaphylactic shock. As another example of a cardiovascular toxidrome, cardiac glycosides, including digoxin, exert efficacy within a narrow therapeutic window. Despite monitoring serum digoxin concentrations, cardiac glycoside toxicity—as evidenced by delirium, fatigue, blurred vision, nausea, and life-threatening cardiac arrhythmias—may be seen in the emergency room. The antidote for digoxin toxicity is intravenous infusion of Digibind, an antidigoxin antibody.

In addition, serum potassium should be measured because hyperkalemia is often present in acute settings and should be promptly corrected to prevent arrythmias. Chronic intoxication with digoxin, on the other hand, may present with hypokalemia and hypomagnesemia. These serum electrolytes should similarly be promptly replaced.

Hepatotoxic Drugs/Poisons

Acetaminophen

Acetaminophen is one of the most commonly used drugs in children (e.g., Tylenol) and is often used in suicide attempts by teenagers and adults. Approximately 100,000 cases of acetaminophen overdose occur annually. It is available in various oral dosage forms and is frequently found in combination with other medications including pain relievers and cough and cold preparations in both prescription as well as

TABLE 3-8. Presentation and Management of Alcohol Poisoning

Agent	Signs/Symptoms	Interventions	Antidotes
Methanol, ethylene glycol	Lethargy Disinhibition Ataxia Nystagmus Miosis Stupor Coma Hypothermia Bradycardia Respiratory failure	Ventilatory support	Ethanol Fomepizole

TABLE 3-9. Presentation and Management of Carbon Monoxide Poisoning

Agent	Signs/Symptoms	Interventions	Antidotes
Carbon monoxide (CO)	Nausea and vomiting Dyspnea Mydriasis Vertigo or syncope Hypotension Tachycardia Arrhythmias	Decontamination	Hyperbaric O_2 (severe cases) Humidified 100% O_2 (mild to moderate cases)

TABLE 3-10. Presentation and Management of Anticoagulant and Cardiac Glycoside Poisoning

Agent	Signs/Symptoms	Interventions	Antidotes
Anticoagulants (e.g., heparin)	Bleeding Osteoporosis HIT Skin necrosis Hypersensitivity	Manage medical condition (e.g., hypertension) to reduce risk of bleeding	Protamine for heparins Vitamin K for warfarin (mild to moderate cases) Fresh frozen plasma (severe cases or rapid correction)
Cardiac glycosides (e.g., digoxin)	Nausea Anorexia Shortened QT interval T wave inversion Disorientation Visual halos Hallucinations Arrhythmias	Manage electrolytes Cardioversion for unstable cardiac arrythmia Cardiac pacing	Digibind (Fab) Potassium (normalize serum levels) Antiarrhythmics

HIT, heparin induced thrombocytopenia.

TABLE 3-11. The Four Stages of the Clinical Course of Acetaminophen Toxicity

Stage	Time Following Ingestion	Characteristics
I	½ to 24 h	Anorexia, nausea, vomiting, malaise, pallor, diaphoresis
II	24 to 48 h	Resolution of above; right upper quadrant abdominal pain and tenderness; elevated bilirubin, prothrombin time, hepatic enzymes; oliguria
III	72 to 96 h	Peak liver function abnormalities; anorexia, nausea, vomiting, malaise may reappear
IV	4 days to 2 wk	Resolution of hepatic dysfunction or complete liver failure

From Behrman RE. *Nelson Textbook of Pediatrics*, 16th ed. Philadelphia: WB Saunders, 2000.

over-the-counter medications. Patients may not realize that acetaminophen is contained in several different products that they are taking; thus, acetaminophen toxicity may be unintentional.

Acute acetaminophen poisoning results in hepatotoxicity and occurs in several stages. Within the first 24 hours of an acetaminophen overdose, toxicity begins with nausea and vomiting. Hepatic necrosis is most likely in those who are malnourished, those who abuse alcohol chronically, and patients who take other hepatotoxic medications (Table 3-11).

Acetaminophen is metabolized in the liver to glucuronide or sulfate conjugates (phase II reactions), which subsequently are excreted renally. A small fraction of acetaminophen, about 5%, is metabolized by P-450 isoenzymes (phase I reactions) to a reactive metabolite N-acetyl-p-benzoquinone-imine (NAPQI). Normally, this metabolite is conjugated with glutathione, a sulfhydryl-containing compound, in the liver and would be excreted in the urine as an inactive mercapturate conjugate. However, in acetaminophen overdose situations, sulfate stores are depleted, thereby depleting glutathione stores. The reactive metabolite NAPQI then reacts with other hepatocellular sulfhydryl groups in the cytosol, cell walls, and endoplasmic reticulum, forming reactive and necrotic tissue adducts and results in hepatotoxicity (Fig. 3-3).

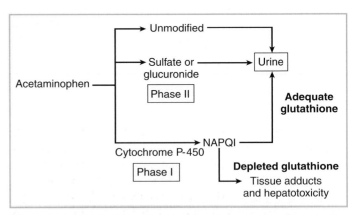

Figure 3-3. Metabolism of acetaminophen. Acetaminophen is degraded by two different pathways. The phase I pathway (cytochrome P-450–mediated) generates a reactive intermediate (N-acetyl-p-benzoquinone-imine [NAPQI]) that damages the liver after exhausting the protective glutathione.

In acetaminophen overdose situations, N-acetylcysteine, a sulfhydryl-containing acetaminophen-specific antidote, replenishes hepatic stores of glutathione by acting as a glutathione surrogate, combining directly with reactive acetaminophen metabolites and preventing hepatic damage. N-acetylcysteine should be initiated within 10 hours of acetaminophen over-

TABLE 3-12. Presentation and Management of Acetaminophen Poisoning

Agent	Signs/Symptoms	Interventions	Antidotes
Acetaminophen	Nausea and vomiting Abdominal pain Hepatic failure	Repeat blood levels to assess for toxicity	*N*-acetylcysteine

TABLE 3-13. Presentation and Management of Heavy Metal Poisoning

Metal	Acute Signs/Symptoms	Chronic Signs/Symptoms	Interventions/Antidotes
Arsenic	GI distress Garlic breath Watery stools Torsades de pointes Seizures	Pallor Skin pigmentation Alopecia Stocking/glove neuropathy Myelosuppression	Charcoal and/or dimercaprol for acute poisoning Penicillamine or succimer for chronic poisoning
Iron	Severe GI distress Hematemesis Bloody diarrhea Necrotic bowel	Dyspnea Shock Coma	Gastric aspiration and carbonate lavage Deferoxamine IV
Lead	Nausea and vomiting GI distress Abdominal pain Malaise Tremor Tinnitus Paresthesias Encephalopathy	Anemia Neuropathy Nephropathy Hepatitis Mental retardation Sterility Stillbirth	Gastric lavage and dimercaprol for severe cases EDTA or succimer Succimer PO in children
Mercury	Chest pain Dyspnea Pneumonitis GI distress GI bleeding Shock Renal failure	CNS effects Ataxia Paresthesias Auditory changes Visual changes	Succimer, PO Penicillamine, PO Add charcoal for orally ingested toxin

dose to achieve optimal results. Although N-acetylcysteine helps prevent liver damage by inactivating reactive acetaminophen intermediates, the antidote does not reverse hepatic injury once it has occurred. Unfortunately, the antidote has an unpleasant odor when administered orally, which often triggers nausea and vomiting and impairs the full course of therapy. For this reason, an injectable form of N-acetylcysteine was recently approved by the U.S. Food and Drug Administration (FDA) (Table 3-12).

Heavy Metal Poisons

Humans are exposed to heavy metals every day, since these elements are used in various industrial processes from which we derive many modern conveniences. For example:

- Arsenic is found in wood preservatives, insecticides, pesticides, ant poisons.
- Iron is found in vitamin supplements.
- Lead is found in tap water, old paint chips, herbal remedies, glazed kitchen-ware.
- Mercury is found in older thermometers, batteries, dyes, electroplating, photography, dental amalgams.

Similarly to drug overdoses, continued exposure to these heavy metals has devastating toxicologic consequences. Treatment of heavy metal toxicity relies on the use of chelating agents. Chelators are organic compounds with two or more electronegative groups that form stable covalent bonds with cationic metal atoms. These stable complexes are readily excreted, thus reducing toxicity associated with heavy metals (Table 3-13).

Arsenic

Acutely, arsenic toxicity causes gastrointestinal distress, "garlic" breath, and watery stools. Chronic exposure causes

Electron Transport Chain

The electron transport chain passes electrons from one protein (cytochrome or flavoprotein) to another in order to capture energy and pump hydrogen ions from the mitochondrion. The potential energy of this hydrogen ion gradient is harnessed to make ATP in oxidative (aerobic) metabolism. This is so named because the final acceptor for the electrons is molecular oxygen with the subsequent production of water. A number of toxic substances interfere with the electron transport chain (e.g., cyanide) or the transport of oxygen (e.g., CO).

alopecia and anemia and may be carcinogenic. Dimercaprol is one chelator used to treat arsenic exposure. It is useful in lead, mercury, and cadmium poisonings as well. Dimercaprol is a chelator (forms two bonds with the metal ion) that is given parenterally as an oily liquid. It is very lipophilic and readily enters cells throughout the body, including the central nervous system. As a result of its permeability, even at therapeutic doses, this chelator is associated with a high incidence of adverse effects including transient hypertension and tachycardia, headache, nausea, vomiting, and paresthesias.

Iron

Iron is the most frequent cause of accidental overdose in children. Iron is irritating to the gastric mucosa, and acute toxicity may cause hemorrhage and gastric perforations. Once absorbed, iron is taken up by tissues, especially the liver, and acts as a mitochondrial poison by perturbing the electron transport chain and inhibiting oxidative phosphorylation. Owing to the pharmacologic characteristics of iron, gastrointestinal distress is common within the first several hours after ingestion of toxic amounts. Within 24 to 36 hours of ingestion, hepatic injury, cardiovascular shock, metabolic acidosis, seizures, and coma may ensue.

Iron overdoses are also common in conditions that require frequent blood transfusions (e.g., hemophilia, thalasemia) and are treated with deferoxamine. Deferoxamine is a chelator with selective affinity for iron. Fortunately, it competes poorly with iron in hemoglobin and the cytochromes. At high doses, deferoxamine may cause visual disturbances including cataract formation and retinal degeneration. Patients should be warned that deferoxamine may change the color of their urine to pink or orange.

Lead

Acute inorganic lead poisoning is not common in the United States at present but may occur in children who have ingested large amounts of lead-containing paint (pica). Signs and symptoms of chronic inorganic lead poisoning include peripheral neuropathies, anorexia, anemia, tremor, weight loss, and gastrointestinal upset. Basophilic stippling of red blood cells is especially common following lead overdose. If encephalopathy occurs, prompt chelation is imperative. Treatment includes dimercaprol, ethylenediaminetetraacetic

Basophilic Stippling

Basophilic stippling is a typical sign of lead poisoning. The term refers to small, blue, dot-like structures scattered uniformly throughout the hemoglobin area of red blood cells. The stippling is derived from nuclear remnants and causes cells to resemble reticulocytes (immature red blood cells).

acid (EDTA), penicillamine, or succimer. Since EDTA also binds to calcium, EDTA is given as a calcium disodium salt to prevent hypocalcemia. Penicillamine is a water-soluble bidentate chelator that is well absorbed from the gastrointestinal tract and is excreted unchanged, although serious toxicities including aplastic anemia, lupus erythematosus, hypersensitivity reactions, and nephrotoxicity have been reported. Succimer is a polar chelator that can be administered orally and is well tolerated. It chelates extracellular but not intracellular arsenic and lead. Gastrointestinal distress, rash, and adverse central nervous system effects have been reported.

Mercury

Mercury poisoning usually occurs via inhalation of elemental mercury. Chest pain, shortness of breath, nausea and vomiting, kidney damage, gastrointestinal distress, and effects on the central nervous system may result. Treatment of mercury intoxication is with penicillamine or succimer. There are significant public concerns that the mercury used as a preservative in pediatric vaccines has contributed to a rise in the prevalence of autism. Even though the U.S. Institute of Medicine reports no link between vaccines and autism, mercury is no longer used as a preservative in new vaccine formulations.

●●● COMPLEMENTARY AND ALTERNATIVE MEDICINES

Patients often utilize natural products mistakenly believing that something "natural" will not be harmful. However, natural products may also produce toxic responses, especially when combined with prescription medications that have narrow therapeutic windows. For instance, a natural compound that interferes with the metabolism of a prescription drug might increase its concentration in the blood and drive it to toxic levels. St. John's wort is frequently used for depression and anxiety. This herbal alternative induces many cytochrome P-450 enzymes and thus affects metabolism of other drugs. In particular, St. John's wort can increase metabolism of sex steroids and render birth control less effective.

●●● TOP FIVE LIST

1. In situations of accidental poisoning or overdose, first stabilize the patient before seeking general or specific antidote therapy.

2. The best antidote for a toxin is an antagonist of the toxic agent. Unfortunately, antagonists are rarely available.

3. Carbon monoxide and methanol poisoning are treated with agents that are themselves considered toxic (high concentrations of oxygen and ethanol, respectively).

4. Antidotes for heavy metals are generally chelators that form stable complexes with the metal and transport them from the body, trapping them in the urine.

5. Hepatotoxicity associated with acetaminophen poisoning is treated by restoring glutathione levels.

Treatment of Infectious Diseases 4

CONTENTS

It's all about death—selective cell death, that is. Agents that kill or inhibit growth of microorganisms are known as antimicrobials. The term *antibiotic* was initially reserved for describing substances produced by microorganisms that killed or inhibited the growth of other microorganisms. However, the terms *antimicrobial* and *antibiotic* are now used interchangeably. Antimicrobial agents used clinically are selectively toxic; i.e., the antibiotics preferentially destroy microorganisms rather than the patient.

Each antimicrobial may be described in terms of whether it has bacteriostatic activity or bactericidal activity. *Bacteriostatic* describes antimicrobials that inhibit growth of microorganisms, while *bactericidal* is a term that describes antimicrobials that kill microorganisms. Additionally, each antimicrobial is associated with a particular spectrum of activity. The *spectrum of activity* describes the number of different types of organisms that are sensitive to the drug. Antibiotics have a broad spectrum if they target many different species of bacteria and a narrow spectrum if they are effective against only a few species of bacteria.

Resistance to antimicrobial agents is becoming increasingly problematic. Numerous antibiotics are no longer able to kill or suppress growth of microorganisms at plasma concentrations that are readily attainable, because the microorganisms are no longer susceptible to the drugs. Microorganisms acquire resistance to antibiotics in numerous ways (Box 4-1).

Another important consideration to keep in mind is that not all bacteria in or on human bodies are disease-causing. In fact, more than 90% of the cells in or on the human body are of prokaryotic origin. In other words, 90% of our bodies are normal flora! Typically, infections from normal flora occur only when our defenses are impaired or these "normal" microorganisms translocate (move) to other parts of the body.

Box 4-1. OVERVIEW OF ANTIBACTERIAL RESISTANCE MECHANISMS

- Alterations in receptor target
  Examples: mutations in penicillin-binding proteins (cell wall synthesis inhibitors); methylation of ribosomal subunits (protein synthesis inhibitors)
- Decreased entry or efflux of drug out of microorganism
  Examples: altered porins (cell wall synthesis inhibitors); efflux pumps to remove drug (tetracyclines)
- Alterations in metabolic pathways
  Example: microorganisms acquire alternative metabolic pathways to bypass a blocked pathway (sulfa drugs)

TABLE 4-1. Microbes Frequently Regarded as Normal at Various Body Locations

Location	Microbe
Skin	Diphtheroids (*Corynebacterium*)
	Propionibacterium
	Staphylococci
	Streptococci
GI tract	*Bacteroides*
	Clostridium
	Diphtheroids
	Enterobacteriaceae (*Escherichia coli*, *Klebsiella*)
	Fusobacterium
	Streptococci (anaerobic)
Upper respiratory tract	*Bacteroides*
	Haemophilus
	Neisseria
	Streptococci
Genital tract	*Corynebacterium*
	Enterobacteriaceae
	Lactobacillus
	Mycoplasma
	Staphylococci
	Streptococci

Box 4-2. FACTORS TO CONSIDER WHEN SELECTING AN ANTI-INFECTIVE

Microorganism Factors

Identification of organism
Susceptibility (MIC, MBC)

Host Factors

Drug allergies
Pharmacokinetic variables
    Effect of food on drug absorption
    Diseases affecting drug absorption
    Impact of other drugs that alter biotransformation
Renal/hepatic function
Pregnancy/lactation
Site of infection
Signs and symptoms
    Fever, malaise, leukocytosis, purulent drainage, etc.

Drug Factors

Economics
    Can patient afford the drug?
Tissue penetration
Drug toxicity
Preventing resistance
    Are combinations of drugs indicated?

Table 4-1 lists microorganisms that are normally found in various sites of the body, although these same bacteria can be pathogens if found in other areas of the body.

To select the most appropriate drug for treating an infection, several factors must be considered, including microorganism factors, host factors, and drug factors (Box 4-2). Briefly, microorganisms should be identified whenever possible utilizing microscopy coupled with Gram's staining or direct culturing. Table 4-2 gives a broad generalization of "suspected" microbes based on site of infection. Typically, empiric antimicrobial therapy against these organisms is initiated even before culture results are complete.

Culturing a microorganism from a site of infection is useful to determine the pharmacologic agents to which the micro-

organism is susceptible. Figure 4-1 depicts the methods by which microbial susceptibility is determined using both quantitative (Fig. 4-1A) and qualitative (Fig. 4-1B) methods. Quantitatively, the minimal inhibitory concentration (MIC) is the lowest concentration of an antibiotic that inhibits microorganism growth in liquid culture. The minimal bactericidal concentration (MBC) is the lowest concentration of an antibiotic that induces bacterial cell death. Qualitatively, disks that are impregnated with antibiotics can be laid onto agar plates that were previously seeded with bacteria. The relative "zone of inhibition" around the drug-impregnated disk gives a general indication of drug-susceptibility. While these susceptibility tests indicate which drugs can prevent growth of an organism in vitro, this information may not always translate to the in vivo situation if the drug cannot reach the site of infection at the necessary concentration.

This chapter describes hundreds of antibacterial, antifungal, antiparasitic, and antiviral agents. For the most part, you should know the mechanisms of actions, contraindications, and side effects for each class of antimicrobials. Rote memorization of each individual organism targeted by each individual drug within each class will not be as effective as simply appreciating the ways in which specific classes of antibiotics target different classes of microorganisms. Many drugs now used may not be used in the near future; it is important to be familiar with the mechanism of action so that when new antibiotics are introduced into clinical practice, you will be comfortable placing them in the appropriate category.

MICROBIOLOGY

Gram's Staining

Microscopy assists in classification of infectious organisms and may tell the shape (coccus, bacillus) of a bacterial species or differentiate bacteria from fungi or spirochetes. Gram's staining with gentian violet is useful to determine whether bacteria are gram-positive or gram-negative. The cell walls of gram-positive bacteria retain a violet color when stained with gentian violet. Cells walls of gram-negative bacteria lose this violet color when de-stained with alcohol but turn red when counterstained with safranin.

TABLE 4-2. Suspected Microorganisms, Based on Site of Infection

Location	Condition	Microorganism
Respiratory tract	Pharyngitis, bronchitis, sinusitis, otitis	Group A streptococci, gonococci
	Pneumonia	H. influenzae, M. catarrhalis, S. pneumoniae, S. aureus
	Community-acquired	
	Normal host	S. pneumoniae, viral, *Mycoplasma*
	Aspiration	Normal aerobic and anaerobic mouth flora
	Pediatric patient	S. pneumoniae, H. influenzae
	COPD	S. pneumoniae, Klebsiella
	Nosocomial	
	Aspiration	Mouth anaerobes, gram-negative aerobic rods, S. aureus
	Neutropenic	Fungi, Pneumocystis, Legionella
	AIDS patient	Nocardia, H. influenzae, pneumococcus
Urinary tract	Community-acquired	E. coli, other gram-negative rods, enterococci
	Hospital-acquired	Resistant gram-negative rods, enterococci
Skin/soft tissue	Cellulitis	Group A streptococci
	IV catheter site	S. aureus, S. epidermis
	Surgical wound	S. aureus, gram-negative rods
	Diabetic ulcer	S. aureus, gram-negative aerobic rods, anaerobes
Intra-abdominal	Gastroenteritis	B. fragilis, E. coli, enterococci
		Salmonella, Shigella, Campylobacter, C. difficile, amoebiasis, Giardia, viral
Skeletal system	Osteomyelitis or septic arthritis	S. aureus, gram-negative aerobic rods
Central nervous system	Meningitis	
	<2 months	Group B streptococci, E. coli, Listeria
	2 months to 12 years	H. influenzae, S. pneumoniae, N. meningitidis
	Adult	S. pneumoniae, N. meningitidis, gram-negative aerobic rods
	Hospital-acquired	S. pneumoniae, N. meningitidis, gram-negative aerobic rods
	Postneurosurgery	Gram-negative aerobic rods, S. aureus

● ● ● ANTIBACTERIALS

In the most simplistic sense, there are four distinct major mechanisms of action by which antibacterial agents work (Fig. 4-2):

- Inhibition of cell wall synthesis.
- Inhibition of protein synthesis.
- Inhibition of folic acid biosynthetic pathways.
- Inhibition of DNA/RNA synthesis.

In some instances, it makes sense to combine drugs that work by different mechanisms of action to achieve synergistic killing effects (Table 4-3).

Cell Wall Synthesis Inhibitors

Multiple drug classes interfere with cell wall synthesis, including the penicillins, the cephalosporins, the carbapenems and the monobactams.

Penicillins

Mechanism of action. Penicillins inhibit cell wall synthesis and destroy existing functional cell walls through autolysin activation (Fig. 4-3). Once penicillins bind to penicillin-binding proteins (PBPs), the transpeptidation reaction that cross-links bacterial cell walls is inhibited and susceptible gram-negative and gram-positive bacterial cells die. Although the exact mechanisms responsible for cell death are unclear, autolysins (carboxypeptidases and endopeptidases that remodel and break down bacterial cell walls) are activated by penicillin-binding to PBPs.

Resistance. For penicillins to gain access to microbial cells, these drugs must first permeate the cell wall. Bacteria may become resistant to penicillins by

- Modification of their PBPs.
- Actively pumping the drugs back out of the cells.
- Cleavage of the β-lactam ring structure of penicillins via β-lactamases (also called penicillinases) within the periplasmic space, rendering the drugs inactive.
- Altered porins (gram-negative bacteria only) that prevent the drugs from reaching the PBP targets.

Figure 4-3 schematically illustrates the layers of a bacterium cell wall, including the peptidoglycan layer with which penicillins interfere, and the periplasmic space where β-lactamases may reside.

Adverse effects. The major adverse effect associated with penicillins is hypersensitivity. Hypersensitivity reactions to

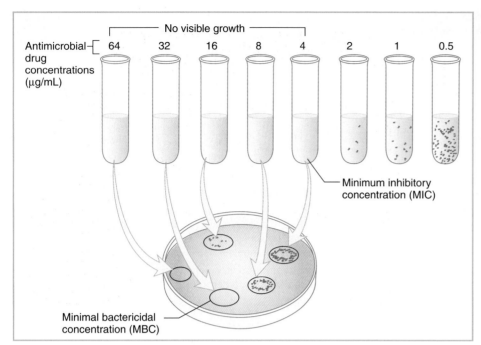

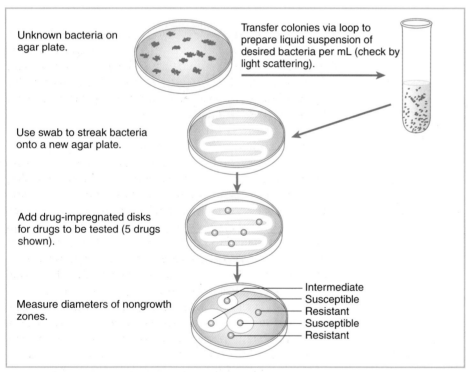

Figure 4-1. Susceptibility testing. **A**, Quantitative method. **B**, Qualitative method.

penicillins range from mild to severe and may include hives, itching, or anaphylaxis. Most penicillins, with the exceptions of nafcillin and oxacillin, are excreted unchanged in the urine; therefore, penicillin dosages must be lowered in patients with renal insufficiency. At high intravenous doses, penicillins may cause seizures or antiplatelet effects. Anemia, thrombocytopenia, and hypoprothrombinemia have also been reported.

It is not uncommon for penicillins, especially broad-spectrum agents, to cause secondary infections by disrupting normal gut flora. This can lead to vaginal yeast infections as well as pseudomembranous colitis caused by overgrowth of *Clostridium difficile* in the gastrointestinal tract.

Drug interactions. When penicillins are combined with drugs that are bacteriostatic (e.g., tetracycline), pharmacologic antagonism results. For penicillins to be effective inhibitors of cell wall synthesis, microorganisms must be actively growing and dividing. Tetracyclines are bacteriostatic; therefore, the growth of microorganisms is inhibited. As a

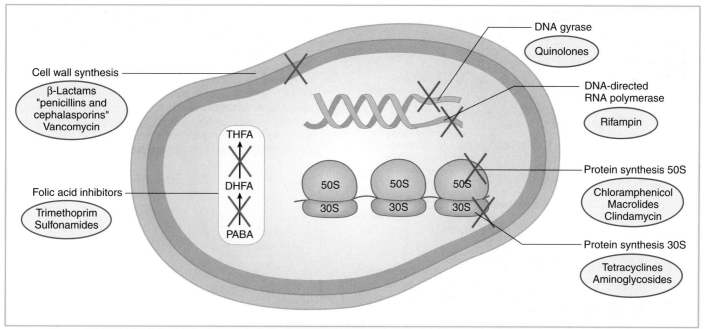

Figure 4-2. The four major mechanisms by which most antibiotics work.

TABLE 4-3. Examples of Synergistic Drug Combinations

Combination	Description
Penicillins + aminoglycosides	This combination is a cell wall synthesis inhibitor plus a protein synthesis inhibitor
Sulfamethoxazole + trimethoprim	These agents act on sequential steps of the same microbial metabolic pathway
Amoxicillin + clavulanic acid	Clavulanic acid inhibits a microbial enzyme that would otherwise inactivate amoxicillin

result, the combination of a bacteriostatic drug like a tetracycline with a bactericidal drug such as penicillin would not be expected to produce synergistic actions.

There has been a long-standing concern that combining penicillins (or any antibiotic) with oral contraceptives may lessen the efficacy of the oral contraceptive. This is because estrogens are recycled via the enterohepatic recirculation pathway. Under normal circumstances, gut bacteria cleave estrogen-glucuronide conjugates, allowing the estrogenic component to be reabsorbed, thereby extending its duration of activity in the body. When antibiotics are given, normal gastrointestinal flora are disrupted, a situation that may impair enterohepatic recirculation of estrogenic compounds, possibly diminishing their half-life. As a result, it is probably wise to warn women relying on oral contraceptives for pregnancy prevention that a back-up method of contraception should be considered while they are taking antibiotics and for 7 days thereafter. More recently, the clinical relevance of this drug-drug interaction has been questioned, yet it is probably better to be "safe" rather than sorry.

Subclassification of Penicillins

The numerous different types of penicillins may be subclassified into four distinct categories: natural penicillins, aminopenicillins, penicillinase-resistant penicillins, and antipseudomonal penicillins. In addition, penicillins may be co-administered with drugs that are irreversible inhibitors of β-lactamase, which broadens the antimicrobial spectrum of coverage to include β-lactamase–producing organisms. As a general and probably oversimplified rule of thumb, natural penicillins and penicillinase-resistant penicillins tend to be used to treat gram-positive microorganisms, whereas aminopenicillins and antipseudomonal penicillins possess activity against gram-negative organisms as well. A list of microorganisms for which natural penicillins are drugs of choice is found in Table 4-4. This table is not an exhaustive list of all microorganisms for which penicillins are effective, and only the "drugs of choice" are listed rather than complete sensitivity data for each penicillin.

Natural Penicillins

Drugs. Penicillin G and penicillin V.
Pharmacokinetics. Since penicillin G is readily destroyed in acidic environments, such as found in the digestive tract, the drug can only be administered intravenously or intramuscularly. Long-acting intramuscular depot injections of penicillin G are sometimes used. Penicillin V is somewhat more stable

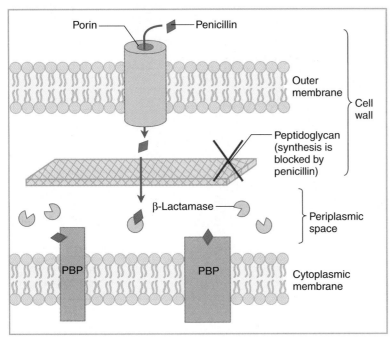

Figure 4-3. A gram-negative bacterial cell wall. Penicillins inhibit synthesis of bacterial cell walls by binding to penicillin-binding proteins (PBPs). PBPs are depicted as different enzymes because they have differing functions. Binding to PBPs leads to (1) inhibition of cell wall synthesis by blocking transpeptidation of peptidoglycan and (2) activation of autolytic enzymes in the cell wall that cause lesions that result in bacterial death. Actions of penicillins may be terminated by β-lactamase enzymes that reside in the periplasmic space. This is a mechanism by which bacteria become resistant to penicillins.

MICROBIOLOGY & IMMUNOLOGY

Cell Walls

Unique to bacteria is a cell wall comprised of a complex peptidoglycan that consists of cross-linked polysaccharides and polypeptides. The polysaccharide contains alternating amino sugars of N-acetylglucosamine and N-acetylmuramic acid, and a short polypeptide is linked to N-acetylmuramic acid. Penicillin-binding proteins (PBPs) catalyze cross-linking of N-acetylmuramic acid with nearby peptides. Such cross-links provide bacterial cell walls with structural rigidity. In addition to the peptidoglycan layer, gram-negative bacteria also possess an outer membrane that is permeated by porins, or channels, that provide access to the cytoplasmic membrane. Gram-positive organisms do not possess an outer membrane but have a much thicker peptidoglycan layer than do gram-negative organisms.

than penicillin G in acidic environments and thus is administered orally; however, the drug still must be given on an empty stomach, 1 hour before meals or 2–3 hours after meals for maximal efficacy.

Clinical use. These antibiotics are primarily used for treating infections caused by susceptible gram-positive microorganisms. Some uses for penicillin G include serious streptococcal infections, neurosyphilis, and endocarditis. Penicillin V is the drug of choice for treating streptococcal pharyngitis. These drugs are inactivated by β-lactamases.

Aminopenicillins

Drugs. These synthetic drugs include ampicillin and amoxicillin.

Pharmacokinetics. Synthetic penicillins such as ampicillin can be administered enterally or parenterally. Like penicillin V, ampicillin may be prescribed orally, but it is best absorbed on an empty stomach. On the other hand, amoxicillin can be taken with or without food, since it is stable even in the presence of gastric acids.

Clinical use. Although used primarily for treating gram-positive bacteria, these antibacterials have a broader spectrum against some gram-negative microorganisms than do the natural penicillins. However, aminopenicillins are ineffective for microorganisms that synthesize β-lactamases (aka penicillinases) and are often used in combination with β-lactamase inhibitors. Aminopenicillins are commonly used to treat infections of the ears, nose, and throat and lower respiratory tract and for prophylaxis against endocarditis.

Adverse effects. A nonallergic "ampicillin rash" is common, even in the absence of hypersensitivity to other penicillins. Ampicillin rashes occur most often in patients with mononucleosis or those using allopurinol concurrently.

Penicillinase-Resistant Penicillins

Drugs. Drugs include dicloxacillin, methicillin, oxacillin, and nafcillin.

Mechanism of action. Chemically, the penicillinase-resistant penicillins contain side groups that protect the drugs from being inactivated by bacterial β-lactamases.

Pharmacokinetics. Methicillin, oxacillin, and nafcillin are usually given parenterally; dicloxacillin is given orally.

Clinical use. Penicillinase-resistant penicillins are useful for treating infections caused by β-lactamase–producing staphylococci. Therapeutic applications for penicillinase-resistant penicillins include treatment or prevention of infections in the upper or lower respiratory tract, skin, bones, and joints. Additionally, these antibiotics are used to treat meningitis, septicemia, and endocarditis.

TABLE 4-4. Microorganisms for Which Penicillins are Drugs of Choice*

Organisms	Natural Penicillins		Aminopenicillins ± β-Lactamase Inhibitors				Penicillinase-Resistant Penicillins	Antipseudomonal Penicillins†
	Penicillin G	Penicillin V	Ampicillin	Ampicillin + Sulbactam	Amoxicillin	Amoxicillin + Clavulanate	Methicillin, Nafcillin, Oxacillin, and Others	Piperacillin and Others
Gram-positive								
Cocci								
E. faecalis, serious infection	X		X					
E. faecalis, urinary tract infection			X		X			
S. aureus, S. epidermis				✓§		✓§	X§	
Streptococcus (groups A, B, C, G, and S. bovis)	X	X	X					
S. pneumoniae, penicillin-sensitive strains	X	X	X					
Streptococcus viridans group	X							
Bacilli								
C. perfringens	X							
Gram-Negative								
Cocci								
M. catarrhalis				X		X		
N. meningitidis	X							
Bacilli								
E. coli			X	✓		X		
H. influenzae				X	X	X		
P. mirabilis			X					
P. aeruginosa								X

*This table is not all-inclusive. It is a representation of *common* infectious microorganisms and the penicillins that are *drugs of choice* to treat a variety of different types of infections.
†Although the antipseudomonal penicillins *could* be used to treat infections caused by most of the microorganisms listed, they are reserved for treating only the infections for which other penicillins would be ineffective.
§Used as long as organism is methicillin-sensitive.
X, drug of choice; ✓, alternative therapy if first-line drugs cannot be used or are ineffective.

TABLE 4-5. Selected Adverse Effects Associated with Penicillinase-Resistant Penicillins

Effect	Drug
Hepatitis	Oxacillin
Nephritis	Nafcillin

It should be assumed that all staphylococci synthesize β-lactamases; hence, staphylococcal infections are best treated with pharmacologic agents that are resistant to the effects of these penicillin-inactivating enzymes.

Adverse effects. Adverse effects that are unique for penicillinase-resistant penicillins are shown in Table 4-5.

Antipseudomonal Penicillins (Extended-spectrum Penicillins)

Drugs. Drugs include carbenicillin, ticarcillin, mezlocillin, and piperacillin.

Pharmacokinetics. These drugs are usually given parenterally. Carbenicillin is the only drug in this class that can be administered orally, but therapeutic levels of this drug are found only in the urinary tract, limiting its enteral utility to treating urinary tract and prostatic infections.

Clinical use. Antipseudomonal penicillins are also called extended spectrum penicillins, since they provide better coverage of gram-negative microorganisms, including *Pseudomonas* and *Enterobacter* species, than other penicillins. These drugs are often reserved for treating serious gram-negative infections of the respiratory tract, soft tissues, bones, joints, and urinary tract as well as for treating sepsis, and these drugs are frequently combined with aminoglycosides for synergistic effects.

CLINICAL MEDICINE

Keys to Prescribing Penicillin

- Amoxicillin/clavulanic acid is particularly effective for ear, nose, and throat infections.
- Nafcillin is the drug of choice for suspected *staphylococcus aureus* infections (unless cultures show methicillin-resistant *S. aureus*, then vancomycin is used).
- Pipercillin/tazobactam is a broad spectrum antibiotic for empiric treatment. The drug combination is also used to treat pseudomonal infections.

Adverse effects. Caution must be utilized when administering carbenicillin or ticarcillin to patients with cardiac disease because these drugs contain large amounts of sodium, which may aggravate hypertension or congestive heart failure. Antipseudomonal penicillins have also been associated with antiplatelet activities.

Irreversible Inhibitors of β-Lactamases

Drugs. Drugs include clavulanic acid, sulbactam, tazobactam.

Clinical use. Irreversible β-lactamase inhibitors have no antimicrobial activity by themselves. However, when these agents are combined with penicillins, expanded coverage against β-lactamase–producing microorganisms is provided. Refer back to Table 4-4 to compare situations in which amoxicillin versus amoxicillin + clavulanic acid might be selected as drugs of choice. Table 4-6 lists some common penicillin + β-lactamase inhibitor products.

Cephalosporins

Cephalosporins structurally resemble penicillins and, like penicillins, possess a β-lactam chemical backbone. Unlike the natural penicillins, cephalosporins are relatively stable to pH changes and may be taken with or without food. Clinical utility of cephalosporins is listed in Box 4-3. Cephalosporins are classified by generation, and in general gram-positive activity is lost while gram-negative activity is gained with each succeeding generation. Table 4-7 lists microorganisms and selected situations in which cephalosporins are drugs of choice.

Mechanism of action. Same as that of penicillins.

TABLE 4-6. Commercially Available Combination Products: Penicillins + β-Lactamase Inhibitors

Penicillin	β-Lactamase Inhibitor
Amoxicillin	Clavulanic acid
Ticarcillin	Clavulanic acid
Ampicillin	Sulbactam
Piperacillin	Tazobactam

Box 4-3. CLINICAL UTILITY OF CEPHALOSPORINS

- Penicillin-allergic patients, when macrolides are not effective
- Drugs of choice for treating gram-negative infections, especially *Klebsiella*
- Drugs of choice for treating the three microorganisms that frequently cause pediatric meningitis (*H. influenzae, S. pneumoniae, N. meningitidis*)
- Polymicrobial infections
- Empiric treatment of infections of unknown etiology
- Prophylaxis during surgery, especially if implants are involved

Resistance. Alterations, mutations, or lack of penicillin-binding proteins are mechanisms by which microorganisms become resistant to cephalosporins. Additionally, alterations in porins may prevent cephalosporins from entering bacteria and may also contribute to resistance, especially among gram-negative species. As a group, cephalosporins are less likely to be degraded by β-lactamases than penicillins are.

Adverse effects. Because of chemical structural similarities between cephalosporins and penicillins, there is a possibility that penicillin-allergic patients may also be hypersensitive to cephalosporins. However, recent data suggest that the incidence of this cross-reactivity is probably much lower than previously believed. As a general rule, it is wise to refrain from prescribing cephalosporins to patients with a documented history of anaphylactic reactions to penicillins.

Gastrointestinal irritation is common with oral cephalosporins, but taking the medications with food may prevent this adverse effect. Parenterally administered cephalosporins cause local irritation at the site of injection. Since many cephalosporins are excreted by the kidneys, renal toxicity is possible; caution should be utilized in patients with pre-existing renal disease (impaired creatinine clearance). As indicated below, some second- and third-generation cephalosporins may cause disulfiram-like reactions and hypoprothrombinemia. Newer cephalosporins, especially those administered parenterally, may cause seizures. Due to disruption of normal flora, secondary infections, including pseudomembranous colitis and vaginal yeast infections, may also occur.

First-Generation Cephalosporins

Drugs. Drugs include cefadroxil, cefazolin, cephalexin, cephradine, and cephapirin. (Note that they all begin with "cef-" or "ceph-.")

Clinical use. As a rule, first-generation cephalosporins possess excellent activity against gram-positive aerobic bacteria but are not effective against many gram-negative microorganisms or anaerobes. Groups A and B streptococcal organisms are typically sensitive to first-generation cephalosporins, but methicillin-resistant staphylococci (MRSA), enterococci, and penicillin-resistant *Streptococcus pneumoniae* are not. Although these drugs have activity against some

TABLE 4-7. Examples of Microorganisms for Which Cephalosporins are Drugs of Choice*†

Organism	First Generation					Second Generation						Third Generation						
	Cefazolin (IM/IV)	Cephalexin (oral)	Cephradine (oral/IM/IV)	Cefadroxil (oral)	Cefazolin (IM/IV)	Cefuroxime (oral/IM/IV)	Cefaclor (oral)	Cefprozil (oral)	Cefoxitin (IV)	Cefmetazole (IM/IV)	Cefotetan (IM/IV)	Cefotaxime (IM/IV)	Ceftriaxone (IM/IV)	Cefixime (oral)	Cefpodoxime (oral)	Ceftibuten (oral)	Cefepime (IM/IV)	Ceftazidime (IM/IV)
Gram-Positive																		
Cocci																		
S. aureus, S. epidermidis, methicillin-sensitive	X	X	X	X														
Streptococcus (groups A, B, C, G and *S. bovis*)	X	X	X	X														
S. pneumoniae, penicillin-sensitive	✓	✓	✓	✓														
S. pneumoniae, intermediate level of resistance to penicillin												X	X					
Streptococcus viridans group	✓	✓	✓	✓														
Bacilli																		
Clostridium perfringens					✓													
Gram-Negative																		
Cocci																		
M. catarrhalis						✓	✓	✓					✓	✓	✓	✓	✓	
N. gonorrhoeae													X	X	X	X		
N. meningitidis												✓	✓					
Bacilli																		
B. fragilis									✓	✓	✓							
Enterobacter spp													✓	✓	✓	✓	✓	X‡
E. coli, meningitis												X	X					
E. coli, systemic infection	✓	✓	✓			✓	✓	✓				X	X					
E. coli, urinary tract infection	X	✓	✓															
H. influenzae, meningitis												X	X					
H. influenzae, other infections						✓												
K. pneumoniae						✓						X	X					
Other																		
Proteus (indole-positive)												X	X	✓	✓		✓	
P. stuartii												X	X					
P. aeruginosa																	✓	X‡
S. typhi												X	X					
T. pallidum (spirochete)													X					
B. burgdorferi				X								✓	X					

*This table is not all inclusive. It is a representation of common infectious microorganisms and the cephalosporins that are the drugs of choice for treatment.
†Third-generation agents are preferred over first- and second-generation agents for most gram-negative infections.
‡Use in conjunction with any aminoglycoside.
X, drug of choice; ✓, alternative.

gram-negative organisms such as *Escherichia coli* and *Proteus mirabilis*, first-generation cephalosporins do not have reliable activity against *Moraxella catarrhalis* (a common culprit in upper respiratory infections). First-generation cephalosporins are frequently utilized for treating uncomplicated skin and soft tissue infections, respiratory infections caused by penicillin-sensitive strains of *S. pneumoniae*, and urinary tract infections.

Second-Generation Cephalosporins

Drugs. Drugs are cefoxitin, cefaclor, cefamandole, cefonicid, cefuroxime, cefmetazole, cefotetan, cefprozil, loracarbef. (Again, notice that most begin with "cef-" or "ceph-" except for loracarbef.)

Clinical use. As a group, second-generation cephalosporins possess wider activity against gram-negative bacteria and anaerobic microorganisms than do first-generation cephalosporins.

Specifically, cefoxitin is effective against *Bacteroides fragilis* and other anaerobic organisms. Additionally, cefuroxime is the only second-generation cephalosporin that enters the central nervous system and can be used to treat meningitis.

Adverse effects. The chemical side chain (N-methylthiotetrazole, or NMTT) on the chemical backbone of cefamandole and cefotetan inhibits aldehyde dehydrogenase; therefore, disulfiram-like reactions may occur if alcohol is consumed within 72 hours of administration of these medications. Disulfiram is a drug that is used to discourage alcohol abuse by elevating plasma aldehyde levels, thereby resulting in unpleasant side effects. The NMTT side chain may also cause hypoprothrombinemia (and associated risk of bleeding). Cefaclor is associated with hypersensitivity including a rash and serum sickness, but these reactions to cefaclor are not contraindications to the use of other cephalosporins or penicillins.

Third-Generation Cephalosporins

Drugs. Drugs include cefoperazone, cefotaxime, cefpodoxime, ceftazidime, ceftibuten, ceftizoxime, ceftriaxone, cefdinir, cefditoren, cefepime, and cefixime. (Again, note that they all begin with "cef-.")

Clinical use. As a group, third-generation cephalosporins have wide activity against gram-negative microorganisms. Additionally, many of the drugs in this class (cefotaxime and ceftriaxone) also possess some coverage against anaerobic bacteria. Activity against gram-positive microorganisms is less reliable with third-generation cephalosporins than with previous generations. Some of these drugs are active against *Pseudomonas* (ceftazidime and cefoperazone), and others cross the blood-brain barrier and can be used to treat meningitis (ceftriaxone). Clinically, third-generation cephalosporins are used to treat infections caused by gram-negative bacteria, especially hospital-acquired infections or complicated community-acquired infections involving the respiratory tract, blood, skin and soft tissues, urinary tract, and intra-abdominal infections. Because of their activity against gram-negative bacteria, third-generation cephalosporins may be an alternative to aminoglycosides.

Adverse effects. Because of the NMTT side chain on ceftriaxone, disulfiram-like reactions and hypoprothrombinemia may occur. Biliary sludging may also occur with third-generation cephalosporins as a result of inhibited bile outflow. Additionally, cefditoren causes renal excretion of carnitine and should be avoided in carnitine-deficient individuals. Cefditoren should also be avoided in patients with a true hypersensitivity to milk (sodium caseinate).

Carbapenems

Drugs. Drugs include imipenem/cilastatin, meropenem, and ertapenem.

Mechanism of action. Like penicillins and cephalosporins, carbapenems are bactericidal and inhibit cell wall synthesis. Unlike penicillins and cephalosporins, carbapenems have a different stereochemical structure in their β-lactam ring that renders them resistant to β-lactamases.

Clinical use. These drugs are broad-spectrum antibiotics and are effective against gram-positive organisms such as staphylococci and streptococci, as well as gram-negative organisms including *Pseudomonas* and anaerobes including *B. fragilis*. Imipenem is always given in combination with cilastatin. Cilastatin does not have antimicrobial activity but, instead, inhibits a renal dehydropeptidase enzyme that inactivates imipenem.

Adverse effects. Seizures have been reported in a small percentage of patients, especially those who are predisposed such as patients with renal insufficiency, a recent history of head trauma, or epilepsy. Pseudomembranous colitis and bone marrow suppression have also occurred. Because of structural similarities, carbapenems should be used cautiously (if at all) in patients who are hypersensitive to penicillins.

Monobactams

Drug. The only choice is aztreonam.

Mechanism of action and clinical use. Currently, aztreonam is the only monobactam approved for use in the United States. Monobactams may be used in penicillin-allergic patients. Aztreonam is relatively resistant to β-lactamases. Aztreonam is a gram-negative specific antimicrobial that interferes with cell wall synthesis. Clinically, aztreonam is used for treating respiratory, urinary, skin, gynecologic, and intra-abdominal infections. Aztreonam may antagonize the efficacy of other β-lactam antibiotics but is often used synergistically with aminoglycosides.

In summary, Table 4-8 lists the major adverse effects associated with antibiotics that possess β-lactam chemical structures.

Other Antibiotics That Disrupt Cell Walls
Vancomycin

Mechanism of action. Vancomycin interferes with cell wall synthesis, alters bacterial cell membrane permeability, and disrupts RNA synthesis.

Clinical use. Although the drug is rapidly bactericidal, it is effective only against gram-positive microorganisms. Vancomycin is used parenterally to treat serious systemic staphylococcal infections (including methicillin-resistant staphylococci [MRSA]), streptococcal, and enterococcal (if susceptible) infections. It is often referred to as the antibiotic of last resort. Vancomycin is also given orally for

TABLE 4-8. Adverse Effects Associated with β-Lactam Antibiotics (penicillins, cephalosporins, monobactams, penems)

Event	Symptom or Condition
Allergic reaction, anaphylaxis, urticaria, serum sickness, rash, fever	Ampicillin rash is common in absence of cross-reactivity to other penicillins; most common in those with mononucleosis or concurrent allopurinol use Cefaclor is associated with a higher-than-expected incidence of hypersensitivity reactions Cross-reactivity between penicillins and imipenem No cross-reactivity between aztreonam and penicillins
Diarrhea	Common with amoxicillin + clavulanic acid, ampicillin, ceftriaxone, cefoperazone Pseudomembranous colitis, caused by *C. difficile* overgrowth, can occur with nearly any antibacterial agent
Anemia, thrombocytopenia, antiplatelet activity, hypoprothrombinemia	Hemolytic anemia is more common at higher doses Antiplatelet activity is most common with antipseudomonal penicillins and high serum levels of other β-lactams
Hepatitis	Most common with oxacillin
Seizure	Associated with high levels of β-lactams, particularly penicillins and imipenem
Sodium load	Carbenicillin, ticarcillin
Nephritis	Most common with methicillin, but reported with all β-lactams
Disulfiram reaction	Cephalosporins with methylthiotetrazole side chains (e.g., cefamandole, cefotetan, cefoperazone, cefmetazole)
Hypotension, nausea	Associated with fast infusion of imipenem

gastrointestinal-specific treatment of *C. difficile*–associated diarrhea and pseudomembranous colitis. Vancomycin is not absorbed systemically when administered orally; therefore, there are few adverse effects with enteral administration.

Adverse effects. A unique adverse effect, termed "red neck syndrome," characterized by itching, rash, fever, and chills, can occur if vancomycin is infused too rapidly. This is not an allergic reaction and is simply an infusion reaction that can be prevented by prior administration of antihistamines or slow administration of the drug. Other adverse effects include the possibilities of nephrotoxicity, cardiac arrest, vascular collapse, and bone marrow suppression. Although current vancomycin formulations are not as nephrotoxic as they once were, it is wise to monitor kidney function, including BUN and serum creatinine, as well as to monitor serum vancomycin (peak and trough) levels. Extra precautions should be utilized to monitor renal function when vancomycin is administered concurrently with other drugs that are also potentially nephrotoxic. Adverse effects associated with vancomycin are listed in Table 4-9. Currently, a concern with use of vancomycin is the potential emergence of vancomycin-resistant enterococci (VRE).

Cycloserine

Mechanism of action. Cycloserine inhibits cell wall synthesis in gram-positive and gram-negative microorganisms, but it is usually reserved for treating *Mycobacterium tuberculosis* infections that are resistant to first-line antitubercular drugs.

Adverse effects. Cycloserine may cause central nervous system toxicities such as psychosis, headaches, visual disturb-

TABLE 4-9. Adverse Effects Associated with Vancomycin

Event	Symptom or Condition
Ototoxicity	Of concern at high serum levels (>50 µg/mL)
Nephrotoxicity	May be increased with concurrent administration of aminoglycosides
Hypotension, flushing	Associated with rapid infusion
Phlebitis	Needs large volume dilution

ances, and seizures; these adverse effects appear to be dose-related. As a result of its side effect profile, cycloserine is contraindicated in patients with seizure disorders, renal disease, alcoholism, depression, and anxiety disorders.

Bacitracin

Due to serious nephrotoxicity, bacitracin is typically reserved for topical use in the treatment of ocular or skin infections. It is available for topical use as a single agent, and it is also one component of "triple antibiotic" ointment, both of which are available without a prescription. In rare circumstances, the antibiotic is used parenterally to treat systemic infections caused by drug-sensitive staphylococci that are *resistant to other, safer antibiotics.*

Polymyxin B

Mechanism of action. This is a drug that is bactericidal to nearly all gram-negative bacilli, with the exception of

Proteus. It is a cationic detergent that disrupts lipoproteins in bacterial cell walls, thus increasing membrane permeability.
Clinical use. Polymyxin B is usually used topically for ocular and otic infections or bladder irrigations. Like bacitracin, polymyxin B is found in "triple antibiotic" ointment. Although rarely used parenterally, it may be used intravenously, intramuscularly, or intrathecally to treat serious infections caused by *Pseudomonas, E. coli, Klebsiella,* or *Haemophilus influenzae* when other antibiotics cannot be used. However, parenteral use of polymyxin B has largely been replaced by aminoglycosides.
Adverse effects. When used parenterally, apnea has occurred, especially when combined with curare-type skeletal muscle relaxants.

Nitrofurantoin

Mechanism of action. The mechanism of action of nitrofurantoin is not entirely clear; however, it appears that this antimicrobial is either converted to reactive intermediates that modify ribosomal proteins or inhibits bacterial carbohydrate metabolism, disrupting cell wall synthesis. At high doses, nitrofurantoin is bactericidal against some strains of bacteria.
Resistance. Because of its unique mechanism of action, nitrofurantoin is not cross-resistant with any other antibiotics.
Clinical use. Nitrofurantoin is excreted unchanged into the urine. This drug only reaches therapeutic concentrations in the urine and is therefore used to treat urinary tract infections.
Adverse effects. Nitrofurantoin may discolor urine, causing it to darken. Gastrointestinal upset may also occur, which is minimized by taking the drug with food. This antibiotic is contraindicated in pregnant women near term and in glucose 6-phosphate dehydrogenase (G6PD)–deficient individuals owing to the risk of hemolytic anemia. Hepatotoxicity and irreversible peripheral neuropathies have also been reported. Nitrofurantoin has also been associated with pulmonary problems, both acutely and chronically (Table 4-10).

Protein Synthesis Inhibitors

In addition to drugs that target bacterial cell walls, other classes of antibiotics target pathways associated with bacterial, but not human, protein synthesis. Drugs that inhibit

TABLE 4-10. Adverse Pulmonary Effects Associated with Nitrofurantoin

Acute	Subacute	Chronic
Dyspnea	Dyspnea	Pulmonary fibrosis
Chills	Tachypnea	Respiratory failure
Fever	Persistent cough	
Angina	Interstitial pneumonitis	
Cough	Chest pain	

Prokaryotic Protein Synthesis

Prokaryotic protein synthesis begins with the initiation phase in which necessary components come together (30S ribosomal subunit, 50S ribosomal subunit, incoming tRNA, mRNA). An incoming tRNA binds to the A site of ribosomal subunits, in response to a codon that it recognizes. The new amino acid is then transferred to the P site, and peptidyl transferase catalyzes formation of a peptide bond between the new amino acid and the growing peptide chain. During the last step, movement of the incoming amino acid from the A site to the P site occurs, a process known as *translocation* (a process catalyzed by an enzyme translocase).

bacterial protein synthesis (aminoglycosides, macrolides, and tetracyclines) exert their effects at different locations along the pathway. These drugs directly interfere with the initiation phase of protein synthesis, the binding of tRNA, and the activities of peptidyl transferase. They also may cause inappropriate amino acid insertions into growing peptide chains (misreading errors), which ultimately interferes with essential protein functions (Fig. 4-4).

Aminoglycosides

Drugs. Amikacin, gentamicin, kanamycin, netilmicin, streptomycin, tobramycin, and neomycin.
Mechanism of action. Aminoglycoside binding to bacterial 30S ribosomal subunits interferes with protein synthesis in at least three ways:
- Aminoglycosides interfere with formation of the initiation complex.
- Aminoglycosides misread mRNA and miscode amino acids in the growing peptide chain.
- Aminoglycosides cause ribosomes to separate from mRNA.

Blockade of movement of the ribosome may occur after formation of a single initiation complex, resulting in an mRNA chain with only a single ribosome, called a *monosome.* This causes inefficient protein synthesis, since many ribosomes (polysomes) typically work together during protein translation.
Pharmacokinetics. Aminoglycosides are too water soluble (because they are highly polar cations) to be absorbed if given orally; therefore, they are usually used parenterally. Except in neonates, aminoglycosides exhibit marginal penetration of the central nervous system because of this high degree of hydrophilicity. Despite short half-lives in systemic circulation, accumulation occurs in the inner ear and renal cortex. Accumulation in these tissues accounts for the nephrotoxic and ototoxic side effects associated with aminoglycosides. Owing to the translational mechanism of action, microorganisms continue to die even as plasma levels of the drug decline, a phenomenon referred to as the "postantibiotic effect."
Clinical use. Aminoglycosides are usually reserved for treating severe gram-negative infections, and they are often

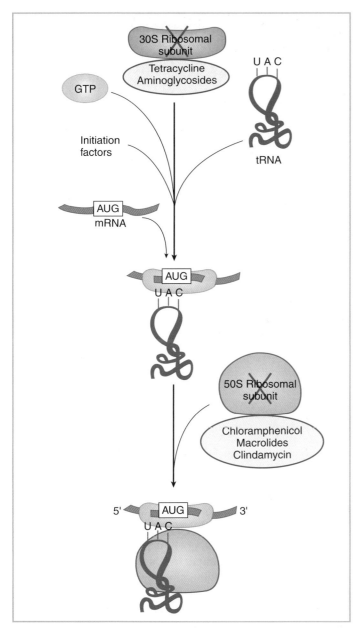

Figure 4-4. Prokaryotic protein synthesis.

TABLE 4-11. Examples of Microorganisms for Which Aminoglycosides are Drugs of Choice*†

Gram-Negative Bacilli	Aminoglycosides
Acinetobacter	✗
Enterobacter	✗
E. coli, urinary tract infection	✓
K. pneumoniae, urinary tract infection	✗
P. aeruginosa	✗
Pseudomonas, urinary tract infection	✗
S. marcescens	✗

*This table is not all-inclusive. It is a representation of *common* infectious microorganisms for which aminoglycosides are the drugs of choice.
†Aminoglycosides are frequently combined with β-lactam antibiotics for treating serious infections caused by gram-negative bacilli.
✗, drug of choice; ✓, alternative choice if first-line agent cannot be used.

Resistance. The aminoglycosides are reliably used only in treating gram-negative infections. Some bacterial species, especially anaerobes, have acquired resistance to aminoglycosides via alterations in receptor proteins on their ribosomes, which prevent aminoglycosides from binding. Additionally, bacteria may enzymatically or posttranslationally alter aminoglycosides through phosphorylation, acetylation, or adenylation, which interferes with the drug's ability to bind efficiently to ribosomal subunits.

Adverse effects. High serum concentrations of aminoglycosides, especially at the nadir (trough) of the dosing cycle, have been associated with serious and irreversible vestibular and auditory ototoxicity as well as nephrotoxicity (usually reversible). Additionally, neuromuscular blockade and acute muscle paralysis may occur, especially in patients with preexisting myasthenia gravis, or when aminoglycosides are used in combination with succinylcholine, or when they are used in dialysis fluid for peritoneal infections. Urinary output and serum peak and trough concentrations should be monitored. Audiometric testing may also be important with chronic therapy. Caution should be used when administering aminoglycosides with other drugs associated with nephrotoxicity (e.g., amphotericin, cephalosporins). Table 4-12 summarizes adverse effects associated with aminoglycoside antibiotics.

added to cell wall synthesis inhibitors for synergistic effects (Table 4-11). Aminoglycosides are used parenterally to treat severe or hospital-acquired infections caused by *Enterobacter, Proteus, Pseudomonas, Klebsiella, E. coli,* and *Serratia* that affect the respiratory system, the gastrointestinal tract, urinary tract, bone, skin, blood, or soft tissues. Gentamicin is usually the parenteral aminoglycoside of choice, although it is available for topical and ophthalmic uses too. Streptomycin may be used in combination with other antibacterials to treat mycobacterial infections. Tobramycin is given via inhalation to treat pseudomonal infections in patients with cystic fibrosis. Neomycin is used for topical skin infections and orally for its "topical" effects in the gastrointestinal tract to eradicate *E. coli, Klebsiella,* and *Enterobacter* prior to surgical bowel procedures.

Tetracyclines

Drugs. Tetracycline, minocycline, doxycycline, demeclocycline, and oxytetracycline.
Note: These drugs end with "-cycline."
Mechanism of action. Tetracyclines inhibit protein synthesis through reversible binding to bacterial 30S ribosomal subunits, which prevents binding of new incoming amino acids (aminoacyl-tRNA) and thus interferes with cell growth (Fig. 4-5). Despite the fact that tetracyclines are bacteriostatic against gram-negative and gram-positive bacteria, the modes of penetration are different: passive diffusion in gram-negative and active transport in gram-positive bacteria.

TABLE 4-12. Adverse Effects Associated with Aminoglycoside Antibiotics (gentamicin, tobramycin, amikacin, netilmicin)

Event	Symptom or Condition
Nephrotoxicity	10% to 15% incidence; generally reversible; usually occurs after 5 to 7 days of therapy Risk factors: advancing age, dehydration, duration of therapy, concurrent nephrotoxins, liver disease
Ototoxicity	1% to 5% incidence; often irreversible; both cochlear and/or vestibular toxicity may occur
Neuromuscular paralysis	Rare; most common with myasthenia gravis

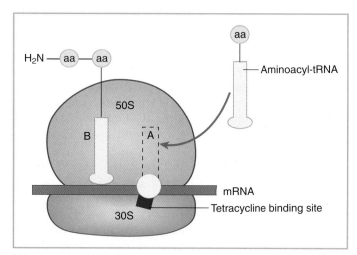

Figure 4-5. Site of action for tetracyclines.

Pharmacokinetics. Gastric absorption of tetracyclines may be inhibited by chelation to divalent cations (iron; aluminum-, magnesium-, or calcium-containing antacids; milk) or to bile acid resins. As a result, it is best to administer tetracyclines on an empty stomach. Of the drugs in this class, doxycycline is metabolized hepatically and excreted in the feces, so it is the safest option in patients with renal dysfunction.

Clinical use. Tetracyclines were the first broad-spectrum antibiotics. These drugs are bacteriostatic against numerous microorganisms (Table 4-13). In addition to susceptible gram-positive and gram-negative microorganisms including *Borrelia burgdorferi* (Lyme disease), tetracyclines are also effective against rickettsia (typhus, Rocky Mountain spotted fever) and *Mycoplasma*. Tetracyclines are also active against *Propionibacterium acnes* and are commonly used to treat inflammatory acne vulgaris.

Resistance. Gram-positive microorganisms acquire resistance to tetracyclines by actively pumping the drugs out of the cells via an efflux pump. Gram-negative bacteria may acquire alterations in their outer membrane proteins that prevent tetracyclines from entering the microorganisms.

TABLE 4-13. Examples of Microorganisms for Which Tetracyclines are Drugs of Choice*†

Organism	Doxycycline
Gram-positive	
Cocci	
E. faecalis	✓
S. aureus, S. epidermis	✓†
Bacilli	
C. perfringes	✓
Gram-negative	
Cocci	
M. catarrhalis	✓
Bacilli	
Legionella spp	✓
P. multocida	✓
Miscellaneous	
C. pneumoniae	✗
C. trachomatis	✗
M. pneumoniae	✓
T. pallidum	✓
B. burgdorferi (Lyme disease)	✗

*This table is not all-inclusive. It is a representation of *common* infectious microorganisms for which doxycycline is the drug of choice.
†Used as an alternative to first-line agents, pending susceptibility.
✗, drug of choice; ✓, alternative choice if first-line agents cannot be used.

Adverse effects. The most notable adverse effects associated with tetracyclines are discoloration of teeth when used in children less than 8 years of age and disturbed fetal bone growth when used during gestation; therefore, tetracyclines should not be used in young children and pregnant women. Photosensitivity, exfoliative dermatitis, secondary super-infections (yeast, pseudomembranous colitis), hypersensitivity, liver disease (jaundice, nausea, vomiting, darkened urine, abdominal pain), renal disease, bone marrow suppression, and pseudotumor cerebri are adverse effects that may be associated with tetracyclines (Table 4-14).

Chloramphenicol

Mechanism of action. Like the tetracyclines, chloramphenicol is bacteriostatic. At the molecular level, chloramphenicol binds to the 50S ribosomal subunit, which prevents peptide elongation by interfering with peptide assembly (Fig. 4-6).

Pharmacokinetics. Chloramphenicol is metabolized via glucuronidation. In infants as well as adults with hepatic disease, the drug accumulates because it is inefficiently glucuronidated, resulting in a "gray baby" (or "gray adult") syndrome in which infants fail to eat, fail to thrive, become pale and cyanotic, have abdominal distention, and may die of respiratory or vasomotor collapse. If any signs of gray syndrome occur, the drug should be discontinued immediately.

Clinical use. Chloramphenicol is used to treat serious infections caused by *Salmonella*, *H. influenzae*, and anaerobic infections including those caused by *B. fragilis*. Chloram-

TABLE 4-14. Adverse Effects Associated with Tetracyclines

Event	Symptom or Condition
Allergic reaction	Rash Anaphylaxis Urticaria Fever
Photosensitivity	
Teeth/bone deposition	Avoid in children and pregnant women
Gastrointestinal upset	Nausea Diarrhea
Hepatitis	Primarily seen with high intravenous doses in the elderly
Renal (azotemia)	Avoid in patients with renal dysfunction Lower incidence with doxycycline
Vestibular toxicity	Associated with minocycline

TABLE 4-15. Adverse Effects Associated with Chloramphenicol

Event	Symptom or Condition
Anemia	Idiosyncratic irreversible aplastic anemia (rare) Reversible dose-related anemia
Gray syndrome	Due to inability of neonates to conjugate chloramphenicol

TABLE 4-16. Microorganisms for Which Clindamycin Is the Drug of Choice*

Organism	Clindamycin
Gram-positive Cocci S. aureus, S. epidermidis, if methicillin-sensitive	✓
Bacilli C. perfringens	✗
Gram-negative Bacilli B. fragilis	✓
G. vaginalis	✓

*This table is not all-inclusive. It is a representation of common infectious microorganisms for which clindamycin is the drug of choice.
✗, drug of choice; ✓, alternative choice if first-line agents cannot be used.

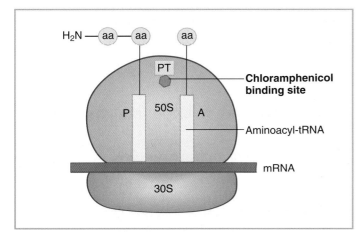

Figure 4-6. Site of action for chloramphenicol and macrolides. PT, peptidyl transferase.

phenicol is also used whenever less dangerous antibiotics are ineffective for meningeal infections, rickettsiae, and gram-negative infections causing bacteremia. In addition to its systemic utility, chloramphenicol is used topically to treat otic and ophthalmic infections. This drug is rarely used in clinical medicine because safer effective antibiotics are usually available.

Adverse effects. Dose-related bone marrow suppression may occur, as well as idiopathic aplastic anemia, which is unrelated to dose and may occur weeks or even months after the drug has been discontinued (Table 4-15). The drug is best avoided in patients with glucose-6-phosphate dehydrogenase (G6PD) deficiency, which is the most commonly inherited red blood cell enzyme deficiency and causes red blood cells to be particularly susceptible to oxidative stress and hemolysis.

Lincosamides

Drug. The common drug is clindamycin. Clindamycin interrupts protein synthesis by binding to 50S ribosomal subunits.
Clinical use. Topically, clindamycin is used to treat acne vulgaris and rosacea and is also used vaginally for bacterial vaginosis. The antibiotic is administered systemically to eliminate numerous species of gram-positive bacteria, and it is the most active antibiotic for treating anaerobic infections, especially *B. fragilis* (Table 4-16). As a result of its broad spectrum, clindamycin is used to treat serious lung abscesses, skin and soft tissue infections, septicemia, intra-abdominal infections, and female pelvic infections. In children, clindamycin may be used for recurrent otitis media when other antibiotics have not been effective.
Adverse effects. Clindamycin potently eliminates numerous anaerobic and gram-positive microorganisms, facilitating opportunistic gastrointestinal infections caused by overgrowth of *C. difficile*. This may lead to pseudomembranous colitis, which is characterized as potentially fatal diarrhea, coupled with abdominal cramping and excretion of blood or mucus (Table 4-17). Additionally, some formulations of clindamycin contain tartrazine (a yellow dye) and should be avoided in patients with asthma or aspirin allergies because of the possibility of allergic responses.

TABLE 4-17. Adverse Effects Associated with Clindamycin

Event	Reason
Diarrhea	High association with pseudomembranous colitis
Allergic hypersensitivities	Tartrazine used as an inactive ingredient

Box 4-4. INDICATIONS FOR MACROLIDES

Amebiasis
Bacterial endocarditis
Chronic bronchitis
Conjunctivitis
Chronic obstructive pulmonary disease (COPD)
Diphtheria
Genital ulcer disease
Legionnaires' disease
Listeria monocytogenes
Otitis media
Pelvic inflammatory disease
Pertussis
Pneumonia
Prevention of disseminated *M. avium-intracellulare* complex in patients with advanced HIV infection
Respiratory tract infections
Rheumatic fever
Sinusitis
Skin and skin structure infections
Syphilis
Urogenital infections

TABLE 4-18. Microorganisms for Which Macrolides are Drugs of Choice*

Organisms	Erythromycin	Azithromycin	Clarithromycin
Gram-positive			
Cocci			
Staphylococcus (groups A, B, C, G, and *S. bovis*)	✓	✓	✓
Streptococcus viridans group	✓	✓	✓
Gram-negative			
Cocci			
M. catarrhalis	✓	✓	✓
Bacilli			
H. influenzae if β-lactamase–negative	✓	✓	✓
Legionella spp		✓	✓
Miscellaneous			
C. pneumoniae	✓	✓	✓
C. trachomatis		✗	
M. pneumoniae	✗	✗	✗
B. burgdorferi		✓	✓

*This table is not all-inclusive. It is a representation of common infectious microorganisms for which a macrolide is the drug of choice.
✗, drug of choice; ✓, alternative choice if first-line agents cannot be used.

Box 4-5. REASONS TO CHOOSE MACROLIDES

- Macrolides are the drugs of choice for penicillin/cephalosporin hypersensitivities
- Macrolides are the drugs of choice for infections caused by atypical microorganisms including *Legionella* and *Mycoplasma pneumoniae*
- Macrolides are the systemic drugs of choice for treatment of impetigo
- Drugs of choice for treating community-acquired pneumonia

Macrolides

Drugs. Drugs include erythromycin base, erythromycin estolate, erythromycin stearate, erythromycin ethylsuccinate (EES), clarithromycin, and azithromycin.

Mechanism of action. Macrolides inhibit protein synthesis by binding to the same site on prokaryotic ribosomal 50S subunits as clindamycin binds. Since they share the same binding site, clindamycin and erythromycin may interfere with one another and cross-resistance may develop between these drugs. Activity may be either bacteriostatic or bactericidal depending on drug concentration.

Clinical use. Indications for macrolides are found in Box 4-4. Macrolides are broad-spectrum antibiotics, active against most gram-positive microorganisms, many gram-negative species, many anaerobes, a variety of mycoplasma species, as well as *Borrelia, Chlamydia, Treponema, Helicobacter pylori,* and *Clostridium tetani* (Table 4-18). Macrolides may be used to treat soft tissue infections, genitourinary infections, Lyme disease, acne vulgaris, and ophthalmic infections. Compared with the erythromycins, clarithromycin has expanded activity, making it a suitable option for eliminating

H. pylori. Similarly, both clarithromycin and azithromycin have expanded gram-negative actions for eliminating *H. influenzae.* These two newer macrolides also have better penetration into lung tissues and macrophages than does erythromycin. Azithromycin is a drug of choice for treating community-acquired pneumonia and is active against *Mycobacterium avium-intracellulare* in immunocompromised individuals. Clarithromycin also is an option for these indications. Additional reasons for selecting macrolides are listed in Box 4-5.

Resistance. Microorganisms become resistant to macrolides when

- Their permeability for macrolides is altered.
- Microorganisms methylate bacterial 50S ribosomal subunits.

TABLE 4-19. Adverse Effects Associated with Erythromycin

Event	Symptom or Condition
Nausea, vomiting, burning stomach	With oral administration
Cholestatic jaundice	Most common with estolate salt
Ototoxicity	Most common with high doses in patients with renal or hepatic failure

Box 4-6. ERYTHROMYCIN MAY INHIBIT THE METABOLISM OF THESE DRUGS

Benzodiazepines
Calcium channel blockers
Carbamazepine
Cyclosporine
Digoxin
Disopyramide
Ergotamine
Glyburide
Nefazodone
Protease inhibitors
Quinidine
Sertraline
Statins
Theophylline
Valproate
Warfarin

Box 4-7. DRUGS WITH WHICH TELITHROMYCIN IS CONTRAINDICATED

Pimozide
Rifampin
Type Ia and type III antiarrhythmics
Simvastatin
Atorvastatin
Lovastatin
Other drugs or risk factors that contribute to QT prolongation

- Bacteria develop mechanisms to enzymatically destroy the drugs.

Adverse effects. Erythromycins are often associated with gastrointestinal distress, which can be minimized if the drugs are taken with food. The estolate salt of erythromycin may cause cholestatic hepatitis, characterized by elevated liver function enzymes, malaise, nausea, vomiting, abdominal cramps, jaundice, and fever. Liver function tests should be monitored if hepatotoxicity is suspected (Table 4-19). Erythromycins may potentiate the actions of other drugs by inhibiting microsomal P-450 3A4 metabolism, leading to toxicity of these other medications (Box 4-6). Erythromycin also prolongs the QT interval on electrocardiograms. This can lead to torsades de pointes, a fatal cardiac arrhythmia, especially when erythromycin is combined with other mediations that also prolong the QT interval. Like erythromycin, clarithromycin also prolongs the QT interval and inhibits P-450 3A4; however, clarithromycin is associated with less gastrointestinal distress than erythromycin is. Unlike clarithromycin and erythromycin, azithromycin does not prolong the QT interval and does not inhibit hepatic microsomal P-450 enzymes. Additionally, azithromycin has only a minimal incidence of diarrhea associated with its use. Because of cross-sensitivity, azithromycin is contraindicated in patients who have a history of allergies to erythromycin.

Ketolides

Drug. Telithromycin.

Mechanism of action. Like the macrolides, telithromycin inhibits protein synthesis by inhibiting the 50S ribosomal subunit. However, telithromycin binds to two separate domains within the 50S ribosomal subunit. This means that two different mutations would be needed in two different domains for bacteria to develop resistance to this drug. Additionally, telithromycin is a very poor substrate for bacterial efflux pumps. Together, these characteristics contribute to the effectiveness of telithromycin, since it is more difficult for bacteria to acquire resistance to this drug.

Clinical use. Telithromycin offers an alternative to fluoroquinolones for treatment of multidrug-resistant streptococci. This ketolide is useful for treating bronchitis, mild-to-moderate community-acquired pneumonia, and sinusitis caused by *S. pneumoniae*, *H. influenzae*, and *M. catarrhalis*.

Adverse effects. Telithromycin is associated with the same concerns as erythromycin and clarithromycin with respect to QT interval prolongation and inhibition of CYP-450 3A4. Drugs that are absolutely contraindicated with telithromycin, because of toxicities that result from P-450 inhibition, are listed in Box 4-7. Additionally, telithromycin is associated with visual disturbances including blurred vision, difficulty focusing, and diplopia. Patients taking telithromycin should be cautioned about these visual disturbances and the dangers of driving while using this antibiotic. New concerns of potentially fatal hepatotoxicity have also emerged.

Mupirocin

Mechanism of action. Available as a topical cream and ointment, mupirocin has a unique mechanism of action that results in no cross-resistance with any other antimicrobials. This antibacterial inhibits the tRNA that transports isoleucine.

Clinical use. Mupirocin is used topically to treat skin infections caused by streptococci or staphylococci (e.g., impetigo, nasal carriers of methicillin-resistant *Staphylococcus aureus*).

Linezolid

Mechanism of action. Linezolid interferes with protein synthesis by binding to a unique RNA site on the 50S subunit.

Clinical use. Linezolid is bacteriostatic against enterococci and staphylococci and is bactericidal for the majority of streptococcal strains. Because of its oral bioavailability, this antibiotic is commonly used for treating vancomycin-resistant *Enterococcus faecium*, methicillin-resistant *S. aureus* (MRSA), and community-acquired *S. pneumoniae*.

Pharmacokinetics. The oral tablet formulation is 100% bioavailable, so it can be used interchangeably with the parenteral form, with no need for dosage adjustments.

Adverse effects. Linezolid inhibits monoamine oxidase; therefore, all tyramine-containing foods (including, but not limited to, beer, wine, cheese, and chocolate) and drugs such as selective serotonin reuptake inhibitors (SSRIs) and pseudo-ephedrine must be avoided. The risk of myelosuppression occurs if linezolid is used for more than 2 weeks, so weekly blood counts are recommended.

Streptogamins

Drugs. Quinupristin/dalfopristin.

Mechanism of action. The quinupristin/dalfopristin combination acts at bacterial ribosomes and interferes with protein synthesis. Quinupristin irreversibly blocks ribosomes and inhibits late phases of protein synthesis, whereas dalfopristin inhibits early phases of protein synthesis. The combination is used to treat life-threatening infections caused by vancomycin-resistant enterococci and complicated skin infections caused by methicillin-resistant *S. aureus* (MRSA).

Adverse effects. Injection site reactions (pain, inflammation, edema) are common, as are muscle/joint pain. Hyperbilirubinemia occurs frequently, and superinfections can occur owing to overgrowth of nonsusceptible microorganisms.

Folic Acid Synthesis Inhibitors

In addition to antibiotics that limit cell wall synthesis or protein synthesis, a third major class of antibiotics targets the synthesis of critical bacterial metabolites. Some antimicrobials capitalize on this fact by inhibiting bacterial folic acid synthesis. Bacteria synthesize their own folic acid. Unlike humans, who obtain this B vitamin from their diets, bacteria cannot utilize folic acid obtained from the environment. Figure 4-7 illustrates the folic acid biosynthetic pathway utilized by bacteria.

Sulfonamides

Drugs. Sulfadiazine, silver sulfadiazine, sulfisoxazole, sulfamethoxazole, sulfacetamide, and sulfasalazine.

Mechanism of action. Sulfonamides compete with para-aminobenzoic acid (PABA) at the first biosynthetic step of the folic acid pathway (see Fig. 4-7).

Pharmacokinetics. Sulfonamides are highly protein-bound, so drug interactions may occur if sulfonamides displace other drugs from plasma protein-binding sites. This can lead to adverse effects when used with drugs such as warfarin, NSAIDs, and sulfonylureas. Sulfonamides are contraindicated in pregnant women near term and in infants less than 2 months of age because these drugs displace bilirubin from protein-binding sites in neonates. Hyperbilirubinemia in neonates

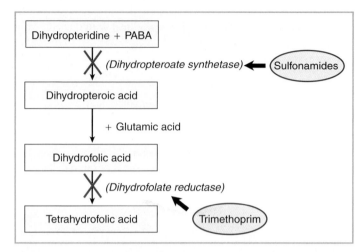

Figure 4-7. Biosynthesis of prokaryotic folic acid and sites of antimicrobial action for sulfonamides and trimethoprim.

Box 4-8. COMMON INDICATIONS FOR SULFONAMIDES

Chancroid
Inclusion conjunctivitis
Malaria
Meningitis, *H. influenzae*
Meningitis, meningococcal
Nocardiosis
Otitis media, acute
Rheumatic fever
Toxoplasmosis
Trachoma
Urinary tract infections (pyelonephritis, cystitis)

---

may cause kernicterus (central nervous system disorders caused by elevated bilirubin).

Clinical use. Sulfonamides have a broad spectrum of activity against gram-positive cocci and gram-negative bacilli; however, antimicrobial resistance is increasingly becoming problematic. Sulfonamides are used to treat urinary tract infections, conjunctivitis, and toxoplasmosis. They also are used to prevent and treat burn-related infections and are used adjunctively with pyrimethamine for malaria. Indications for some sulfonamides are listed in Box 4-8.

Individual sulfonamides have unique actions. Sulfadiazine distributes widely to the central nervous system. Sulfisoxazole may be used to treat urinary tract infections and is also an option for prophylaxis of rheumatic fever if the child is allergic to penicillin. Sulfisoxazole is also administered in a formulation that is combined with erythromycin. Sulfamethoxazole is commonly used in conjunction with trimethoprim for synergistic effects in the treatment of urinary tract infections. Sulfacetamide is used topically in the eyes for treating conjunctivitis or corneal ulcers. Sulfasalazine is used as a treatment for inflammatory bowel disease. Silver sulfadiazine is available as a topical cream for treating burn patients.

CLINICAL MEDICINE

Stevens-Johnson Syndrome

Stevens-Johnson syndrome is a type III immunocomplex-mediated hypersensitivity that usually begins within 2 weeks of taking a drug. Variable lesions, including macules, papules, vesicles, urticarial plaques, and confluent erythema, develop but usually do not itch. The palms of the hands, soles of the feet, corneas, and mucosa are most often affected. Mucosal involvement may include erythema, edema, sloughing of skin, blistering, ulceration, and necrosis. A sore throat, fever, chills, headache, and malaise usually occur coincidentally. Patients often suspect they have influenza, and chickenpox initially may be misdiagnosed in children. This is a potentially life-threatening reaction, and pathologically, the exfoliative dermatitis that accompanies Stevens-Johnson syndrome is similar to a burn.

TABLE 4-20. Adverse Effects Associated with Sulfonamides

Event	Symptom or Condition
Gastrointestinal	Nausea Diarrhea
Hepatic	Cholestatic hepatitis Increased incidence in AIDS
Rash	Exfoliative dermatitis Stevens-Johnson syndrome (more common in AIDS)
Bone marrow	Neutropenia Thrombocytopenia (more common in AIDS)
Kernicterus	Sulfonamide displaces bilirubin from protein, resulting in excessive free sulfonamide and kernicterus

Resistance. Bacteria develop resistance to sulfonamides in several ways including

- Reduced bacterial uptake of the drugs.
- Development of alternative metabolic pathways to synthesize folic acid.
- Production of excessive amounts of PABA (up to 70 times normal) to compete with the sulfonamides for folic acid synthesis.
- Alterations or mutations in dihyropteroate synthase, the enzyme that catalyzes the rate-limiting step of folate synthesis.

Pharmacokinetics. Sulfonamides are metabolized hepatically via acetylation, oxidation, and/or glucuronidation. Individuals who are genetically "slow acetylators" may be at an increased risk of hypersensitivity reactions. Oxidation of sulfonamides likely is responsible for many of the adverse effects associated with sulfonamides. After hepatic biotransformation, sulfonamide metabolites are excreted renally.

Adverse effects. Sulfonamides predispose patients to photosensitivity. Bone marrow suppression, including hemolytic anemia, leukopenia, and thrombocytopenia may occur. There is an increased risk of adverse hematologic effects in patients who are genetically deficient in G6PD. Sulfonamides may precipitate in the kidneys, causing renal stones; good hydration prevents this. Other miscellaneous effects include hepatotoxicity, pseudomembranous colitis, and hypersensitivity reactions, including Stevens-Johnson syndrome (Table 4-20). Because of chemical similarities, patients who are allergic to sulfonamides may also be hypersensitive to sulfonylureas, thiazide diuretics, and sunscreens that contain PABA.

Trimethoprim

Mechanism of action. Trimethoprim inhibits dihydrofolate reductase, the enzyme that catalyzes the last step of bacterial folic acid synthesis (see Fig. 4-7).

Clinical use. Trimethoprim, though available as a single agent, is seldom used this way. Instead, trimethoprim is nearly always used in combination with sulfamethoxazole for synergistic effects. This antibacterial also possesses antimalarial properties. When used alone, trimethoprim is bacteriostatic, but it is bactericidal when combined with sulfonamides. Trimethoprim is used in combination with sulfonamides to treat urinary tract infections, prostatic infections, otitis media in children, elimination of *Shigella*, and treatment of *Pneumocystis carinii* pneumonia. When combined with polymyxin B, trimethoprim is also used for acute conjunctivitis. Although rarely used alone, trimethoprim may be used to treat uncomplicated urinary tract infections caused by *E. coli*, *P. mirabilis*, *Klebsiella pneumoniae*, *Enterobacter* species, and coagulase-negative *Staphylococcus*. Despite interfering with bacterial folate synthesis, patients taking trimethoprim (and sulfonamides) may use folic acid supplements without the supplements interfering with the activity of the antimicrobials.

Resistance. Bacteria may become resistant to trimethoprim through

- Reduced bacterial uptake.
- Alterations or mutations in dihydrofolate reductase.
- Overproduction of dihydrofolate reductase.

Adverse effects. Trimethoprim is associated with adverse effects similar to those of the sulfonamides, including pruritic rashes, gastrointestinal distress, hematologic abnormalities, and fever. Patients with HIV who take trimethoprim have an unusually high incidence of rash and fever.

Inhibitors of DNA/RNA Synthesis

This is the fourth and final major mechanism by which antibacterial agents work.

Fluoroquinolones

Drugs. Ciprofloxacin, gatifloxacin, levofloxacin, lomefloxacin, moxifloxacin, norfloxacin, ofloxacin, sparfloxacin, trovafloxacin, and gemifloxacin.

Mechanism of action. Fluoroquinolones are bactericidal and interfere with bacterial DNA synthesis by inhibiting one of two enzymes. Some fluoroquinolones inhibit DNA gyrase, the enzyme responsible for relaxing supercoiled DNA. This enzyme is essential for replication, transcription, and DNA repair. Other fluoroquinolones inhibit topoisomerase IV, an enzyme involved with separating DNA into daughter cells during replication. One fluoroquinolone, gemifloxacin, is especially effective at inhibiting both enzymes; therefore, for resistance to develop to this antibiotic, bacteria must acquire mutations in two different enzymes.

Pharmacokinetics. Food or cations such as calcium, iron, aluminum, magnesium, and zinc may impair absorption of fluoroquinolones. Additionally, sucralfate interferes with fluoroquinolone absorption.

Although drug penetration into the central nervous system is minimal, fluoroquinolones distribute to nearly all other body compartments including the lungs, gallbladder, sputum, bronchi, bones, muscle, genitourinary tissues, lymph, skin, and prostate.

Clinical use. Early fluoroquinolones, such as ciprofloxacin, predominantly possessed coverage for gram-negative microorganisms such as Enterobacteriaceae, *Pseudomonas aeruginosa*, *H. influenzae*, and *M. catarrhalis* and were used primarily for treating urinary tract infections. However, newer fluoroquinolones have a wider spectrum of activity, with actions against gram-positive microorganisms such as *Streptococcus* and atypical bacteria such as *Mycoplasma pneumoniae*, *Chlamydia pneumoniae*, and *Legionella pneumoniae*. As a result of their expanded coverage, newer fluoroquinolones may also be used treat respiratory infections. Additionally, fluoroquinolones are used to treat infections of the skin, bone and joints, and prostate, as well as intra-abdominal infections, infections caused by *Salmonella* or *Shigella*, and inhalational anthrax. Several fluoroquinolones are also available as ophthalmic drops for treating conjunctivitis and otic drops for external otitis; however, it is probably best to reserve use of these agents to prevent or delay emergence of fluoroquinolone-resistant strains.

Resistance. Microorganisms develop resistance to fluoroquinolones via altered membrane permeability or through mutations in the DNA-binding region.

Adverse effects. Photosensitivity, rash, and rarely, Stevens-Johnson syndrome may occur with fluoroquinolones. (Rash is most common with gemifloxacin.) Additionally, some patients experience dysgeusia, an unpleasant taste in the mouth (Table 4-21).

Fluoroquinolones, especially moxifloxacin, prolong the QT interval and should be used cautiously in patients with risk factors for prolonged QT syndrome (Box 4-9) and patients who are taking medications that also prolong the QT interval (Box 4-10). Elderly patients seem to be particularly susceptible to the central nervous system side effects (psychosis, tremor, stimulation, bad dreams, confusion, seizures, elevated intracranial pressure) of fluoroquinolones. Central nervous system adverse effects may occur because fluoroquinolones prevent γ-aminobutyric acid (GABA) from binding to its receptors. There are also increasing numbers of reports of peripheral nervous system effects (tingling, numbness, twitching pain, spasms) associated with fluoroquinolones.

Fluoroquinolones frequently cause tendinitis, muscle or joint pain, and tendon rupture, which may be apparent immediately after therapy begins or may not appear for up to 90 days afterward. Typically, tendon and joint problems resolve after the drugs are discontinued, but pain and discomfort may last for up to 3 months. Because of possible cartilage damage, fluoroquinolones are contraindicated during pregnancy, lactation, and in children under 17 years of age.

Lipopeptides
Daptomycin

Mechanism of action. The mechanism of daptomycin differs from that of all other antibacterials. Daptomycin binds to bacterial membranes, causing rapid depolarization of the cell.

TABLE 4-21. Adverse Effects Associated with Fluoroquinolones

Event	Symptom or Condition
Gastrointestinal upset	Nausea, vomiting, diarrhea
Central nervous system disorder	Altered mental state, confusion, seizures
Cartilage toxicity	Teratogenic; avoid in children

Box 4-9. RISK FACTORS FOR PROLONGED QT SYNDROME

Advanced age	Hypomagnesemia
Anorexia nervosa	Hypothermia
Bradycardia	Hypothyroidism
Female gender	Infection
Genetic predisposition	Liquid protein diets
Hemodialysis	Major psychiatric problems
Hemorrhage	Pheochromocytoma
Hepatic failure	Stroke
History of cardiac problems	Use of multiple medications
Hypoglycemia	Trauma
Hypokalemia	Tumor

Box 4-10. DRUGS THAT PROLONG QT INTERVAL

Amiodarone	Quetiapine
Cisapride	Quinidine
Clarithromycin	Risperidone
Erythromycin	Telithromycin
Flecainide	Thioridazine
Fluoroquindones	Ziprasidone
Procainamide	

Loss of membrane potential brings DNA, RNA, and protein synthesis to a halt, resulting in cell death.

Clinical use. Daptomycin is approved for parenteral treatment of staphylococcal (including methicillin-resistant *S. aureus*), streptococcal, and enterococcal (vancomycin-susceptible strains) infections.

Adverse effects. Some patients experience muscle pain and weakness associated with elevations of creatine phosphokinase (CPK). Thus, CPK levels should be monitored. As a result of muscular adverse effects, it is best to temporarily discontinue statin therapy in patients who are taking daptomycin.

Metronidazole

Mechanism of action. Metronidazole inhibits DNA synthesis, degrades existing DNA, causes DNA strand breaks, and inhibits nucleic acid synthesis, all of which lead to bacterial cell death. Because of its actions, metronidazole may be mutagenic and possibly carcinogenic. Its use is contraindicated during the first trimester of pregnancy. Interestingly, metronidazole is unique because this drug is not only an antibacterial but is also effective against parasites (e.g., *Giardia*, amoebiasis).

Pharmacokinetics. Metronidazole penetrates the central nervous system and can be used to treat meningitis and brain abscesses caused by anaerobes. Absorption through skin or mucus membranes is low when used topically.

Clinical use. Metronidazole is used topically to treat acne or rosacea; bacterial vaginosis caused by *Trichomonas*, *Gardnerella vaginalis*, or other anaerobic infections; and orally or intravenously to treat *H. pylori* (peptic ulcer disease), amebiasis, *Giardia*, *C. difficile* (pseudomembranous colitis), or *Bacteroides* species.

Adverse effects. It is common for patients to experience peripheral neuropathies and a metallic taste in the mouth. Severe disulfiram-like reactions may occur, and alcohol must be strictly avoided during therapy and for at least 3 days afterward. Metronidazole may cause urine to darken in color.

● ● ● ANTIMYCOBACTERIALS

Mycobacterial are rod-like gram-positive aerobic bacteria that can form filamentous branching structures. Infections caused by mycobacteria (e.g., tuberculosis, leprosy) are notoriously difficult to treat for a variety of reasons including the following:

- Mycobacteria grow slowly. Even during periods of active growth, they may take 18 hours or longer to divide.
- Mycobacteria can lie dormant.
- Mycobacterial cell walls are thick and impermeable; therefore, it is difficult for antibiotics to attain access intracellularly.
- Mycobacterium can reside inside host cells, making it even more difficult to reach therapeutic drug levels inside the mycobacterial cells.
- Mycobacteria become resistant to antibiotic therapies rather quickly.

For these reasons, it is necessary to treat mycobacterial infections for long periods of time, with several different antibiotics simultaneously, to prevent emergence of resistant strains. It is important to eradicate the organisms to obtain a cure. The drugs that treat mycobacterial infections work by several different mechanisms and include isoniazid, rifampin, pyrazinamide, ethambutol, and clofazimine.

Treatment Options

Isoniazid

Mechanism of action. Isoniazid inhibits synthesis of mycolic acids, essential components of mycobacterial cell walls.

Pharmacokinetics. Isoniazid diffuses throughout total body water, even the central nervous system. Metabolism of isoniazid occurs by acetylation. In patients who are genetically "fast acetylators," isoniazid may not reach therapeutic levels and will have a short plasma half-life compared with that of "slow acetylators." Slow acetylators are at a greater risk for drug-related toxicities because of the drug's long half-life.

Clinical use. At therapeutic levels, isoniazid is bactericidal against actively growing intracellular and extracellular *M. tuberculosis*; therefore, the drug is primarily used in treatment or prophylaxis of tuberculosis.

Adverse effects. Neuropathies may occur with isoniazid as a result of pyridoxine (vitamin B_6) deficiency, but supplementation with vitamin B_6 often prevents or minimizes this. Severe, even fatal, hepatitis may occur, and patients should avoid taking acetaminophen or drinking alcohol when taking isoniazid.

Rifampin

Mechanism of action. Rifampin inhibits bacterial RNA polymerase, which prevents transcription by suppressing initiation of RNA chain formation.

Pharmacokinetics. Rifampin is a potent inducer of drug metabolism and alters the plasma levels of many drugs (digoxin, quinidine, warfarin, oral contraceptives, methadone, theophylline, antifungals, β-blockers, calcium channel blockers, and others.) Thus, drug-drug interactions are a major concern.

Clinical use. At therapeutic levels, rifampin is bactericidal against intracellular and extracellular *M. tuberculosis* organisms and is used in combination with other antimycobacterials to treat tuberculosis. Rifampin is effective against many gram-positive and gram-negative microorganisms. This antimicrobial is the drug of choice for prophylaxis of meningococcal meningitis. Rifampin is used prophylactically in close contacts of patients who are affected by epiglottitis or meningitis caused by *H. influenzae*. The drug is also used prophylactically against leprosy, and is used in combination with other drugs for treating *Legionella*.

Adverse effects. Hepatotoxicity may occur with rifampin. For this reason, acetaminophen should be avoided. Rifampin also discolors body fluids, turning urine, sweat, saliva, and tears reddish orange. Contact lenses may be permanently stained. Oral contraceptive efficacy may be severely lessened by induction of hepatic P-450 microsomal enzymes, and patients should consider alternative contraceptive measures.

Pyrazinamide

Mechanism of action. The mechanism of action of pyrazinamide is unclear. It may be that pyrazinamide lowers the pH in the tubercle cavity and inhibits growth of mycobacterium.
Clinical use. This drug is often added to isoniazid and rifampin when treating tuberculosis.
Adverse effects. Pyrazinamide is associated with gastrointestinal distress, elevated uric acid, and hepatotoxicity. Patients should be monitored for hyperuricemia and signs of hepatotoxicity.

Ethambutol

Mechanism of action. Ethambutol inhibits RNA synthesis and decreases replication of tubercle bacilli.
Clinical use. This drug may be added as a fourth drug to the antitubercular cocktail while awaiting drug-susceptibility data in patients with tuberculosis. Ethambutol is also used to treat *M. avium-intracellulare* infections in patients with AIDS.
Adverse effects. Ethambutol may cause optic neuritis, which decreases visual acuity. Additionally, ethambutol may lead to an inability to see the color green. For these reasons, eye examinations are recommended every 2 to 3 months. Gout, joint pain, liver impairment, and cataracts may also occur.

Clofazimine

Mechanism of action. Clofazimine binds to mycobacterial DNA and inhibits RNA polymerase actions. The bactericidal activities of this drug are very slow, and patients are treated for a minimum of 2 years and possibly for life.
Clinical use. Clofazimine is used to treat leprosy, but it should always be used in combination with other antimycobacterial drugs to prevent emergence of resistant strains.
Adverse effects. Clofazimine colors body secretions red-brownish-black, which may last for years after the drug is discontinued. The drug has been associated with gastrointestinal intolerance and dry skin.

●●● ANTIFUNGALS

Although their mechanisms of action differ slightly, antifungals often interfere with lipid biosynthesis and therefore integrity of the fungal membrane. A variety of antifungals are used to treat fungal infections, depending on whether the infection is cutaneous or systemic. Major antifungals include the polyenes (amphotericin B, nystatin) and the "azoles" (voriconazole, ketoconazole, and fluconazole).

Polyenes

Amphotericin B

Mechanism of action. Amphotericin B is an example of a "polyene" type of antifungal. Polyenes bind to fungal ergosterol (the primary sterol in fungal cell membranes). This

---

Box 4-11. TOXICITIES ASSOCIATED WITH AMPHOTERICIN B

Liver disease
Renal failure
Hypokalemia
Hypomagnesemia
Hypersensitivity including anaphylaxis
Phlebitis
Cardiac arrest
Cardiac arrhythmias
Seizures
Intra-alveolar hemorrhage
Blood dyscrasias
Fever, chills, headache in 50% (prevented by premedicating with acetaminophen)

---

alters cell membrane permeability, and intracellular components leak from the cell. Depending on the concentration attained in the body, amphotericin B can be either fungistatic or fungicidal.
Pharmacokinetics. Amphotericin B does not penetrate the central nervous system well. This drug has a very long half-life.
Clinical use. Amphotericin B may be used to treat serious, life-threatening systemic fungal infections. It is administered intravenously or intrathecally for systemic fungal infections including systemic *Candida*, *Cryptococcus*, blastomycosis, and histoplasmosis.
Adverse effects. Numerous toxicities are attributed to amphotericin B (Box 4-11). Serum creatinine, blood urea nitrogen, complete blood counts, serum potassium, serum sodium, serum magnesium, and liver function tests must be monitored. When amphotericin B is used with aminoglycosides or neuromuscular blockers, prolonged skeletal muscle paralysis may result.

Nystatin

Mechanism of action. Nystatin is a polyene antifungal that is effective only against *Candida*.
Clinical use. It is poorly absorbed, and thus it is reserved for topical treatment of oral thrush, vaginal infections, intestinal infections, and cutaneous infections.
Adverse effects. Gastrointestinal upset is common when nystatin is taken orally.

Natamycin

Mechanism of action. Natamycin is a polyene antifungal that is used for ocular infections.

"Azoles"

"Azole" antifungals (imidazoles and triazoles) work by slightly different mechanisms but they all inhibit the biosynthesis of ergosterol, the main sterol in fungal cell membranes. Disruption in ergosterol synthesis ultimately increases cellular permeability and causes cell leakage. Some of these drugs (e.g., ketoconazole) also interfere with human cortisol and testosterone biosynthesis, which explains side effects like gynecomastia in men and menstrual irregularities in women. "Azoles" are potent inhibitors of P-450 hepatic metabolism and have the potential to cause many severe and even life-threatening drug interactions. Additionally, all "azoles" have been associated with liver toxicity when used systemically.

Voriconazole

Pharmacokinetics. Voriconazole is metabolized hepatically and inhibits P-450 enzymes.

Clinical use. Voriconazole is an option for treating serious fungal infections including those caused by *Aspergillus* and *Scedosporium*.

Adverse effects. Visual disturbances and hallucinations may occur; therefore, patients are warned not to drive at night. Some patients experience a rash. Liver function tests may be elevated and should be monitored periodically. Overall, voriconazole is better tolerated than amphotericin B.

Ketoconazole

Pharmacokinetics. Ketoconazole requires an acidic environment for dissolution and systemic absorption. It does not enter the central nervous system. Ketoconazole is potent inhibitor of hepatic P-450 enzymes, thus dosage adjustments may be necessary to prevent adverse drug interactions. Table 4-22 contains a partial listing of potentially serious drug interactions.

Clinical use. Ketoconazole is used to treat severe recalcitrant infections such as mucocutaneous candidiasis, histoplasmosis, coccidioidomycosis, and chromomycosis. It is not active against *Aspergillus*. In addition to systemic formulations, ketoconazole is available as a topical cream and shampoo.

Adverse effects. Ketoconazole may cause hepatotoxicity. Because of the risk of liver toxicity, liver function tests should be monitored. Gynecomastia and impotence may occur in men (Table 4-23).

Fluconazole

Pharmacokinetics. A single dose of fluconazole has a long half-life; this property allows a one-time oral dose to be used for treating vaginal yeast infections. Eighty percent of the drug is cleared from the body renally. The drug also penetrates the central nervous system and is used prophylactically in immunocompromised patients. Numerous drug interactions are likely, since fluconazole inhibits P-450 hepatic enzymes.

Clinical use. Fluconazole has a greater activity and spectrum than other "azoles" (Box 4-12). Owing to its penetration of the central nervous system, fluconazole may be used to treat cryptococcal meningitis.

Adverse effects. Toxicities associated with fluconazole include hepatic disease and exfoliative skin disorders.

Itraconazole

Pharmacokinetics. Like ketoconazole, itraconazole is best absorbed in an acidic environment. By inhibiting P-450 hepatic enzymes, numerous severe drug interactions may occur.

Clinical use. Itraconazole was initially used orally for treating fungal infections of the nails; however, parenteral forms are also available for treating life-threatening infections caused by blastomycosis, histoplasmosis and aspergillosis. This drug may be an alternative to amphotericin B. Itraconazole has greater activity against *Aspergillus* than either ketoconazole or fluconazole.

Adverse effects. Itraconazole may exacerbate preexisting congestive heart failure and may cause liver failure.

Other "Azole" Antifungals

Other "azole" antifungals include clotrimazole, miconazole, butoconazole, tioconazole, and terconazole. These drugs may be used topically to treat tinea pedis, tinea cruris, tinea

TABLE 4-23. Adverse Effects Associated with "Azole" Antifungals (ketoconazole, fluconazole, itraconazole, and others)

Event	Symptom or Condition
Hepatitis	Ranges from mild liver dysfunction to fatal hepatitis
Gynecomastia	More common with high doses of ketoconazole (>400 mg/d) due to decreased testosterone synthesis; decreased libido and azoospermia

TABLE 4-22. Partial Listing of Serious Drug Interactions Associated with Ketoconazole

Interacting Drug	Adverse Reaction
Statins	Rhabdomyolysis
Alcohol	Disulfiram-like reactions
Warfarin	Increased bleeding
Cyclosporine	Potential nephrotoxicity
Sulfonylureas	Hypoglycemia

Box 4-12. SPECTRUM OF ACTIVITY FOR FLUCONAZOLE

Aspergillus
Blastomyces dermatitidis
Candida albicans
Candida kefyr
Candida tropicalis
Coccidioides immitis
Cryptococcus neoformans
Histoplasma capsulatum
Torulopsis glabrata

versicolor, tinea corporis, and candidal infections of the vagina, vulva, and throat.

Other Antifungal Agents

Caspofungin and Micafungin (β-[1,3]-D-Glucan Inhibitors)

Mechanism of action. Caspofungin is the first in a new class of antifungals, the glucan synthesis inhibitors, which inhibit the synthesis of β-(1,3)-D-glucan, a necessary component of fungal cell walls.

Clinical use. Caspofungin is effective for treating invasive aspergillosis in patients who cannot tolerate, or who are refractory to, other therapies. In clinical studies, caspofungin appears to have a lower incidence of adverse effects compared with amphotericin B. Micafungin may be used to treat patients with esophageal candidiasis and used prophylactically in patients at risk of developing *Candida* infections while undergoing hematopoietic stem cell transplantation.

Adverse effects. Serious hypersensitivity reactions (rash, itching, facial swelling, vasodilation) and elevated bilirubin levels have been reported with micafungin.

Griseofulvin

Mechanism of action. Griseofulvin deposits in the stratum corneum layer of skin, hair, and nails. It inhibits fungal mitosis by blocking assembly of microtubules. The drug is gradually exfoliated and replaced by uninfected tissues.

Clinical use. Griseofulvin is used to treat infections of the hair, nails, and skin.

Adverse effects. The most common side effects are hypersensitive skin reactions and hives. Although rare, more serious reactions may occur including angioneurotic edema, gastrointestinal bleeding, leukopenia, menstrual irregularities, and hepatotoxicity. The drug is contraindicated in patients with liver disease and should not be used in pregnant women owing to carcinogenic and teratogenic effects in animal studies. Griseofulvin may decrease the efficacy of warfarin and oral contraceptives.

Terbinafine

Mechanism of action. This drug inhibits an enzyme (squalene epoxidase) that is required for sterol synthesis.

Pharmacokinetics. Terbinafine undergoes extensive first-pass metabolism in the liver. Owing to its inhibition of hepatic P-450 enzymes, numerous drug interactions are possible.

Clinical use. Terbinafine has a spectrum of action similar to that of griseofulvin and is used to treat nail fungus.

Adverse effects. Terbinafine may cause patients to temporarily lose their sense of taste.

Ciclopirox

Mechanism of action. Ciclopirox chelates polyvalent cations (aluminum, iron), resulting in inhibition of metal-dependent enzymes that are responsible for degrading peroxides inside fungal cells.

Clinical use. Ciclopirox is an option for treating topical fungal infections. The drug is formulated as a topical cream, gel, and solution. The topical solution is applied daily (like nail polish) to fingernails and toenails that are affected by fungus. Each day, a new layer of drug is applied over existing layers; once a week, previous layers of drug are removed. Although it takes a year for ciclopirox to eliminate the nail fungus, it is an option for patients who are unable or unwilling to tolerate the potential hepatotoxicity of "azoles."

●●● ANTIPARASITICS

Antimalarials

Malaria is a mosquito-transmitted illness caused by parasitic protozoans that is mainly found in tropical and subtropical areas. Transmitted via a variety of *Plasmodium* species, the illness is characterized by bouts of shivering, fever, sweating, and red blood cell lysis. Once a diagnosis of malaria has been confirmed, the infecting species of *Plasmodium* must be identified so that an appropriate therapy can be selected. Therapy is based on (1) the clinical status of the patient and (2) the drug susceptibility of the parasite as determined by the geographic area where the infection was acquired. Treatments include chloroquine, mefloquine, primaquine, atovaquone-proguanil, and quinine, as well as some antibacterials that have already been discussed (Table 4-24 presents an overview). The latest treatment guidelines compiled by the U.S. Centers for Disease Control and Prevention (CDC) can always be found at http://www.cdc.gov. Therapeutic recommendations change regularly, as *Plasmodium* resistance patterns to antimalarial drugs constantly change.

Chloroquine and Hydroxychloroquine

Mechanism of action. Chloroquine and hydroxychloroquine are taken up more readily into affected cells than non-

TABLE 4-24. Treatment Options for Malaria

Plasmodium Species	Drug Options
P. falciparum, *P. malariae*	Chloroquine *or* Quinidine sulfate plus doxycycline, tetracycline, or clindamycin *or* Atovaquone-proguanil *or* Mefloquine
P. vivax, *P. ovale*	Chloroquine plus primaquine *or* Quinidine sulfate plus either doxycycline or tetracycline plus primaquine *or* Mefloquine plus primaquine

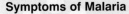

MICROBIOLOGY & IMMUNOLOGY

Symptoms of Malaria

Malaria is transmitted by mosquitoes in tropical areas. Early symptoms are nonspecific and include malaise, headache, fatigue, abdominal discomfort, muscle aches, fever, nausea, vomiting, orthostatic hypotension, and anemia. These symptoms are followed by the classic symptoms of malaria, which include high fever, chills, and rigors occurring at regular intervals. Four different species of *Plasmodium* may cause malaria. *P. falciparum* can rapidly progress to severe illness or death, whereas the other species (*P. vivax*, *P. ovale*, and *P. malariae*) rarely cause severe illness. *P. vivax* and *P. ovale* infections may require treatment for the hypnozoite forms that lie dormant in the liver and cause relapsing infections.

infected cells. Their exact mechanism is unknown. Inside cells, the antimalarials may raise the internal pH inside parasite vesicles and may also interfere with parasite nucleoprotein synthesis.

Clinical use. These drugs are used for prophylaxis and acute attacks of malaria. They are effective for treating the erythrocytic (blood) stage of malaria; however, they have no effect on exoerythrocytic (tissue) forms of malaria.

Adverse effects. Resistance to these drugs is increasing in many parts of the world. These drugs may cause hemolysis in patients with G6PD deficiency. Additionally, these drugs have been associated with seizures, electrocardiographic changes, agranulocytosis, and irreversible retinal damage. Ophthalmic examinations are recommended.

Mefloquine

Mechanism of action. The mechanism of mefloquine is unknown.

Clinical use. Mefloquine is used for treatment and prevention of malaria.

Adverse effects. Mefloquine is associated with gastrointestinal upset, circulatory disturbances, rash, and musculoskeletal weakness and cramps. Additionally, disorientation or confusion as well as psychiatric symptoms of depression, hallucinations, or suicidal thoughts may occur.

Primaquine

Mechanism of action. Primaquine disrupts parasitic mitochondria and binds to DNA.

Clinical use. Primaquine is used to treat tissue (exoerythrocytic) and blood (erythrocytic) forms of *Plasmodium vivax* malaria.

Adverse effects. Primaquine causes drug-induced hemolysis and gastrointestinal upset.

Atovaquone-Proguanil

Mechanism of action. Atovaquone-proguanil interferes with two different pathways in pyrimidine biosynthesis that are required for parasitic nucleic acid replication.

Clinical use. This combination of drugs is used to treat and prevent malaria.

Adverse effects. Of all the antimalarials, atovaquone-proguanil is probably the safest, although it is also the most expensive.

Quinine

Mechanism of action. The precise mechanism of quinine is unknown but may involve elevating the pH of intracellular organelles inside parasites.

Adverse effects. A conglomeration of symptoms called cinchonism (headache, tinnitus, nausea, blurred vision, diplopia, disturbed color vision) may occur, as well as hepatitis and other gastrointestinal disturbances and cardiac arrhythmias. This drug is contraindicated in patients with G6PD deficiency owing to the risk of hemolysis.

Antihelmintics

Numerous types of helminths (flatworms, round worms, flukes, and tapeworms) exist and are particularly problematic in areas of the world where sanitation is poor. In addition, some worm infections may be obtained by eating poorly cooked pork. Drugs of choice are listed in Table 4-25. Note that some of these medications are available only outside the United States or through the CDC. The following discussion features a few of the medications used to treat worm infections.

Mebendazole

Mechanism of action. Mebendazole and thiabendazole block assembly of tubulin polymers. By disrupting microtubule assembly, the formation of mitotic spindles is disrupted. Additionally, glucose uptake into the parasite is disrupted with mebendazole, causing worms to starve to death.

Clinical use. These drugs may be used to treat the enteric stages of pinworm, roundworm, hookworm, and whipworm infections but not larvae once they have migrated to muscle tissues.

TABLE 4-25. Parasitic Infections and Drugs of Choice

Infection (Common Name)	Drugs of Choice
Intestinal nematodes	Mebendazole, pyrantel pamoate, albendazole, or diethylcarbamazine
Tissue nematodes	Thiabendazole, albendazole, flubendazole, mebendazole, ivermectin, suramin, or diethylcarbamazine
Cestodes	Praziquantel, niclosamide, or albendazole
Trematodes	Praziquantel, oxamniquine, or bithionol

Adverse effects. These drugs may cause gastrointestinal upset. Additionally, these agents are embryotoxic and should be avoided during pregnancy.

Ivermectin

Mechanism of action. Ivermectin causes a tonic paralysis of worms, probably by activating a glutamate-activated chloride channel. This leads to hyperpolarization of invertebrate nerve and muscle cells, which causes paralysis. Fortunately, ivermectin does not cross the mammalian blood-brain barrier.
Clinical use. Ivermectin is effective for treating nematodes.
Adverse effects. Because of its rapid killing effects, an inflammatory response termed the *Mazzotti reaction* (itching, rash, fever, swollen lymph nodes, and arthralgias) may occur as the worms are eliminated.

Praziquantel

Mechanism of action. Praziquantel increases cell membrane permeability, causing a loss of intracellular calcium, massive contractions, and paralysis.
Clinical use. Praziquantel is effective against a broad spectrum of helminths, including cestodes and many flukes.
Adverse effects. Adverse effects generally involve gastrointestinal discomfort and are short-lived.

Head Lice Medications

Other than the common cold, head lice affect more school-aged children than any other communicable illness.

Lindane

Adverse effects. Although the gold standard for many years in treatment of head lice was lindane, a drug that is ovicidal by absorbing directly into the parasites and their ova, this drug has been banned from use in many countries and even in some states of the United States because of possible neurotoxicity (seizures and death). As a result, lindane is rarely used, and if it is prescribed, it should definitely not be used in persons with a history of seizure disorders. Additionally, it should never be applied more than one time.

Permethrin

Mechanism of action. Permethrin keeps sodium channels opened for prolonged periods of time, thus delaying repolarization, resulting in paralysis of scabies.
Clinical use. Permethrin is a safer alternative to lindane. It is available over-the-counter as a lotion and cream rinse and is available with a prescription in a more concentrated cream formulation. Unfortunately, permethrin may not kill lice eggs, called nits. Nits are best removed with special combs. Permethrin may be applied again 2 weeks following initial use, but excessive application contributes to lice resistance (which may be as high as 50% to 98%).
Adverse effects. Permethrin is contraindicated in patients allergic to ragweed and chrysanthemums. Irritation at the site of application may occur.

Other Options

Other alternatives for treating head lice include malathion, ivermectin, and even sulfamethoxazole/trimethoprim, all of which are covered elsewhere in this book.

●●● ANTIVIRALS

It is important to keep in mind that antivirals are not a cure! Antivirals simply shorten the duration, decrease the severity, and reduce the sequelae associated with viral infections. Antivirals are most efficacious when they are initiated at the first sign of infection.

Several classes of antivirals that work through distinct mechanisms have been approved (Fig. 4-8). Antivirals inhibit viral replication by
- Inhibiting viral uncoating
- Inhibiting viral neuraminidase
- Serving as "foreign" or nonfunctional analogs of DNA/RNA nucleotides
- Interfering with viral penetration of the host cell, or inhibiting fusion of viral or host membranes
- Inhibiting reverse transcriptases
- Inhibiting proteases responsible for cleaving viral precursor proteins

Some antiviral drugs assure specificity of the response by becoming "activated" only inside virally infected cells. For example, some drugs that are analogs of nucleosides are administered in an unphosphorylated form. When these drugs are taken up by infected cells, the viral enzyme, thymidine kinase, phosphorylates the drug. (Note that because the host enzyme does not add the first phosphate, the drug does not

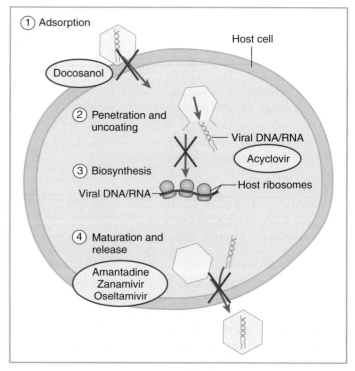

Figure 4-8. Drug targets for viral infection and replication.

become activated in unifected cells.) The host cell subsequently adds two additional phosphates to the virally produced monophosphorylated drug. The triphosphorylated drug may now be incorporated into DNA or RNA as a "nucleic acid." When the drugs have been incorporated into viral DNA or RNA, the end result is chain termination and disrupted viral replication (see Fig. 4-8).

Inhibitors of Viral Uncoating

Amantadine and Rimantadine

Mechanism of action. Amantadine and rimantadine appear to work, at least in part, by preventing viral nucleic acid from being released into the host cell (see Fig. 4-8).

Clinical use. Amantadine and rimantadine are effective for reducing the duration of influenza A if given within 24 hours of symptom onset and may prevent the infection in close contacts of affected individuals.

Adverse effects. Amantadine is associated with central nervous system side effects (nervousness, lightheadedness, insomnia, and seizures), especially in the elderly. Additionally, amantadine is associated with anticholinergic side effects and may promote dopamine release. Because of these additional mechanisms, amantadine is sometimes used for managing symptoms associated with Parkinson's disease. Use caution and consider dose reductions in patients with renal impairment.

Inhibitors of Viral Neuraminidase

Zanamivir and Oseltamivir

Mechanism of action. Zanamivir and oseltamivir inhibit viral neuraminidase, an enzyme that is essential for release of newly formed virus particles from infected cells and further spread of the infectious virus.

Clinical use. Zanamivir and oseltamivir are effective for reducing the duration of influenza A and B if administered within 48 hours of symptom onset and may prevent viral infection in close contacts of affected individuals.

Adverse effects. Oseltamivir is not recommended in infants less than 1 year of age owing to fatalities in mice. Zanamivir

---

MICROBIOLOGY & IMMUNOLOGY

Mechanics of Viral Infection

Viruses are obligate intracellular parasites that usurp the metabolic processes of the hosts they invade for their own replication purposes. Briefly, viruses must attach to and penetrate susceptible host cells—that is, cells that have appropriate receptors for viral binding and the necessary intracellular machinery for viral replication. Next, the virus uncoats, a process by which the viral DNA/RNA separates from the viral capsid. The virus then exploits the host's RNA/DNA/protein synthesis machinery. Viral subunits are then assembled, allowing the progeny viruses to be released, as the host cell disintegrates.

---

should be avoided in those with asthma or COPD because it can cause bronchospasm.

Inhibition of Intracellular Synthesis by Analogs of Viral Nucleic Acids

Ribavirin, Acyclovir, Valacyclovir, Ganciclovir, Valganciclovir, Famciclovir, Penciclovir, and Foscarnet

Note: Many antivirals end in "-ovir."

Mechanism of action. Ribavirin and the other drugs interfere with intracellular viral replication processes. Most of these drugs are guanosine analogs (acyclovir, valacyclovir, ganciclovir, valganciclovir, famciclovir, and penciclovir). The exact mechanism of ribavirin is not known, but it may act as an analog of guanosine or xanthosine. These drugs are first phosphorylated by a viral thymidine kinase and subsequently phosphorylated by the host cell, prior to drug incorporation into viral nucleic acids. When the phosphorylated drugs are encountered by viral polymerases, the drugs are recognized as "foreign" and viral polymerase action is halted.

Unlike other antivirals in this class, foscarnet, although still an inhibitor of viral DNA polymerases, does not need to be "activated" (or phosphorylated) for its activity. Foscarnet binds directly to viral DNA polymerases and inhibits their activity.

Pharmacokinetics. Valacyclovir, valganciclovir, and famciclovir are simply pro-drugs of acyclovir, ganciclovir, and penciclovir, respectively, with superior bioavailability over the parent compounds. These antivirals are excreted renally, so dosage adjustments are necessary at low glomerular filtration rates.

Clinical use. Ribavirin is approved as an aerosol for treating respiratory syncytial virus (RSV), a leading cause of pneumonia in infants; however, the aerosolized drug has cumbersome requirements (e.g., endotracheal intubation) because sometimes patients, especially infants, suddenly get worse with inhalation. Additionally, strict isolation is necessary to prevent drug exposure to pregnant visitors and caregivers. This drug is also used in combination with peg-interferon α-2b for treatment of hepatitis C in patients with decompensated liver disease.

Penciclovir is available only as a topical cream for treating oral cold sores caused by the herpesvirus. Acyclovir is used to treat herpes simplex virus (mucosal, cutaneous, encephalitis, recurrent genital infections, shingles, and varicella); the drug may also be used to reduce the risk of cytomegalovirus in high-risk patients. When used to treat chickenpox, acyclovir reduces the number of lesions, shortens the healing time, and decreases the duration of fever. The drug does not appear to have any pain-relieving properties when used for management of shingles. Famciclovir and valacyclovir are also used in treatment and management of herpes infections. Ganciclovir and valganciclovir are used to treat life-threatening or sight-threatening cytomegalovirus infections, and foscarnet is also used to treat herpes infections as well as cytomegalovirus in immunocompromised patients.

TABLE 4-26. Adverse Effects Associated with Common Antivirals

Medication	Symptom or Condition
Acyclovir	Phlebitis: 15% to 20% incidence; due to poor solubility Renal failure: dehydration predisposes to toxicity CNS: 1% incidence (confusion, headache, lethargy, seizures, disorientation)
Ganciclovir	Neutropenia, thrombocytopenia: increased incidence in AIDS Hepatitis: usually mild to moderate increase in liver function tests

CLINICAL MEDICINE

Human Immunodeficiency Virus (HIV)

HIV is the retrovirus that causes acquired immunodeficiency syndrome (AIDS). Lymphocytes are infected first. Initially, patients may experience mononucleosis- or influenza-like symptoms while the virus spreads to lymphoid and other body tissues. It may take years before the patient becomes clinically ill. During this time, CD4+ T-cell numbers decline and patients become highly susceptible to opportunistic infections. Patients are monitored for CD4+ T-cell counts as well as the level of HIV RNA in plasma. Viral replication rates predict what will happen to CD4+ cell counts in the future.

Adverse effects. The primary toxicity associated with ribavirin is hemolytic anemia, which may worsen cardiac disease, even leading to death. The drug is mutagenic, carcinogenic, and teratogenic and should not be administered via the inhalation route by pregnant health care workers. Acyclovir is associated with rashes and photosensitivity. Granulocytopenia, anemia, and thrombocytopenia are limiting side effects of ganciclovir and valganciclovir, and these drugs are also thought to be carcinogenic and teratogenic (Table 4-26). Foscarnet may cause nephrotoxicity and electrolyte imbalances, so close monitoring is essential.

Antivirals That Interfere with Viral Penetration into Host Cells

Docosanol

Mechanism of action. Docosanol interferes with viral penetration of host cells and subsequent migration of the virus to the nucleus (see Fig. 4-8).

Clinical use. This agent is available over-the-counter, without a prescription, as a cream that is applied topically to external cold sores.

●●● MANAGEMENT OF HUMAN IMMUNODEFICIENCY VIRUS

Currently, four classes of antiretrovirals are used to manage human immunodeficiency virus (HIV):

- Nucleoside-dependent reverse transcriptase inhibitors
- Non-nucleoside reverse transcriptase inhibitors
- Protease inhibitors
- Fusion inhibitors

Combinations of drugs are always used to delay the emergence of drug-resistant viral strains. Regimens can be very complicated, with some patients ingesting 15 pills daily. Some medications must be taken with food, while other medications cannot be taken with food and should only be taken with an antacid. Numerous drug interactions and contraindications are associated with these drugs, and

clinicians prescribing these medications must be thoroughly versed in these interactions, with appropriate safeguards in place. This brief review chapter is not intended to provide a detailed discussion of each antiretroviral drug but instead provides an overview of each of the four major drug classes.

Nucleoside/Nucleotide Reverse Transcriptase Inhibitors

Zidovudine, Zalcitabine, Stavudine, Lamivudine, Emtricitabine, Didanosine, Abacavir, and Tenofovir

Note: Tenofovir is the only nucleo*tide* reverse transcriptase inhibitor.

Mechanism of action. These drugs are structurally related to the sugars and nucleotides that comprise nucleic acids. Like many other antivirals, these drugs are phosphorylated and inserted as nonfunctional nucleotides. They inhibit viral DNA polymerase (reverse transcriptase), so that viral DNA synthesis is inhibited and viral replication is decreased.

Clinical use. Frequently, two nucleoside reverse transcriptase inhibitors are combined with a protease inhibitor to prevent development of resistant strains. The only indication for monotherapy is when the drugs are used to prevent perinatal transmission of the virus from mother to infant during labor and delivery. These drugs may also be used prophylactically to prevent infection in healthcare workers who have experienced accidental needle sticks.

Adverse effects. Adverse effects associated with this class of medications are listed in Box 4-13.

Non-Nucleoside Reverse Transcriptase Inhibitors

Nevirapine, Delavirdine, and Efavirenz

Mechanism of action. These drugs are direct noncompetitive inhibitors of HIV-1 reverse transcriptase. Non-nucleoside reverse transcriptase inhibitors block RNA-dependent and DNA-dependent polymerase activities by inducing a conformational change that disrupts the enzyme's catalytic site. Unlike the nucleoside reverse transcriptase inhibitors, these drugs do not require intracellular phosphorylation for

Box 4-13. ADVERSE EFFECTS ASSOCIATED WITH NUCLEOSIDE REVERSE TRANSCRIPTASE INHIBITORS

Pancreatitis
Peripheral neuropathy
Granulocytopenia
Myopathy
Lactic acidosis with hepatic steatosis (rare, but potentially fatal)

their actions. These drugs potentiate the actions of other antiretroviral drugs.

Clinical use. Non-nucleoside reverse transcriptase inhibitors are used in combination with other antiretroviral agents to treat HIV infections.

Pharmacokinetics. These drugs are metabolized by the P-450 enzymes and are susceptible to numerous drug interactions by drugs that induce or inhibit the hepatic P-450 microsomal enzymes.

Adverse effects. All drugs may cause potentially fatal hepatotoxicity. Severe, life-threatening skin rashes, including Stevens-Johnson syndrome and toxic epidermal necrosis, may also occur.

Protease Inhibitors

Saquinavir, Ritonavir, Indinavir, Nelfinavir, Amprenavir, Lopinavir/Ritonavir, Atazanavir, and Fosamprenavir

Note: These drugs end in "-avir."

Mechanism of action. These drugs inhibit the protease that is responsible for cleaving viral precursor proteins, which are essential for HIV maturation, replication, and infection of new cells. Inhibition of the protease enzyme produces immature viral particles. When used in combination with other anti-retroviral drugs, protease inhibitors lead to clinical improvements and prolonged patient survival. Rapid HIV resistance emerges if protease inhibitors are used as monotherapy.

Clinical use. Protease inhibitors are used in combination with other antiretrovirals for treating HIV infections.

Pharmacokinetics. All drugs in this class are metabolized by hepatic microsomal enzymes and are susceptible to many severe, even life-threatening drug interactions.

Adverse effects. All protease inhibitors can cause gastrointestinal intolerance, increased bleeding, hyperglycemia, insulin resistance, hyperlipidemia, and hepatitis. As a result of the "metabolic syndrome" associated with these drugs, some practitioners suggest delaying administration of these drugs rather than using them as part of initial treatment regimens.

Fusion Inhibitors

Enfuvirtide

Mechanism of action. Enfuvirtide interferes with entry of HIV-1 into CD4$^+$ cells by inhibiting fusion of viral and cellular membranes.

Pharmacokinetics. Enfuvirtide is a 36-amino-acid synthetic peptide that is administered twice daily by subcutaneous injections into the arm, thigh, or abdomen.

Adverse effects. Adverse effects include hypersensitivity reactions and injection site discomfort. Overall, enfuvirtide may have an improved safety profile compared with other antiretrovirals because it doesn't exert its effects inside host cells. Since the drug is metabolized to individual amino acids, there are no interactions with other medications or with the P-450 hepatic enzymes. Adverse effects are primarily gastrointestinal (diarrhea, nausea).

●●● COMPLEMENTARY AND ALTERNATIVE MEDICINE

Treatment of Antibiotic-Associated Diarrhea

Nearly all antibacterials disrupt normal gastrointestinal flora. This can lead to overgrowth of undesirable species including *C. difficile*. The incidence of severe, life-threatening diarrhea caused by overgrowth of *C. difficile* is increasing, and some estimates from the CDC indicate that the incidence doubled between 2000 and 2002 in the United States.

Probiotic supplements that replace the "good" gastrointestinal flora have been shown to prevent antibiotic-associated diarrhea and "cure" severe *C. difficile* diarrhea even in patients who are refractory to therapy with metronidazole and vancomycin. Most often, the bacterial species contained in probiotic supplements belong to members of the *Lactobacillus* or *Bifidobacterium* genera.

It is becoming increasingly apparent that for maximal benefit probiotic supplements must remain refrigerated, must contain tens or hundreds of billions of "good" bacteria, and are more likely to exert beneficial effects when multiple species are contained in a single product. These healthy bacterial supplements eliminate harmful *Clostridia* species via several mechanisms including competitive exclusion for space and nutrients, production of short-chain fatty acids, production of peroxides and bacteriocins, and stimulation of IgA secretion.

Numerous probiotic products are available. Recommend products that have been shown effective in clinical trials, and shy away from products that have no data to back up their claims.

Another type of probiotic that has been shown extremely beneficial for preventing and treating *C. difficile* diarrhea is the yeast strain *Saccharomyces boulardii*. Although not normally part of our endogenous flora, this strain of yeast secretes an enzyme that selectively inactivates *C. difficile* toxins.

Treatment of Yeast Infections

For difficult-to-eradicate yeast infections, especially thrush in infants, a 0.5% gentian violet solution, painted onto affected oral tissues with a cotton-tipped swab twice daily for 5 days can be effective at eradicating the infection. If the infant is breast-fed, the mother's nipples may also require treatment. Alternatively, if the baby is bottle-fed, nipples and bottles

TABLE 4-27. Common Pharmacologic Options for Various Microorganisms (Grouped by Morphology and Gram Staining)

Microbe	Option
Gram-positive Cocci	
Staphylococci (Assume all make β-lactamases)	Penicillinase-resistant penicillins (e.g., nafcillin, methicillin, dicloxacillin) Amoxicillin/clavulanic acid Cephalosporins Vancomycin Imipenem Clindamycin Fluoroquinolones
Group A streptococci (*S. pyogenes*) (Cause of "pink eye" and "strep throat")	Penicillin Amoxicillin Clindamycin Macrolides
Group B streptococci (Possibly problematic for babies whose mothers are vaginal carriers)	Penicillin Ampicillin Cephalosporins Vancomycin
S. viridans (Cause of bacterial endocarditis, persistent urinary tract infections)	Penicillin Cephalosporins Gentamicin Vancomycin
Gram-negative Cocci	
M. catarrhalis (One of three major causes of otitis media Secrete β-lactamases)	Amoxicillin/clavulanic acid Cephalosporins Macrolides Fluoroquinolones
N. gonorrhoeae	Ceftriaxone Cefixime Spectinomycin (An aminoglycoside reserved for gonorrhea)
Gram-positive Bacilli	
B. anthracis (anthrax)	Penicillin G Ciprofloxacin
C. perfringens and *C. tetani*	Penicillin G
C. diphtheriae (diphtheria)	Macrolides
Gram-negative Enteric Microorganisms	
Bacteroides	Metronidazole Clindamycin
Enterobacter	Imipenem or meropenem
E. coli	Third-generation cephalosporin Gentamicin
Klebsiella (Almost always acquired from hospital)	Third-generation cephalosporin
P. mirabilis (Frequent cause of urinary tract infections)	Ampicillin Cephalosporins
Salmonella	Fluoroquinolones Ceftriaxone

should be boiled daily to prevent reinfection at subsequent feedings.

Probiotics containing *Lactobacillus acidophilus* may also be effective at preventing chronic, recurrent vaginal yeast infections, including those that occur secondarily to antibiotic use. These probiotic supplements can be taken orally or inserted vaginally.

Treatment of the Common Cold

There is some evidence that *Echinacea* may shorten the duration of upper respiratory tract infection symptoms; however, there is no evidence that it *prevents* colds. Furthermore, some studies suggest that repeated use of *Echinacea* may actually suppress the immune system. Adverse reactions are rare, although people with allergies may be more susceptible to allergic effects (bronchospasm; itchy, watery eyes; hives). Recent evidence suggests that *Echinacea* may decrease fertility and should not be used by couples who are trying to conceive.

●●● TOP FIVE LIST

Although at first glance, memorization of the antibiotics seems a daunting task, the most important thing to learn is to match the drug with the bug. Remember that antibacterials can be divided into four major categories: those that interfere with cell wall synthesis, those that interfere with folic acid synthesis, those that interfere with protein synthesis, and those that interfere with transcription of DNA/RNA.

1. Understanding the mechanism of action allows for the rational combination of antibiotics to synergistically treat infections.
2. When selecting an antibacterial agent, always choose the most narrow spectrum agent that is likely to eliminate the infecting microorganism. This practice helps decrease antibacterial resistance. Table 4-27 lists drugs of choice.
3. Emerging antimicrobial resistance is a major health concern in hospitals and the community (leading to secondary and *nosocomial* infections). Physicians should be wary of prescribing third-generation cephalosporins and immediately using latest generation antibiotics as first-line therapies.
4. Secondary yeast infections (thrush and vaginal) often follow antibiotic therapy.
5. The major adverse effects or toxicities for antibacterials, antifungals, and antivirals are diarrhea, nephrotoxicity, hypersensitivity, and myelosuppression.

Cancer and Immunopharmacology

5

●●● ANTINEOPLASTIC CHEMOTHERAPY

It's all about combinatorial therapy—the use of multiple antitumor drugs that have different mechanisms of action. In addition, combinatorial treatment regimens often combine drugs that target different phases of the cell cycle. Optimal treatment protocols combine drugs that have nonoverlapping toxicities. In this way, overall toxicity can be minimized, despite the use of a synergistic cohort of cytotoxic drugs. These cytotoxic cocktails provide maximal cell killing efficacy and may slow or prevent resistant cancer cells from developing.

Often, acronyms are used to describe these combinatorial treatment protocols. For example, MOPP, originally developed for Hodgkin's lymphoma, uses *m*echlorethamine, *O*ncovin™ (trade name for vincristine), *p*rocarbazine and *p*rednisone. More current combinatorial protocols are abbreviated FOLFOX, FOLFIRI, ABVD, and CHOP. However, memorizing these detailed protocols is not so important as understanding the overarching mechanisms of action of the drugs that preferentially target proliferating cancer cells. In fact, treatment protocols are continually modified or changed as more specific chemotherapeutics are developed and validated. Physicians often utilize the National Comprehensive Cancer Network (NCCN) (www.NCCN.org) as a site to find clinical consensus guidelines and treatment protocols that are updated annually for treatment of all cancers.

Despite intense efforts over the last few decades, cancer continues to be a leading cause of death in the Western world. In the United States, lung neoplasms account for the largest percentage of cancer deaths among both males and females, although prostate and breast cancer are highest in incidence, respectively. Smoking, a modifiable risk factor, remains the single most common cause of cancer worldwide. At present, a curative or palliative approach to the treatment of cancer patients comprises five modalities: surgery, radiotherapy, chemotherapy, gene therapy, and immunotherapy. Often, two or more modalities may be combined in the hope of better clinical outcomes. When antineoplastic chemotherapy is given after surgery or irradiation (to diminish the risk of relapse from foci of microscopic lesions left behind by the initial therapy), the drug therapy is termed *adjuvant chemotherapy*.

The goal of antineoplastic therapy is to kill cancerous cells or inhibit their growth, with minimal effects on normal cells. Cancer cells differ from regular cells in one striking fashion—unlike untransformed cells, which undergo apoptosis (programmed cell death) after some finite number of cell divisions, cancer cells do not undergo apoptosis and are immortal. The rate of cellular division for cancer cells may also be unregulated. Antineoplastic drugs exploit this unchecked and possibly rapid rate of cell growth at the molecular level, allowing these drugs to work with some specificity. However, the same molecular mechanisms by which proliferative cancer cells are targeted also make normal cells with rapid turnover susceptible to cytotoxic actions of antineoplastic drugs. In fact, the hallmark toxicities of cytotoxic drugs—hair loss, neutropenia, and thrombocytopenia—are directly linked to the rapid growth rate of hair follicles and bone marrow. Additional common adverse side effects of cytotoxic drugs, including sterility and nausea, are listed in Table 5-1.

●●● CANCER DRUG RESISTANCE

Similarly to bacteria and antibiotic resistance, some tumors are also relatively resistant to antineoplastic agents. Extra-

TABLE 5-1. General Adverse Effects of Cytotoxic Drugs

Tissue	Side Effects
Bone marrow	Myelosuppression 　Leukopenia 　　Infection 　Thrombocytopenia 　Anemia 　　Hemorrhage Immunosuppression 　Secondary cancers
Gastrointestinal tract	Decreased mucosal cell division 　Anorexia 　Ulceration 　Diarrhea 　Nausea/vomiting
Skin	Alopecia Impaired wound healing
Reproductive organs	Sterility Teratogenesis Mutagenicity

TABLE 5-2. Distinctive Organ Toxicities of Cytotoxic Agents

Organ or System Affected	Drugs
Pulmonary	Bleomycin, procarbazine, busulfan
Cardiac	Doxorubicin, daunorubicin
Renal	Cisplatin, methotrexate
Hepatic	Mercaptopurine, cyclophosphamide, busulfan
Neurologic	Vincristine, cisplatin, paclitaxel
Immune	Cytarabine, dactinomycin, methotrexate, cyclophosphamide
Bladder	Cyclophosphamide
Leukocyte	Procarbazine
Pancreas	Asparaginase

cellular factors that account for such behavior include the location of tumors within "safe havens" in the body, where large solid tumors are protected from the actions of drugs by a necrotic core and a dysfunctional capillary network, as well as physiologic barriers, such as the blood-brain barrier. In addition, tumor resistance to anticancer drugs is often the result of "selection" for resistant clones; i.e., antineoplastic drugs kill off the sensitive clones in the tumor, leaving behind resistant, virulent cells. Again, the major rationale for combinatorial drug therapies is to evade cancer cell resistance and minimize dose-limiting toxicity.

At the intracellular level, tumors can utilize numerous mechanisms to reduce their sensitivity to chemotherapeutic agents, such as

- Decreased drug influx due to diminished binding affinity to receptors or decreased membrane permeability
- Increased drug efflux due to increased expression of the multidrug resistance (MDR) P-glycoproteins that actively pump drug out of the cells
- Increased expression of enzymes that metabolize the drugs
- Abnormal intracellular binding to target proteins
- Enhanced nucleic acid repair mechanisms
- Diminished activation of pro-drugs

In general, chemotherapeutic drugs exert their effects via one of three mechanisms:

- Cytotoxic actions (the vast majority)
- Endocrine activities
- Immunotherapy

Each of these classes of chemotherapeutics, as well as their major organ-specific side effects (Table 5-2), are reviewed in the following sections.

●●● CYTOTOXIC DRUGS

Cytotoxic drugs work by affecting DNA synthesis and are classified according to their site of action within the cell cycle. As shown in Figure 5-1, some agents kill cells only during specific parts of the cell cycle as the cells replicate (these drugs are referred to as *phase-specific*), while other drugs work throughout the cell cycle (*phase-nonspecific*).

Cytotoxic agents usually follow first-order kinetics and, as a result, affect a fixed percentage of tumor cells per cycle. This is known as the *log-kill hypothesis*, and it provides another rationale for drug combinations; i.e., multiple drugs lead to a greater percentage of neoplastic cell death. A one-log drug kills 90% of the cells, a two-log drug kills 99%, and a three-log drug kills 99.9%.

By far, the majority of antineoplastic agents used in clinical practice today achieve their desired effects through cell cytotoxicity. This group of drugs can be further subdivided into four distinct categories (Fig. 5-2):

- Alkylating agents
- Antimetabolites
- Cytotoxic antibiotics
- Mitotic inhibitors

Alkylating Agents

Altretamine, Busulfan, Carboplatin, Carmustine, Chlorambucil, Cisplatin, Cyclophosphamide, Dacarbazine, Estramustine, Ifosfamide, Lomustine, Mechlorethamine, Melphalan, Mitomycin, Oxiliplatin, Procarbazine, Streptozocin, Temozolomide, Thiotepa, and Uracil mustard

Mechanism of action. Yes, there are a lot of alkylating agents. However, the main critical mechanism of action is that these drugs possess a reactive alkyl group that forms covalent bonds with nucleic acids, resulting in either DNA cross-

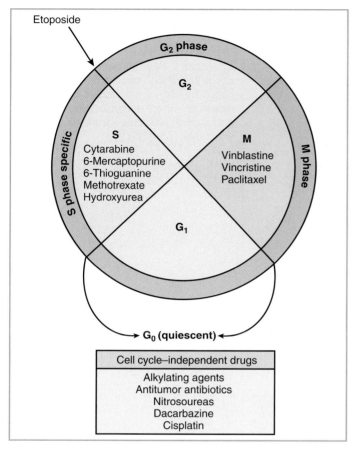

Figure 5-1. Sites of action of cell cycle phase–specific drugs.

EMBRYOLOGY

The Cell Cycle

The G_1 phase is associated with synthesis of DNA, while the S phase is associated with increased activity of DNA-replicating enzymes, including thymidine kinase, DNA polymerase, dihydrofolate reductase, ribonucleotide reductase, RNA polymerase II, and the topoisomerases. Synthesis of machinery needed for mitosis (M phase) occurs during the G_2 phase. Mitosis divides the two sets of chromosomes. For rapidly dividing embryonic stem cells, the G_1 phase is minimized or significantly shortened. For dormant, nondividing cells, the G_1 phase is lengthened and is referred to as G_0. Cyclin-dependent kinases modify the phosphorylation state of cyclins to control the cell cycle.

BIOCHEMISTRY

Checkpoint Control and Telomerases

A hallmark of tumorigenic cells is increased proliferation as a result of loss of regulatory control and regulatory proteins. For example, many cancers are classified as p53 negative. p53 is a protein that extends the G_1 phase (growth arrest) to allow DNA repair or apoptosis to remove damaged cells. Thus, these p53-negative cancers have lost control of the mechanisms to rid the body of transformed cells. Cancer cells may also lose the ability to repair damaged DNA during the G_2/M transition (checkpoint). In several types of hereditary colon cancers, mutations in and/or loss of DNA repair genes that correct for mismatched base pairs are often observed.

Telomerases protect and maintain the structure of the telomere at the end of chromosomes, which is essential for chromosomal alignment during mitosis. All non–germ cells lose a portion of the telomere structure during cell division owing to diminished telomerase activity during growth and development. This leads to normal cellular senescence. Most cancer cells can reexpress telomerase, leading to cellular immortality. Often, the loss of checkpoint control mechanisms, including p53, leads to overexpression of telomerase.

EMBRYOLOGY

Angiogenesis

Solid tumors and their metastases must develop and maintain an adequate blood supply for rapid growth. Activation of tyrosine kinase receptors by vascular endothelial growth factor or fibroblast growth factor is a crucial step in angiogenesis (formation of new blood vessels). Understanding the molecular mechanisms of angiogenesis offers new therapeutic targets for chemotherapy.

linkage or strand breakage, both of which prevent further replication of nucleic acids. In fact, these cytotoxic drugs damage all cellular molecules (including proteins and RNA). However, it is the DNA damage (exceeding repair mechanisms) that kills the cells. For example, the nitrosoureas (carmustine and lomustine) and platinum compounds, such as cisplatin and carboplatin, directly interact with DNA to prevent proliferation. Cisplatin directly binds to guanine in DNA and RNA. Alkylating agents are phase-nonspecific.

Clinical use. As examples of the wide use of alkylating agents for the treatment of multiple cancers, melphalan, cyclophosphamide, chlorambucil, and cisplatin will be discussed. Melphalan is typically used in the treatment of chronic leukemias, myelomas, and some solid tumors, whereas cyclophosphamide and chlorambucil are used to treat a variety of leukemias and lymphomas. Cyclophosphamide can be helpful in treating a variety of solid tumors and non-Hodgkin's lymphoma and is also used to treat non-neoplastic diseases like nephritic syndrome or severe rheumatoid arthritis. Cisplatin is used to treat lung, bladder, and testicular or ovarian carcinoma.

Adverse effects. The usual dose-limiting toxicity for alkylating agents is myelosuppression. These drugs may also be emetogenic. In addition to general side effects (see Table 5-1), the urinary metabolite of cyclophosphamide and ifosfamide, acrolein, is associated with serious hemorrhagic cystitis, which is prevented by adequate hydration or by administering MENSA (the Na^+ salt of methylethylsulfonate), which binds acrolein. Development of secondary acute nonlymphocytic

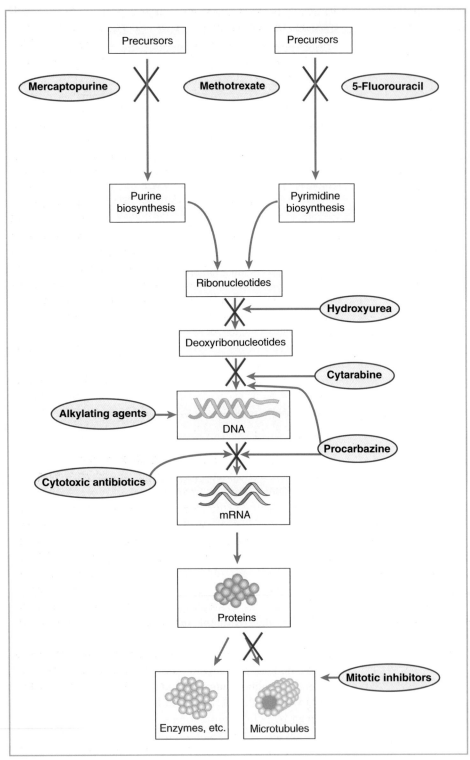

Figure 5-2. Site of action of four classes of cytotoxic drugs. These classes include: antimetabolites (mercaptopurine, methotrexate, 5-fluorouracil, hydroxyurea, cytarabine), DNA alkylating and modifying drugs (cisplatin, mechlorethamine, procarbazine), antibiotics (daunorubicin, doxorubicin, actinomycin, bleomycin), and natural products (vinblastine, vincristine, paclitaxol).

leukemias and temporary sterility are also common problems associated with alkylating agents. Secondary malignancies and leukemia-related toxicities are not unexpected, since alkylating agents interact with DNA in highly proliferative noncancer cells also. Note that the dividing cells are most at risk because they have little time to repair DNA damage before mutations are passed to daughter cells. Nondividing cells have more time to repair alkylating damage. Cisplatin

and carboplatin are associated with cumulative nephrotoxicity and ototoxicity.

Multiple alkylating agents are administered as pro-drugs. These pro-drugs include procarbazine and dacarbazine. Procarbazine is metabolized in the liver into an alkylating azoxy intermediate, while dacarbazine is metabolized to release an alkylating methyl diazonium ion. Procarbazine also inhibits monoamine oxidase; thus, tyramine-containing foods must be avoided, since patients could be put at risk of a hypertensive crisis. Additionally, disulfiram-like adverse reactions occur when procarbazine is used in combination with alcohol.

Antimetabolites

Azacitidine, Capecitabine, Cladribine, Cytarabine, Floxuridine, Fludarabine, Fluorouracil, Gemcitabine, Mercaptopurine, Methotrexate, Pentostatin, Tegafur, Thioguanine, and Trimetrexate

Note: Most, but not all, of these drug names end in "-bine" or "-dine."

These drugs are structural analogs of naturally occurring substances or metabolites within the body and thus compete with the endogenous metabolite, consequently interfering with specific cellular processes. For the most part, these drugs are mimetics of nucleotides, but because of their slightly altered structures they are actually inhibitors of purine or pyrimidine metabolism. These antimetabolites are cell cycle–specific drugs, and the major side effects are myelosuppression, diarrhea, and mucositis.

Fluorouracil, a pyrimidine (thymine) analog, acts via its conversion to a pseudopyrimidine nucleotide (fluorodeoxyuridine monophosphate), which inhibits thymidylate synthetase and impairs DNA synthesis. The difference between fluorouracil and thymidine is replacement of a fluorine atom with a methyl group. Fluorouracil is helpful for solid tumors and is used topically for some malignant skin conditions.

Cytarabine (ara-C) is a pyrimidine (cytosine) analog, which undergoes intracellular conversion to a triphosphate form and competes with cytosine triphosphate for DNA polymerase. Cytotoxicity occurs when the mimetic is inappropriately incorporated into DNA. Again, the drug takes advantage of a subtle change in structure as the ribose sugar is replaced by D-arabinose in cytarabine. Gemcitabine also is a cytidine analog, with slightly better pharmacokinetic and pharmacodynamic parameters. Cytarabine is used in treatment of various leukemias, whereas gemcitabine is used in solid tumors.

Mercaptopurine and thioguanine are converted to pseudopurine nucleotides that feed back to inhibit the first step of *de novo* purine biosynthesis (glutamine 5-phosphoribosylpyrophosphate amino transferase). In addition, these drugs inhibit conversion of the purine precursor, inosinate, to adenylate or xanthylate, the precursor of guanylate. Dysfunctional RNA and DNA synthesis results. These drugs are also used to treat a variety of leukemias.

Methotrexate is structurally related to folic acid and competitively inhibits dihydrofolate reductase, preventing regeneration of tetrahydrofolate. Because tetrahydrofolate is an essential cofactor for synthesis of both purines and pyrimidines (thymidylate synthase), cellular DNA synthesis is diminished (Fig. 5-3). Methotrexate is used in the treatment of acute lymphoblastic leukemia (ALL) and non-Hodgkin's lymphoma. Interestingly, the drug is also used for symptomatic control of psoriasis and management of severe rheumatoid arthritis. Leucovorin, a derivative of folic acid, can be used as a "rescue therapy" to counteract adverse and sometimes life-threatening effects that high doses of methotrexate cause on the bone marrow. Methotrexate also has nephrotoxic effects at high doses, which can be minimized with good hydration and alkalinization of the urine to increase renal excretion of the drug.

Hydroxyurea, while not strictly a purine or pyrimidine analog, inhibits ribonucleotide reductase and prevents conversion of ribonucleotides to deoxyribonucleotides. Hydroxyurea is used to treat chronic myelogenous leukemia (CML).

Cytotoxic Antibiotics

Bleomycin, Dactinomycin, Daunorubicin, Doxorubicin, Epirubicin, Idarubicin, Mitomycin, Streptozocin, Valrubicin

Although each antibiotic in this category has a unique mechanism of action, they are cell cycle–specific in their cytotoxicity, disrupting DNA function. In contrast to alkylating agents, these antibiotics *indirectly* damage DNA.

Dactinomycin interferes with RNA polymerase and thus prevents transcription. Dactinomycin is primarily used in the pediatric population and is approved for the treatment of Wilms' tumor, rhabdosarcoma, testicular carcinoma, and choriocarcinoma.

Bleomycin binds reduced iron and forms an intercalating complex with DNA; i.e., it inserts (intercalates) between adjacent bases in the double-stranded DNA. Upon oxidation

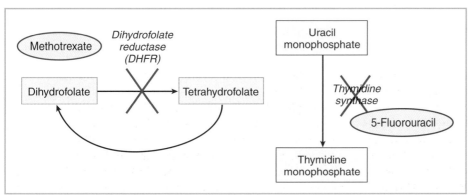

Figure 5-3. Multiple drugs inhibit thymidine synthesis. Tetrahydrofolate is a cosubstrate required for purine and pyrimidine biosynthesis (pyrimidine is shown here).

of the iron complex, superoxide and hydroxyl radicals are formed that result in DNA strand breakage. Bleomycin is used for lymphomas, testicular carcinoma, and squamous cell carcinomas. In addition to general side effects (see Table 5-1), bleomycin is associated with the development of pulmonary fibrosis as well as hyperpigmentation of the hands. Bleomycin differs from most antineoplastic agents in that it rarely causes myelosuppression, but the drug does cause a high incidence of fever and chills.

Doxorubicin belongs to a class of antibiotics known as the *anthracyclines*, which inhibit transcription by impairing topoisomerase II, as well as by intercalating into DNA.

Doxorubicin and other anthracycline-like antibiotics (including daunorubicin, idarubicin, epirubicin) intercalate nonspecifically between adjacent DNA pairs, thereby blocking DNA and RNA synthesis. Intercalation interferes with the normal DNA repair mechanisms of topoisomerase II. Doxorubicin is used widely in the treatment of acute leukemias, lymphomas, and various solid tumors. Doxorubicin (and other anthracyclines), at high doses, can produce irreversible, dose-dependent cardiotoxicity as a result of free radical damage. Idarubicin is a semisynthetic analogue of daunorubicin and has been approved as an oral formulation outside the United States.

Mitotic Inhibitors

Docetaxel, Paclitaxel, Vincristine, Vinblastine, and Vinorelbine

Vincristine, vinblastine, and vinorelbine, often referred to as *Vinca* alkaloids, are metabolites derived from the periwinkle plant (*Vinca rosea*). These drugs inhibit polymerization of microtubules by binding to tubulin, leading to late G_2 growth arrest by disrupting mitotic filaments required for nuclear and cellular division. In contrast, paclitaxel, isolated from tree bark, enhances and stabilizes microtubule assembly. However, paclitaxel is equally cytotoxic, since it disrupts the dynamic equilibrium between tubulin monomers and dimers.

Vinca alkaloids are useful in management of acute leukemias, lymphomas, and some solid tumors. Vincristine is

the "O" (for Oncovin, the trade name) in the MOPP (mechlorethamine plus vincristine plus procarbazine plus prednisone) and CHOP (cyclophosphamide plus hydroxy-daunorubicin plus vincristine plus prednisone) therapeutic regimens. Vinblastine is frequently used in combination with bleomycin and cisplatin for metastatic testicular carcinoma. Paclitaxel is used as primary or adjuvant therapy for ovarian and breast cancers.

In addition to myelosuppression and nausea and vomiting, *Vinca* alkaloids can cause phlebitis and cellulitis. Additionally, peripheral neuropathy resulting in paresthesias, areflexia, or weakness occurs with vincristine. These neurologic and neuromuscular side effects, although reversible, often resolve very slowly. Interestingly, compared with most antineoplastic agents (including vinblastine), vincristine is associated with unusually low levels of bone marrow suppression. Paclitaxel can induce neutropenia and neuropathy. Hypersensitivity and cardiac reactions may also occur, caused by the excipient (polyoxyl castor oil), which solubilizes the intravenous formulation of the drug. Fortunately, this adverse effect can often be controlled with glucocorticoids or antihistamines.

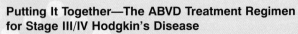

●●● ENDOCRINE THERAPY

Some cancers are hormone dependant, and the growth of such tumors can be inhibited by surgically removing the source of the stimulating hormone. However, to avoid complications associated with surgical interventions, the use of hormonal antagonists (antihormones) is gaining preference (Table 5-3). Endocrine therapy can cause side effects, which generally are characterized by physiologic effects of the hormone being administered or antagonized. In general, side effects associated with endocrine therapy are considerably milder than those associated with cytotoxic agents.

As a case in point, patients with estrogen receptor–positive breast cancers have an approximately fivefold better outcome than patients with estrogen receptor–negative breast cancer. Tamoxifen, a selective estrogen receptor modulator (SERM), acts primarily as an estrogen receptor *antagonist* that competes for and blocks the promitogenic actions of endogenous estrogen. Through undefined mechanisms, tamoxifen may exert *agonistic* estrogen-like actions after long-term use (2 to 5 years) and is usually discontinued.

Circulating levels of estrogen can be maintained in postmenopausal women by a cytochrome P-450 enzyme known as *aromatase*, which converts adrenal steroids (androstenedione and testosterone) to estrogens. Since breast cancer patients often have evidence of enhanced aromatase activity in tumors, drugs that inhibit aromatase are gaining popularity. Aromatase inhibitors (anastrazole, letrozole, exemestane) often are first-line therapies and have a lower risk of venous thromboemboli than does tamoxifen.

As another example of effective endocrine therapy, prostate tumors are particularly sensitive to antiandrogens or therapeutics that diminish endogenous concentrations of androgens. Flutamide is an androgen receptor antagonist that blocks androgen receptor function in the prostate, resulting in diminished DNA synthesis. Alternatively, subcutaneous administration of leuprolide or goserelin, synthetic peptide analogs that act as luteinizing hormone–releasing hormone (LHRH) agonists, chronically down-regulate LHRH receptors, resulting in low levels of testosterone and causing prostate-specific apoptosis. The adverse side effects associated with leuprolide and goserelin therapy include impotency and loss of bone mass.

Glucocorticoids are often integral components of combinatorial chemotherapeutic regimens (the final "P" in the CHOP and MOPP protocols is prednisone). For the most part, they are included as an immunosuppressant of white cells (Hodgkin's disease). Moreover, they have ancillary effects, including diminished inflammation, allergic reactions, neurologic side effects, and emesis.

●●● INTRODUCTION TO IMMUNOPHARMACOLOGY

Relatively new in the arsenal against cancer, immunotherapy gained attention when it was observed that bacterial infections sometimes provoked regression of certain tumors. This is presumed to be due to indirect immunostimulation provided by the infection. Such observations have led to various immunologic approaches for cancer therapy, such as immunostimulatory cytokines, the use of tumor-specific monoclonal antibodies, and the potential of vaccines prepared from tumor cells.

Specifically, interferon-α has been used as an adjunctive therapy for chronic myelogenous leukemia and T-cell lymphomas. Immunostimulation may be mediated by an increase in major histocompatibility complex expression, as well as by an increase in immune effector T and NK cells. In addition to immunostimulation, interferon-α may stimulate ribonucleases via 2′5′-oligoadenylate synthase activity. Major side effects of interferon therapy are malaise, fatigue, and fever. Interleukin 2 (aldesleukin) is also being used for melanoma and renal cell carcinoma.

Use of monoclonal antibodies as therapeutics has revolutionized pharmacology, and these antibodies are being exploited as cancer therapies (Table 5-4). Gemtuzumab induces selective cytotoxicity of myelogenous leukemia cells by specifically interacting with the CD33 antigen, which is overexpressed on these cells. In a similar fashion, alemtu-

TABLE 5-3. Hormonal Agonists and Antagonists in Endocrine Therapy

Hormone	Clinical Use
Estrogen antagonists (e.g., tamoxifen)	Competitive inhibition of estrogen receptors impairs stimulatory effect of estrogen on breast cancer cell division
Androgen antagonists (e.g., flutamide)	Useful in androgen-dependent prostate cancers
Estrogens (e.g., diethylstilbestrol)	Antiandrogenic effects can be used to suppress androgen-dependent prostate cancers
Progesterone derivatives	Useful in endometrial, prostate, and breast cancers
LHRH (luteinizing hormone–releasing hormone)/ GnRH (gonadotropin-releasing hormone) agonist (e.g., leuprolide)	Used in androgen-dependent prostate cancers for their ability to inhibit LHRH/GnRH receptors via negative feedback
Adrenocortical steroids (e.g., prednisone)	Inhibits growth of lymphoid tumors and hematologic neoplasms

TABLE 5-4. Clinical Uses of Monoclonal Antibodies (Mabs)

Mab	Clinical Utility	Target
Trastuzumab	Breast cancer	Her2/neu receptor
Rituximab	Non-Hodgkin's lymphoma	Surface protein
Gemtuzumab	Myeloid leukemia	CD33
Alemtuzumab	Chronic lymphocyte leukemia	CD52
Infliximab	Rheumatoid arthritis and Crohn's disease	TNF
Abciximab	Antiplatelet therapy	IIb/IIIa receptors
Daclizumab	Transplant rejection	IL-2 receptor
Muromonab	Transplant rejection	CD3

TABLE 5-5. Clinical Uses of Recombinant Cytokines

Cytokine	Clinical Utility
G-CSF (filgrastim)	Bone marrow suppression; increases granulocytes
GM-CSF (sargramostim)	Bone marrow suppression, increases granulocytes
Thrombopoietin	Thrombocytopenia
Erythropoietin (epo)	Anemias
Interferon-α	Leukemias, melanoma, hepatitis B and C
Interferon-β	Multiple sclerosis
Interferon-γ	Chronic granulomatous disease
Interleukin-2 (aldesleukin)	Renal cell carcinoma and melanoma
Interleukin 11	Thrombocytopenia

zumab interacts with CD52 antigen to treat B cell chronic lymphocyte leukemia (CLL). Rituximab targets non-Hodgkin's lymphoma cells, whereas trastuzumab targets overexpressed Her2/neu, a growth factor receptor for breast adenocarcinomas. (All the monoclonals end in "-mab" for monoclonal antibody.) Drug discovery has also begun to identify selective small molecule inhibitors of dysfunctional signaling targets in cancer cells. As an example, imatinib binds to and inhibits the ATP-binding site on c-abl, a critical promitogenic kinase for certain types of chronic myelogenous leukemia.

Interestingly, recombinant human granulocyte colony–stimulating factor (rh-G-CSF; filgrastim), and granulocyte-macrophage colony–stimulating factor (GM-CSF; sargramostim) are now being used to reduce the severity and duration of neutropenia following successful cytotoxic therapy. In addition, interleukin 11 (oprelvekin), thrombopoietin, and erythropoietin are being evaluated to maximize platelet and RBC counts after chemotherapy (Table 5-5).

Immunosuppressive Agents

Cyclosporine, Tacrolimus, and Sirolimus

Suppression of the immune system via pharmacologic agents is not only helpful for cancer therapy but also is used to treat autoimmune diseases, preventing host immune rejection to donor organ or transplant and suppressing donor immune responses against host antigens (graft-versus-host disease). For the most part, these agents (monoclonal antibodies, immunoglobulins, antibiotics, recombinant proteins, or receptors) restrict the proliferation or differentiation of B lymphoid cells, mediators of antibody formation and humoral immunity, as well as T lymphoid cells, responsible for cellular immunity. Various agents modulate components of the immune system as their primary targets, and an even larger number of drugs list "altered immune function" in their side

effect profiles. Commonly used immunosuppressive agents include cyclosporine derivatives, mycophenolate mofetil, glucocorticoids, and modulators of tumor necrosis factor (TNF) activity.

Cyclosporine is a cyclic peptide derived from fungi that selectively inhibits T-cell receptor–mediated signal transduction (and therefore T-cell function). Cyclosporine enters T cells and specifically binds to cyclophilin, which leads to inhibition of a calcium-regulated cytoplasmic phosphatase known as calcineurin (Fig. 5-4). The resultant inhibition of the phosphatase leaves transcription regulators like NFAT (nuclear factor for activated T cells) in a phosphorylated/inactive state (i.e., retained in cytosol), which can no longer facilitate the nuclear transcription of genes regulating the production of T-cell activators such as IL-2, IL-3, and interferon-γ. Since it suppresses overall T-cell function, the net impact of cyclosporine is impaired cell-mediated and antibody-specific immune responses. Tacrolimus functions similarly to cyclosporine to inhibit calcineurin, but its intracellular binding protein is known as FK-BP. The tacrolimus/FK-BP complex directly inhibits calcineurin. (This notation is derived from an earlier tacrolimus derivative, FK-506, which bound and activated a heat-shock protein, given the name FK-binding protein). Sirolimus also binds to FK-BP but through undefined mechanisms does not inhibit calcineurin, instead inhibiting the promitogenic kinase m-TOR, which itself is regulated by IL-2.

Cyclosporine analogs are the drugs of choice to prevent graft or transplant rejection and graft-versus-host disease (GVHD). Tacrolimus and pimecrolimus are also used topically to treat eczema. As an aside, sirolimus and paclitaxel have recently been approved as adjuvants to coronary stents for local drug delivery to limit vascular smooth muscle proliferation at the sites of coronary stent–induced re-stenosis (reblockage).

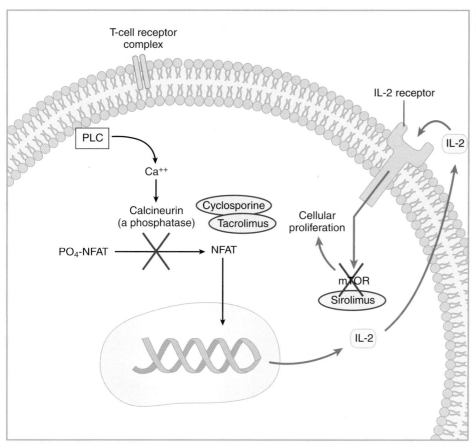

Figure 5-4. T-cell suppression by cyclosporine analogs.

In contrast to most other immune suppressants, cyclosporine and tacrolimus do not cause myelosuppression. They do, however, exhibit marked nephrotoxicity (proximal tubule). Sirolimus can induce hyperlipidemia. Caution must be used if cyclosporine is administered in conjunction with other immunosuppressants because of increased susceptibility of infections and possible development of lymphoma. Cyclosporine analogs sold by different manufacturers are not bioequivalent and cannot be used interchangeably. Chronic topical use of tacrolimus and pimecrolimus appear to be associated with an increased risk of cancer.

Mycophenolate, Mofetil, and Azathioprine

Mechanism of action. These immunosuppressive drugs diminish B- and T-cell proliferation by inhibiting purine metabolism. Mycophenolate inhibits inosine monophosphate dehydrogenase, whereas azathioprine, through its metabolite mercaptopurine, impairs DNA replication by inserting itself into the replication fork as a pseudonucleotide.

Clinical use. Mycophenolate is one of the main drugs used to prevent transplant rejection, whereas azathioprine is used to treat various autoimmune illnesses.

Adverse effects. Myelosuppression is a major side effect with these drugs. Fortunately, the combination of mycophenolate with cyclosporine permits dosage of both drugs to be lower than if monotherapy were utilized, thus reducing the incidence of cyclosporine-induced nephrotoxicity.

Etanercept and Infliximab

Mechanism of action. Both these immunosuppressive agents decrease TNF activity and resultant activation of B and T cells. Etanercept is a circulating recombinant TNF receptor that serves as a reservoir to bind up circulating TNF. Infliximab is a neutralizing monoclonal antibody that targets TNF.

Clinical use. Both agents are used to treat rheumatoid arthritis patients, and infliximab is also used to treat patients with Crohn's disease.

Adverse effects. Both drugs can predispose patients to severe infections, cancers, or hypersensitivity reactions.

Glucocorticoids

A detailed discussion of glucocorticoids is found in Chapter 10. In terms of the immune system, glucocorticoids are used as adjunctive therapies in organ transplantation and autoimmune diseases. Glucocorticoids reduce activity of immune cells by inhibiting proinflammatory phospholipase A_2 products, including prostaglandins, thromboxanes, and leukotrienes.

A summary of the use of monoclonal antibodies and recombinant cytokines in immune modulation was presented earlier in Tables 5-4 and 5-5.

●●● COMPLEMENTARY ALTERNATIVE MEDICINE FOR CANCER PREVENTION

The verdict is still out on the true effectiveness of complementary alternative medicines for cancer prevention. However, the following agents are routinely used by patients as putative preventative measures: garlic, green tea, folic acid, lycopene, saw palmetto, selenium, soy, St. John's wort, flax seed, and wheat bran.

●●● TOP FIVE LIST

1. Most antineoplastic agents target dividing cells.
2. Therapeutic regimens are often combinatorial, targeting multiple mechanisms of action to evade cancer cell resistance and dose-limiting toxicities.
3. Cancer cells have evolved multiple cellular mechanisms to evade the toxicities of antineoplastic agents.
4. Cytotoxic drugs damage DNA (mitigating DNA synthesis, replication, or repair) as well as alter microtubule function.
5. Immunotherapy is a double-edged sword: immunosuppression can be effective for myeloproliferative neoplastic disorders, whereas immunostimulation can be effective to reduce the severity of cytotoxic drug–induced neutropenia.

Autonomic Nervous System 6

CONTENTS

It's all about diversity—diversity of receptors, that is. Similar receptor subtypes can produce differential effects if they are hard-wired to different intracellular effectors and second messengers. In this way, the same neurotransmitter can have differing pharmacologic effects on target organs. This allows for specific drugs to target unique receptor subtypes. Nowhere is this more important than in the autonomic nervous system (ANS).

The ANS is the control mechanism for all automatic functions of the body. In essence, the ANS controls all the muscles of the body except skeletal muscles (the somatic nervous system). The difference between autonomic and somatic nervous systems is that the former controls functions that do not require conscious control (e.g., heart rate, blood pressure, gastrointestinal functions), while the latter is responsible for conscious control of movement (e.g., walking, driving, writing). Our minute-to-minute survival relies on coordinated control of autonomic functions; note that because the cranial nerves (representing a portion of the ANS) are intact, quadriplegic patients survive despite having no voluntary control from the neck down.

In general, there are two branches of the ANS that either speed or slow biologic processes. The *sympathetic* nervous system generally speeds things up ("fight or flight" functions), whereas the *parasympathetic* nervous system often slows things down ("rest and digest" functions). Key contrasting factors in the two branches of the ANS are summarized in Table 6-1.

It should be apparent from Table 6-1 that the branches of the ANS are fundamentally different in structure and function. In fact, the anatomy, neurochemistry, physiology, and pharmacology are distinct for each of the branches. Many of the neuropharmacologic and anatomic aspects of the ANS are summarized in Figures 6-1 and 6-2.

In general, both branches of the ANS are composed of a series of two nerve cells (a presynaptic neuron and a post-synaptic neuron) connected to each other at a ganglion synapse and connected to effector organs by another synapse. The key points to remember are (1) the specific neurotransmitter released at each anatomic location and (2) the corresponding receptor subtype to which neurotransmitters bind. With these pieces of information, the pharmacologic responses of organs can generally be predicted in light of the facts summarized in Table 6-1.

●●● ORGANIZATION OF THE AUTONOMIC NERVOUS SYSTEM

Neurochemical Organization

Figure 6-2 summarizes the structural organization of the ANS. Anatomic compartments of the ANS can be defined by the neurotransmitter used at each location. Surprisingly, there

TABLE 6-1. Autonomic Nervous System

Sympathetic	Parasympathetic
Fight or flight	Rest and digest
Stress responder	Resting homeostasis
"Whip" ("driving" the system)	"Reins" (tonic control)
Systemic fire alarm	Discrete localization of control

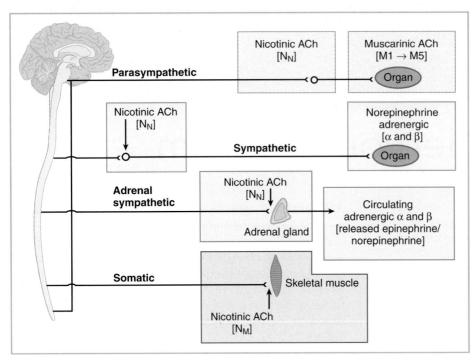

Figure 6-1. Autonomic and somatic physiology and pharmacology: neuroanatomic compartments. Note that the sympathetic and parasympathetic systems have two nerve components: presynaptic and postsynaptic. The adrenal gland functions as a neurohormone system that releases norepinephrine and epinephrine into the circulation where the neurotransmitters elicit the system-wide "fight or flight" response. The somatic nervous system employs a single, long motor neuron that is functionally similar to a presynaptic autonomic neuron. ACh, acetylcholine; N_N, neuron-type nicotinic receptor; N_M, neuromuscular-type nicotinic receptor; M, muscarinic receptor (five subtypes); α/β, alpha-type and beta-type adrenergic receptors. Note: A reduced version of this figure is used throughout the chapter to illustrate the locations of various autonomic components.

ANATOMY

Central Nervous System

Recall that the nervous system is composed of unique cell types. Whereas the typical liver cell might be 20 μm on a side, a single autonomic cell might be 10 μm across at the cell body, but it sends a long fiber called an axon (less than 1 μm in diameter) literally tens of centimeters away. The sympathetic nervous system originates from the thoracolumbar regions of the spinal cord and travels a short distance to the paravertebral chain ganglia. Following neurochemical communication from presynaptic fibers, a long axon from a postsynaptic cell travels to innervated organs where it synapses with muscle. Because there is signal amplification as the cells leave these ganglia (few preganglionic fibers in and many fibers out) and go out to numerous organs, the sympathetic nervous system has very global effects on physiology (a global fire alarm). On the parasympathetic side, cells originate from craniosacral regions of the spinal cord and send long fibers to synapse in organ-specific ganglia where short postganglionic fibers innervate target organs. This specific innervation of a particular organ provides for point-to-point, discrete regulation of physiology by the parasympathetic nervous system. The adrenal medulla can be considered a specialized version of the sympathetic nervous system; signals from a long presynaptic axon trigger the release of a circulating hormone from the specialized ganglion-like cell in the gland.

are only two major neurotransmitters at end organs in the ANS (acetylcholine [ACh] and norepinephrine). There is a single neurotransmitter at every autonomic ganglion in the body (regardless of whether it is parasympathetic or sympathetic)—the neurotransmitter is ACh. This includes the "ganglion" that is the adrenal medulla. In addition, the neurotransmitter at parasympathetic effector organs is also ACh. Although it is not the subject of the present chapter, we will also briefly consider the somatic motor nervous system because the neurotransmitter at the neuromuscular junction is also ACh. How can so many different physiologic functions be "driven" by the same simple neurochemical—ACh? This critical question can be answered by the various ACh receptor subtypes that receive this chemical signal.

The preceding paragraph deals with the preganglionic fibers and postganglionic parasympathetic fibers. On the other hand, the neurotransmitter at most sympathetic effector synapses is the chemical norepinephrine (or epinephrine in the case of the neurohormone released from the adrenal medulla). Note that specialized exceptions exist in the case of certain sweat glands (sympathetic ACh innervation) and renal vasculature (sympathetic dopamine).

Neuroreceptor Organization

There are essentially three different classes of neurotransmitter receptors in the ANS, with a number of different receptor subtypes (Table 6-2):

- Nicotinic ACh
- Muscarinic ACh
- Adrenergic norepinephrine/epinephrine

For ACh, there are nicotinic receptors (defined by a prototypical agonist that activates these receptors—nicotine) and muscarinic receptors. Nicotinic receptors come in two types: (1) ganglionic nicotinic receptors found in ganglia/

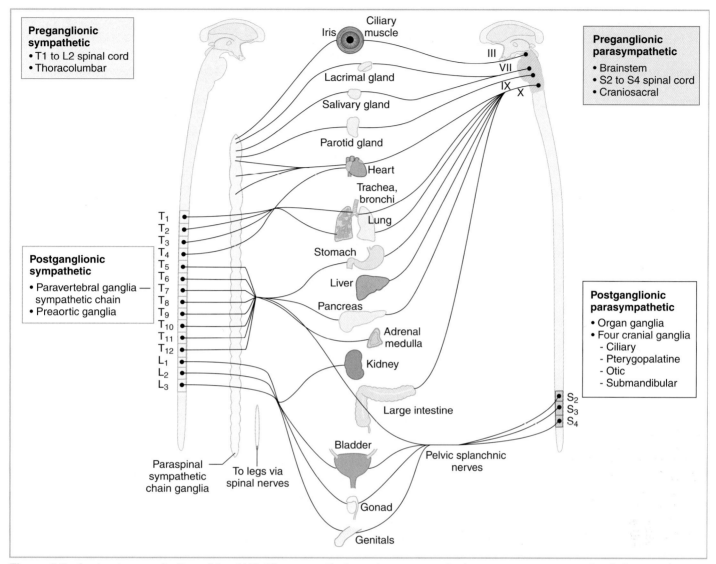

Figure 6-2. Anatomic organization of the ANS. The sympathetic and parasympathetic systems are structurally distinct.

TABLE 6-2. Autonomic Receptor Subtypes

Receptor Class	Receptor Subtypes
Nicotinic	1. Ganglionic (N_N; neuronal) 2. Neuromuscular junction (N_M; muscle)
Muscarinic	1. M_2 and M_4 (M_{even}) 2. M_1, M_3, M_5 (M_{odd})
Adrenergic	1. Alpha (α_1 and α_2) 2. Beta (β_1, β_2, and β_3)

adrenal gland and (2) neuromuscular nicotinic receptors found at the end-plate of the somatic (voluntary) motor nervous system. Parasympathetic end-organs contain different ACh receptors that are stimulated by the prototypical agonist muscarine; thus, these receptors are called *muscarinic cholinergic receptors.*

Finally, the sympathetic nervous system contains two kinds of adrenergic receptor subtypes: (1) α-adrenoceptors and (2) β-adrenoceptors. Each of these classes has several receptor subtypes. Luckily for the clinician, although this seems to be a dizzying array of different receptor subtypes, a set of "rules" will assist in mastering their underlying physiology and pharmacology.

Physiologic Responses

Table 6-3 is a simplified summary of organ responses to sympathetic and parasympathetic stimulation. Understanding this table helps us predict pharmacologic responses to autonomic agonists and antagonists. For example, consider the heart—one of the simplest organs from an autonomic standpoint. The heart functions with an intrinsic pacemaker function. The ANS either speeds or slows this rhythm depending on need. Stimulation of the parasympathetic nervous system slows the heart and decreases contractility.

TABLE 6-3. Physiologic Response to Autonomic Nerve Activity

Organ or System	Dominant Tone	Cholinergic Response (Receptor)	Adrenergic Response (Receptor)
Heart	Parasympathetic	Decreased rate (M_2) Decreased force (M_2)	Increased rate (β_1) Increased force (β_1)
Blood vessels	Sympathetic	Dilation Muscarinic receptors are present but not innervated Dilation mediated by nitric oxide (NO)	Biphasic • Constriction (α_1): Resting tone increases blood pressure • Dilation (β_2): decreases TPR and blood pressure
Bronchial tree	Parasympathetic	Bronchoconstriction	Bronchodilation β_2 receptors are present but not innervated
Eye			
Iris, radial muscle	Sympathetic	—	Contraction (mydriasis; α_1)
Iris, sphincter	Parasympathetic	Contraction (miosis)	—
Ciliary muscle	Parasympathetic	Contraction (near vision)	Relaxation (β_2) (allows for far vision)
Gastrointestinal			
Motility	Parasympathetic	Increased motility	Decrease motility (α_1)
Sphincters	Parasympathetic	Relaxation	Constrict (α_1)
Secretions	Parasympathetic	Stimulation	Decrease (α_1)
Urinary bladder			
Detrusor	Parasympathetic	Contraction	Relaxation (via β_2)
Trigone and sphincter	Sympathetic	Relaxation	Contraction (via α_1)
Sweat and salivary glands	Parasympathetic	Increased secretion	Increased secretion (via α_1)

Conversely, stimulation of the sympathetic nervous system increases heart rate and increases the force of contraction—to effectively increase cardiac output (CO). Injection of epinephrine, a sympathetic agonist, increases CO, whereas administration of propranolol, a nonselective β-adrenergic blocker (sympathetic antagonist), decreases CO. Table 6-3 therefore is an important resource for understanding underlying mechanisms that modulate autonomic function.

An important aspect of Table 6-3 is the designation of the autonomic branch that exerts the dominant tone at rest. Not surprisingly, this is generally the parasympathetic nervous system ("rest and digest"). However, there are several noteworthy exceptions. Foremost is the control of peripheral resistance and blood pressure. The dominant tone for blood pressure regulation is mediated via the sympathetic nervous system. This is because there is *no* parasympathetic regulation of the peripheral vasculature. There are no parasympathetic nerves that communicate with receptors on the vasculature. On the other hand, there are sympathetic nerves that communicate with vasculature receptors (α_1) to constrict the vessels and increase peripheral resistance and blood pressure. In adults this is how blood pressure is regulated in a resting state. In times of great stress, however ("fight or flight"), circulating epinephrine binds to a different set of receptors—the noninnervated β-receptors—leading to decreased resistance and greater delivery of blood and O_2 to the peripheral muscles. These important pharmacologic and physiologic concepts are explored in greater detail below.

Thus, in order to review autonomic pharmacology, it is essential to begin by reviewing the underlying autonomic physiology to understand the following:
- What are the responses to sympathetic and parasympathetic stimulation?
- Which autonomic system exerts dominant neural control in various tissues?
- What types of receptors are present in each organ?

Indeed, this last question provides the opportunity to design and develop selective pharmacotherapeutic agents.

●●● CHOLINERGIC SYSTEMS

Biochemistry of Cholinergic Systems

The synthesis and degradation of ACh are the same at all locations. Indeed, the synthesis/metabolism of ACh is elegant in its simplicity. Figure 6-3 describes the creation and destruction of ACh. This neurotransmitter is generated by a simple chemical condensation between choline (a chemical constituent of diet-derived lecithin [phosphatidyl choline]) and acetyl-CoA (a ubiquitous energy source derived from glycolysis via the pyruvate dehydrogenase complex reaction).

Choline and acetyl-CoA are condensed in neurons via the enzyme, choline acetyltransferase (CAT), and packaged as the neurotransmitter ACh. Neurons release the neurotransmitter on demand and a physiologic response is stimulated, depending on the type of postjunctional receptor and its anatomic

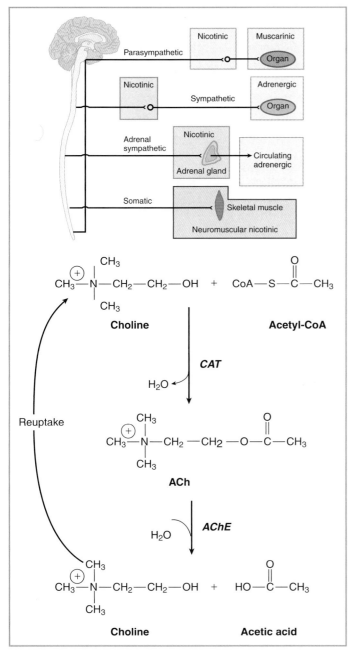

Figure 6-3. ACh synthesis and degradation. ACh is synthesized from choline and acetyl-CoA, a reaction that is catalyzed by choline acetyltransferase (CAT). Once released into the synapse, ACh is degraded by acetylcholinesterase (AChE) into choline (which gets recycled for reuse) and acetate.

BIOCHEMISTRY

The Two Forms of Acetylcholinesterase

An important pharmacologic aspect of the cholinergic system is that there are two forms of acetylcholinesterase (AChE). The first is a "true" cholinesterase that resides in the synapse and serves no role other than to break down the acetylcholine neurotransmitter. On the other hand, there is also a nondiscriminating circulating esterase that has broad substrate specificity and essentially cleaves any ester bond. This latter enzyme appears to function as a detoxifying enzyme and efficiently scavenges any circulating acetylcholine. It is so efficient, in fact, that it prevents detection of naturally circulating ACh and, more importantly, eliminates the possibility of using acetylcholine directly as a pharmacologic agent. Any exogenous ACh injected is eliminated almost instantaneously.

location. When the neuron completes its required stimulation —presumably after eliciting a physiologic response—further release of ACh is terminated. Neurotransmitter in the synapse is rapidly degraded by a very efficient hydrolase, acetylcholinesterase (AChE). The products of hydrolysis are choline and acetate, which can both be reutilized. Both elegant and simple, this is the biological equivalent of on-demand synthesis. It is worth noting that confusion commonly arises, at this point, from the unfortunate similarity in synthetic and degradative enzymes (choline acetyltransferase and acetyl-

cholinesterase). Recall that the latter is an esterase that *degrades* ester bonds, whereas the former transfers a choline onto an acetate group (*creating* an ester bond).

Cholinergic Receptor Subtypes

Given the universal and widespread distribution of the ACh system, how does the body generate diversity in physiologic responses? The answer resides in the diversity of ACh receptor subtypes. Specifically, there are two major classes of ACh receptors (muscarinic and nicotinic) having different functions, different signal transduction mechanisms, and, significantly, differing pharmacologic characteristics (see Table 6-2). As noted in Figure 6-1, the neuronal synapse found at a ganglion contains one type of nicotinic receptor (N_N). The neuromuscular junction (NMJ) at the skeletal muscle within the somatic (voluntary) nervous system contains a different, but related, nicotinic receptor (N_M). Finally, parasympathetic end-organs synthesize and express muscarinic ACh receptors with fundamentally distinct pharmacologic and cell biological characteristics. Specifically, five different subtypes of muscarinic receptors (designated M1 through M5) are found in the end-organs innervated by the parasympathetic system.

Nicotinic Receptors

We will begin to explore the pharmacologic profiles of the receptors that reside in different anatomic compartments within the ANS. When a neuronal action potential arrives at the nerve terminal, there is Ca^{++}-mediated release of ACh into the cleft. Target cells (postganglionic nerve cell or muscle) express nicotinic receptor subtypes. These receptors derive their name from the fact that they are stimulated by the tobacco plant alkaloid nicotine. Nicotinic ACh receptors (nAChR) form a pore and serve as ligand-gated ion channels (Fig. 6-4). When the nicotinic AChR is stimulated, the channel opens and allows Na^+ to rush into the cell. This triggers depolarization of the cell and elicits a neuronal action potential (in a postganglionic nerve) or muscle contraction (in

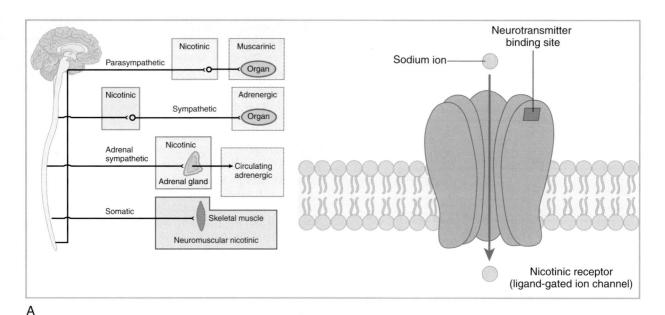

Figure 6-4. Schematic diagrams of the ACh receptors. **A**, Nicotinic receptors (N_N or N_M) are ligand-gated ion channels. Following stimulation, the resulting depolarization in neurons (N_N-type) leads to a neuronal action potential, while depolarization in muscles (N_M-type) leads to muscular contraction. **B**, ACh muscarinic receptors are 7-transmembrane domain G protein–coupled receptors (7TM-GPCR) found at postganglionic terminals, representing the parasympathetic innervation of an end-organ.

skeletal muscle). While the receptors on skeletal muscle and ganglionic nerves are both nicotinic, they are genetically different, being composed of different subunits. As distinct entities, they are, therefore, designated as neuronal (in this case ganglionic) nicotinic receptors (N_N AChR) or skeletal muscle nicotinic receptors (N_M AChR). Their physiologic functions are identical, but their pharmacologic responses can be discriminated through the use of selective ligands or through differential adaptations to stimulation.

Muscarinic Receptors

Upon reexamination of Figure 6-1, it is apparent that there are yet other forms of ACh receptors—the muscarinic receptors—present on postganglionic target organs of the parasympathetic nervous system. These receptors are superficially different from nicotinic receptors because they are stimulated by the plant alkaloid muscarine instead of by nicotine. On a more fundamental level, however, these receptors act in a different manner from nicotinic receptors and elicit different kinds of physiologic effects. First, rather than being multimeric receptors that form ion channels, the muscarinic receptors are classical single subunit, 7-transmembrane-spanning domain, G protein–coupled receptor proteins (7TM-GPCR) (see Fig. 6-4B). This information points out that these are proteins that elicit their actions through guanosine triphosphate-binding protein (GTP) signal transduction (camp AMP [cAMP] vs phosphatidylinositides) (for review, see Chapter 2).

TABLE 6-4. Nicotinic Versus Muscarinic Receptors

Receptor	Structure	Function	Mechanism	Agonist	Antagonist
Nicotinic	Multisubunit channel (five subunits)	Excitatory	Ligand-gated Opens sodium channel	ACh; nicotine	Curare (neuro-muscular only)
Muscarinic	Seven transmembrane receptor (7TM; one subunit)	Excitatory or inhibitory (depends on subtype and mechanism)	G protein–couple receptor (GPCR) stimulates PLC [M1/M3/M5] or inhibits cAMP and calcium, while stimulating potassium channel [M2/M4]	ACh; muscarine	Atropine

ACh, acetylcholine; PLC, phospholipase C.

Studying the pharmacologic nature of muscarinic receptors is simultaneously a good news/bad news situation. The bad news is that there are five distinct subtypes of muscarinic receptors, termed M1 through M5 AChR (named according to the order in which they were discovered). These receptors have different signal transduction mechanisms based on the G protein to which they are coupled. However, the good news is that they fall into two broad categories: M1/M3/M5 stimulate inositol trisphosphate (IP_3) production while M2/M4 inhibit cAMP production. Finally, although muscarinic receptors have differential anatomic distribution and physiologic functions, we have yet to develop discriminating agonists and antagonists (i.e., there are very few drugs currently in clinical use that selectively interact with one muscarinic receptor over another).

To summarize before moving on to specific pharmacologic therapies, there are two broad classes of ACh receptors—nicotinic and muscarinic (Table 6-4). Nicotinic receptors are found in (1) the autonomic ganglion and (2) the neuromuscular junction. Nicotinic receptors are always excitatory (they are ligand-gated Na channels that cause depolarization). Although there are two distinct types of nicotinic AChR (N_N and N_M), they share the following pharmacologic features: they are stimulated by the prototypical agonist nicotine.

At parasympathetic end-organs, ACh receptors are of the muscarinic type (with five subtypes: M1 through M5). These are all 7TM-GPCRs and couple either to phospholipase C (M1/M3/M5, leading to Ca^{++} mobilization and contraction; Fig. 6-5) or the inhibitory G protein (M2/M4, leading to decreased cAMP and decreased activity; Fig. 6-6). As a result of their coupling mechanisms, muscarinic receptors can be either stimulatory or inhibitory. The muscarinic receptors are defined pharmacologically by the fact that they are stimulated by muscarine and blocked by the antagonist atropine.

Now we will begin to consider various pharmacologic compounds that interact with and modulate the cholinergic aspects of the ANS. Prototypical agonists at nicotinic and muscarinic receptors are listed in Table 6-5.

Nicotinic Drugs

Drugs that modulate nicotinic receptors have very limited applications because of the anatomic localization of these receptor subtypes (see Fig. 6-1). Specifically, pharmacologic stimulation of ganglionic neuronal AChR (N_N) has limited utility because this receptor affects both branches of the ANS, eliciting opposing effects. Intentional stimulation would, therefore, be counterproductive. Moreover, any agent that lacks specificity for the N_N receptor and crosses, pharmacologically, to the N_M version of the receptor would have untoward side effects in terms of skeletal muscle stimulation.

In spite of these considerations, one nicotine agonist is among the most widely used drugs in the world—i.e., nicotine itself. Despite significant side effects and reinforcing/rewarding aspects of nicotine use, social pressures drive individuals to use this drug via tobacco to the point where side effects become minimal because of tolerance. Pharmacologically, nicotine patches, inhalers, gums, and lozenges are used by patients in attempts to wean themselves from cigarette dependence.

Nicotinic Agonists
Nicotine

Stimulation of nicotinic receptors can be accomplished in two ways: direct or indirect agonists. In the former case, nicotine can be administered as a direct pharmacologic agonist. In the latter case (indirect agonists), agents that inhibit degradation of ACh (acetylcholinesterase inhibitors) are powerful agents. Cholinesterase inhibitors will be considered as a separate drug class because of their clinical uses and their potential uses as biochemical weapons and because they have both muscarinic and nicotinic activities. In general, with the exception of recreational use of nicotine in tobacco (or its use in tobacco cessation), there are few applications for direct-acting nicotinic ganglionic (N_N) agonists. No matter how they are stimulated, nicotinic stimulation has a variety of side effects including nausea, vomiting, diarrhea, salivation, sweating, and dizziness.

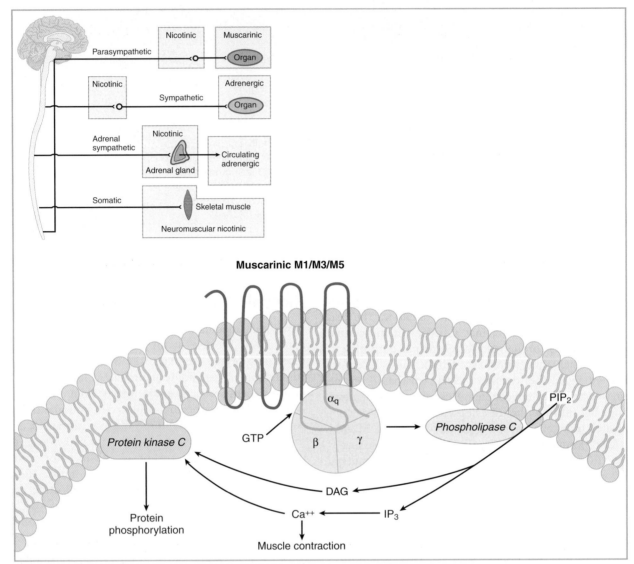

Figure 6-5. Muscarinic M1/M3/M5 ACh receptors. The "odd" class of muscarinic receptors works through an α_q G protein to activate a membrane-associated phospholipase C.

TABLE 6-5. Pharmacology of Acetylcholine-like Agonists

Agonist	Degradation by Cholinesterase	Muscarinic Receptor Activity	Atropine Antagonism	Nicotinic Receptor Activity
Acetylcholine	+++	++	+++	++
Methacholine	+	++	+++	+
Carbachol	—	++	+	+++
Bethanechol	—	+++	+++	—
Muscarine	—	+++	+++	—
Pilocarpine	—	+++	+++	—

+++, strong effect; ++, moderate effect; +, low effect; —, no effect.

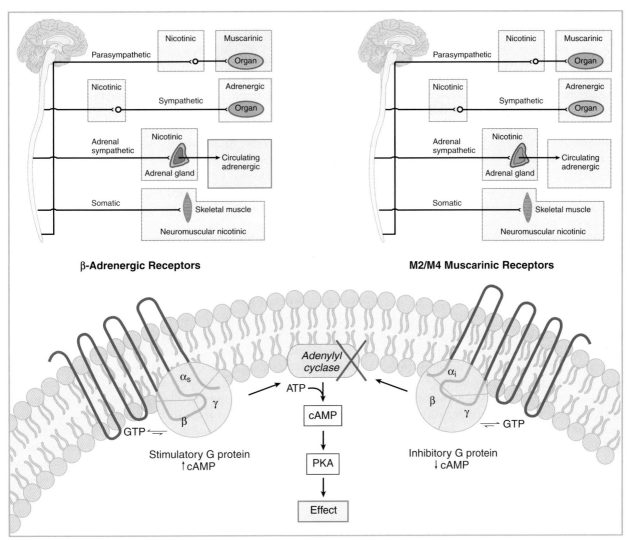

β-Adrenergic Receptors

M2/M4 Muscarinic Receptors

Figure 6-6. Reciprocal regulation of adenylyl cyclase by muscarinic and adrenergic receptors. **A**, The M2/M4 "even" class of muscarinic receptors works through an α_i- inhibitory G protein to reduce synthesis of cAMP. This inhibition results in reduced intracellular signaling. **B**, The β-adrenergic receptors work through an α_s-stimulatory G protein to activate adenylyl cyclase and increase the production of cAMP from ATP. These receptors frequently reside on the same organs to provide reciprocal regulation. PKA, protein kinase A.

Nicotinic Antagonists

Mecamylamine, Trimethaphan, Curare, Succinylcholine, Atracurium, Mivacurium, Pancuronium, Vecuronium, and Rocuronium

Nicotinic antagonists discriminate between the ganglionic (neuronal, N_N) and the neuromuscular nicotinic AChR (N_M) receptors. There are several agents (mecamylamine, trimethaphan) that act as ganglionic receptor antagonists (N_N) (see Fig. 6-1). Curare shows selectivity for the N_M neuromuscular junction receptor. (Note: Historically, South American Indians used curare on the tips of their arrows while hunting, to paralyze their prey if the piercing arrow was insufficient to kill the animal.) There are very few uses for ganglionic antagonists at present; they are used only to elicit controlled hypotension during surgery or manage some cases of hypertensive crisis.

The N_M nAChR is an important target for inducing skeletal muscle paralysis for surgery and/or endrotracheal intubation.

With skeletal muscle paralysis induced, less general anesthetic may be required during surgery, which can reduce postoperative respiratory and cardiovascular depression. Two classes of N_M antagonists (succinylcholine and curare-like compounds) are used to induce paralysis (1) in situations in which controlled ventilation is needed and (2) to eliminate the muscular manifestations of tonic clonic seizures. Remember that these agents cause paralysis but have no analgesic properties.

Blockade of neuromuscular junction ACh receptors (N_M AChR) can be achieved with succinylcholine. This drug is essentially a tail-to-tail condensation of two ACh molecules. There is a two-phase response when succinylcholine binds to N_M AChR. Phase I involves stimulation of receptors, with associated muscle contraction. Continued stimulation, however, is followed fairly rapidly by phase II blockade. This produces a desensitization of receptors, making them refractory to subsequent stimulation. For this reason, succinylcholine is often referred to as a depolarizing muscle relaxant. When using succinylcholine, it is important to remember that the drug has a very short half-life (less than 8 minutes) so it is used only for very short procedures. Skeletal muscle blockade with succinylcholine first affects muscles that move rapidly (e.g., eye, jaw), with limbs and diaphragm affected last. Recovery from blockade occurs in the reverse order (i.e., the diaphragm recovers first).

Succinylcholine has been associated with transient hyperkalemia and malignant hyperthermia. Because of the risk of hyperkalemia, succinylcholine should be used cautiously in patients with electrolyte imbalances or those using certain antiarrhythmic drugs. Malignant hyperthermia can be managed by administration of dantrolene sodium, which uncouples excitation-contraction coupling in muscle cells by preventing release of Ca^{++} from the sarcoplasmic reticulum. Patients taking aminoglycosides may be at greater risk of prolonged paralysis. On the other hand, patients with myasthenia gravis may be resistant to the effects of succinylcholine.

Whereas succinylcholine binds to N_M AChR in a *noncompetitive* fashion (the drug cannot be displaced by increasing ACh concentrations), curare-like direct-acting N_M AChR antagonists (atracurium, mivacurium, pancuronium, vecuronium, and rocuronium) are *competitive* antagonists (effects of the drugs can be reversed by increasing ACh in the synapse). Compared with succinylcholine, the curare-derivatives have longer half-lives. Atracurium is somewhat unique in that it is spontaneously hydrolyzed. Likewise, mivacurium is inactivated by plasma cholinesterase. Therefore, the actions of these two drugs are terminated regardless of hepatic or renal function.

Muscarinic Drugs

While nicotinic agents do not enjoy widespread clinical use, there are several important applications for muscarinic agents. However, there is a major limitation to the use of these drugs, since relatively few are selective for M2/M4 versus M1/M3/M5 receptor subclasses.

Muscarinic Agonists
Muscarine, Pilocarpine, Carbachol, and Bethanechol
Muscarine is the prototypical agonist for all muscarinic receptors (muscarine is an alkaloid derived from mushrooms and is associated with toxicity when poisonous mushrooms are ingested). A few drugs that are derivatives of ACh have proven effective as therapeutic agents, in part because of their resistance to degradation by acetylcholinesterase (see Table 6-5).

Because of limitations in receptor specificity, there are limited applications for muscarinic agonists. Notably, pilocarpine and carbachol are used ocularly to treat glaucoma because these drugs facilitate the outflow of aqueous humor, thereby reducing intraocular pressure. Pilocarpine is also used orally to treat xerostomia (dry mouth). Bethanechol is used to treat urinary retention (because it stimulates detrusor contraction [muscle of the bladder wall] and relaxes the

trigone/sphincter) and nonobstructive gastrointestinal hypomotility.

However, muscarinic agonists have serious side effects including SLUD syndrome (*s*alivation, *l*acrimation, *u*rination, *d*efecation). Moreover, they are contraindicated in patients with asthma because they cause bronchoconstriction and increase mucous secretions. Muscarinic-induced hypotension can lead to serious problems associated with reduced coronary blood flow. Additionally, these drugs are contraindicated in patients with hyperthyroidism because the body reacts to hypotension by releasing norepinephrine. Patients with hyperthyroidism are very sensitive to norepinephrine and can develop atrial fibrillation.

Muscarinic Antagonists
Atropine, Scopolamine, Ipratropium, Tiotropium, Oxybutynin, Tolterodine, Trospium, Solifenacin, Darifenacin, Dicyclomine, Hyoscyamine, Benztropine, and Glycopyrrolate
Atropine, scopolamine, and the related muscarinic antagonists work by competitive antagonism. That is, they bind to muscarinic receptors, have no intrinsic activity following this binding, and block the ability of the endogenous ligand—ACh—to bind. However, few of these drugs demonstrate selectivity for any of the five muscarinic receptor subtypes. Interestingly, in spite of being similar in structure, atropine has fewer central nervous system (CNS) effects than scopolamine and is favored for peripheral applications. However, scopolamine continues to be used as a transdermal patch in the treatment of motion sickness and in postoperative nausea and vomiting.

A major use for muscarinic antagonists is in the treatment of acetylcholinesterase poisoning (see the next section), which produces a dramatic increase in ACh. In fact, atropine is the drug of choice for treating accidental poisoning (typically due to accidental insecticide or pesticide exposure or mushroom poisoning). In addition, it has been issued in battlefield settings (both Gulf Wars) for use in the event of nerve agent attacks employing anticholinesterase agents. Clinically, drugs that work by this mechanism may also be used in ophthalmology to produce mydriasis (dilatation of the pupil) and cycloplegia (loss of accommodation, or inability to focus).

In the respiratory system, ipratropium and tiotropium are used to block bronchoconstrictive muscarinic tone in the lungs and reduce bronchial secretions. These drugs are used in management of chronic obstructive pulmonary disease.

Numerous muscarinic receptor antagonists are also available to treat overactive bladder episodes. Antimuscarinic drugs reduce the number of incontinent episodes, increase the amount of urine the bladder can hold, reduce the frequency of urination, and decrease urgency. Drugs include oxybutynin, tolterodine, trospium, solifenacin, and darifenacin. Each of these drugs is available in oral dose forms. Additionally, oxybutynin is available as a transdermal patch. The patch appears to have fewer adverse effects compared with the oral formulation, probably as a result of lower blood levels of the active metabolite that causes the "anticholinergic" adverse effects. The newest agents—solifenacin, trospium, and darifenacin—are said to be specific antagonists at M3 receptors. Note: Since each of these agents slows voiding, they are not appropriate for individuals prone to urinary retention (e.g., men with benign prostatic hypertrophy).

Other muscarinic receptor antagonists include dicyclomine and hyoscyamine, which are used to treat the irritable bowel syndrome type of gastrointestinal hypermotility and spasticity. Benztropine, which crosses the blood-brain barrier, may be used to decrease tremors in Parkinson's disease, while glycopyrrolate is used to dry glandular secretions (e.g., during surgical procedures, cerebral palsy).

Adverse effects of muscarinic receptor antagonists include dry mouth, mydriasis (causes blurred vision), tachycardia, hot and flushed skin, agitation, urinary retention, constipation, and delirium. To remember these side effects, think: red as a beet, dry as a bone, blind as a bat, mad as a hatter.

Acetylcholinesterase Inhibitors: Indirect-Acting Muscarinic and Nicotinic Receptor Agonists

Edrophonium, Ambenonium, Neostigmine, Physostigmine, Pyridostigmine, Echothiophate, Sarin, Soman, Tabun, Tacrine, Donepezil, Rivastigmine, and Galantamine

Another potent class of muscarinic mimetics includes the cholinesterase inhibitors that block the breakdown of ACh. For the effects of ACh to be rapidly and exquisitely regulated, the actions of the neurotransmitter need to be terminated by acetylcholinesterase. The inhibition of AChE results in the indirect increase in ACh, so these drugs are termed indirect-acting cholinomimetics.

There are two classes of anticholinesterases. The first class is composed of *reversible* compounds that have significant clinical utility (edrophonium, ambenonium, neostigmine, physostigmine, and pyridostigmine). The second class is largely *irreversible* agents that often have more "toxic" roles as insecticides and chemical weapon agents (nerve gases). Members of this latter class share the characteristic of being reactive organophosphates and include echothiophate (used ocularly for treatment of glaucoma) and nerve gas agents such as sarin, soman, and tabun.

Endogenous acetylcholinesterase is susceptible to these pharmacologic inhibitors. ACh binds to the active site of AChE, where the acetyl group of ACh is transferred to a serine hydroxyl residue within the enzyme's active site. Then, H_2O rapidly cleaves the acetate and regenerates the active enzyme. For the anticholinesterase pharmacologic agents, a reactive group is transferred to the serine that is slower to come off. With the *irreversible* organophosphates, the phosphorylated serine is very slowly reversed and, if given time, "ages" into a permanent modification that cannot be reversed and hence inactivates the enzyme. With acetylcholinesterases inactivated, large excesses of cholinergic activity occur that can kill the affected individual.

Treatment of AChE inhibition toxicity or poisoning relies on the use of atropine antagonists. However, in the case of nerve gas poisoning, rapid intervention with an additional substrate called *pralidoxime* (abbreviated 2-PAM) provides a strong nucleophilic center that strips the phosphate moiety from the enzyme. However, pralidoxime needs to be administered within several hours of the exposure (before it "ages"); otherwise, the acetylcholinesterase enzyme cannot be regenerated.

Clinically, the most common use for anticholinesterase agents is in diagnosis and treatment of myasthenia gravis, a neuromuscular disease in which the body makes antibodies against the N_M AChR. Of the various neuromuscular disorders presenting as muscle weakness, myasthenia gravis is the one that responds to anticholinesterase therapy. Therefore, diagnosis is made with a short-acting "challenge" (called the "Tensilon test") using ultra-short-acting edrophonium (half-life in minutes). Following definitive diagnosis, treatment is initiated with the use of longer-acting agents such as pyridostigmine, neostigmine, or ambenonium. Use of these drugs causes local synaptic concentrations of ACh to increase within the neuromuscular junction of the skeletal muscle, which increases the activity at the remaining functional receptors.

Several of the newest acetylcholinesterase inhibitors do not *covalently* bind to the acetylcholinesterase; rather, they bind as *noncovalent*, competitive inhibitors, and these drugs are used to treat Alzheimer's disease (tacrine, donepezil, rivastigmine, and galantamine). Observations in brains affected by Alzheimer's disease reveal that cholinergic neurons are among the earliest to be lost. Thus, the rationale for this treatment is that administration of anticholinesterase inhibitors increases central cholinergic tone to partially reverse the effects of lost cholinergic neurons. Unfortunately, these drugs have only modest effects in improving overall cognition in patients with Alzheimer's disease and all are associated with adverse gastrointestinal symptoms (e.g., diarrhea) because of excess ACh activity.

●●● ADRENERGIC SYSTEMS
Biochemistry of Adrenergic Systems

The term *adrenergic* refers to the fact that these neurotransmitters are found in the adrenal medulla, where epinephrine content predominates over that of norepinephrine. As shown in Figure 6-7, these neurotransmitters are synthesized from the amino acid precursor tyrosine. This single precursor (tyrosine) gives rise to three different catecholamine neurotransmitters: dopamine (primarily in the kidney and CNS), norepinephrine (autonomic sympathetic nerves and CNS), and epinephrine (primarily adrenal gland with a small CNS component). Therefore, the biosynthetic enzymes described in Figure 6-7 are differentially expressed in different cells of the body.

Termination of adrenergic neuronal signals is not mediated by a simple hydrolysis reaction. Rather, at the neuron-organ

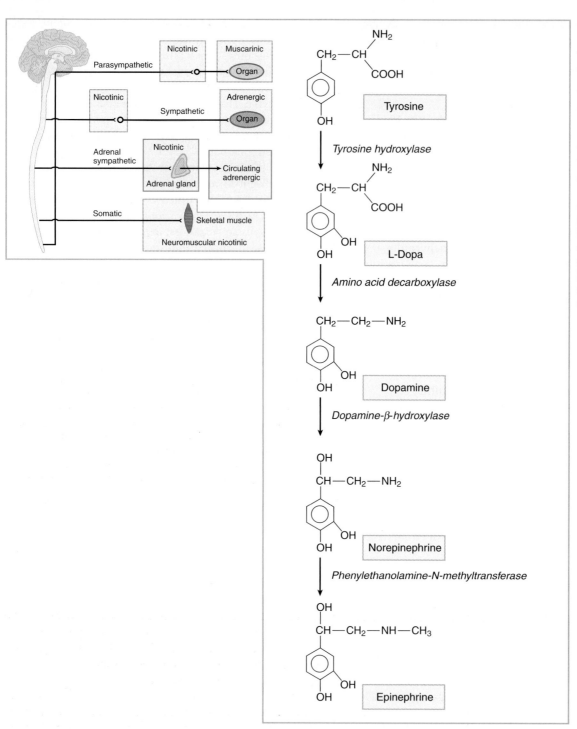

Figure 6-7.
Catecholamine biosynthesis. Adrenergic biosynthesis begins with an essential amino acid—tyrosine—and its hydroxylation by the rate-limiting enzyme tyrosine hydroxylase. This reaction produces a benzene ring with neighboring hydroxyl groups. This chemical is called "catechol" and is the reason this class of molecules (all of subsequent molecules in the pathway) is collectively referred to as the catecholamines.

synapse, 60% of norepinephrine is taken back into the nerve via an Na^+-dependent "pump" (Fig. 6-8A). (This reuptake transporter also happens to be the molecular target of cocaine.) Neurotransmitters can then be directly packaged for re-release. Of the remaining neurotransmitter in the synapse, 20% simply diffuses from the site of action, and 20% is degraded *in situ*. Degradation results in destruction of neurotransmitter function and excretion of metabolic products (Fig. 6-8B). As discussed in Chapter 13, drugs that inhibit

catecholamine metabolism are utilized to treat several CNS disorders.

Adrenergic Receptor Subtypes

As is the case for the cholinergic system, specific neurotransmitter receptor subtypes are found at various anatomic locations. In this case, there are again five different receptor subtypes: α_1, α_2, β_1, β_2, and β_3. Luckily, these receptors serve

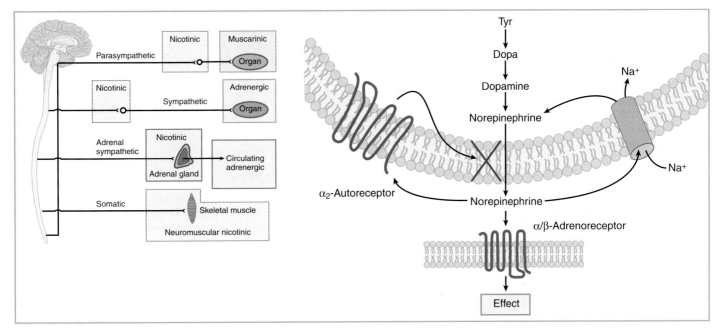

A

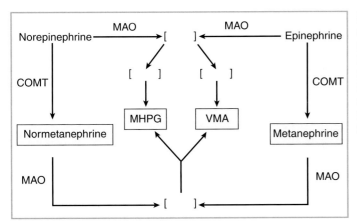

B

Figure 6-8. Termination of adrenergic responses. **A**, Most sympathetic signaling is terminated through reuptake (and repackaging and reuse) via a norepinephrine transporter. **B**, Enzymatic degradation of the catecholamines, a minor mechanism for signal termination, is also involved in terminating norepinephrine actions. The empty brackets represent unimportant chemical intermediaries. COMT, catechol-O-methyltransferase; MAO, monoamine oxidase; MHPG, 3-methoxy-4-hydroxyphenylglycol; VMA, vanillomandelic acid.

fairly discrete functions and can be functionally summarized by a relatively simplified table (Fig. 6-9). Moreover, they are all 7TM-GPCRs.

Alpha Receptors

The adrenergic receptors are classified into two main subgroups: alpha (α) and beta (β). In the case of the α-receptors, there are α_1 and α_2 (Figs. 6-8A, 6-9, and 6-10). These receptors conveniently assume different functions and have different subcellular localizations. Adrenergic α_1-receptors are found on innervated organs and elicit a physiologic response to nerve signals (see Fig. 6-8A). In contrast, α_2-receptors are found primarily on *pre*synaptic cells. That is, α_2-receptors are located on nerve cells and function there as autoreceptors (see Fig. 6-8A). The functional role of these α_2 autoreceptors is to "sense" synaptic activity and "dampen" activity in situations where there may be too much neurotransmitter in the synapse. Because they have different functions and anatomic locations, α_1- and α_2-receptors also display differing pharmacologic characteristics (see Fig. 6-10; see also Tables

6-6 and 6-7). Adrenergic α_1-receptors are coupled to the α_q-type subunit of G protein and stimulate phospholipase activity to release IP_3 and DAG, which ultimately trigger Ca^{++} release and cell stimulation (muscle contraction) (much like the M1/M3/M5 muscarinic receptors).

Adrenergic α_2-receptors, as noted above, often function as autoreceptors. Working through a G_i/G_0 G protein, these receptors inhibit adenylyl cyclase (much like the M2/M4 muscarinic receptors; see Fig. 6-10) and decrease cAMP levels. This produces a cascade of downstream events that ultimately results in decreased catecholamine neurotransmitter synthesis, as well as decreased neurotransmitter release (see Fig. 6-8).

Beta Receptors

The β-receptors, like the α-receptors, are 7TM-GPCRs and are coupled to G proteins. However, they are linked to G_s proteins that stimulate adenylyl cyclase activity and ultimately increase cAMP levels. Depending on the cell type being innervated, stimulation of β-receptors produces vastly different results (see Table 6-6; see also Figs. 6-9 and 6-11).

BIOCHEMISTRY

Role of Amino Acids and Metabolic Intermediaries

Amino acids and metabolic intermediaries serve a variety of functions, in addition to being the building blocks of proteins and providing sources of energy, respectively. In the present context, acetyl-CoA is normally considered to be a product of glycolysis, and choline is a dietary molecule that becomes a part of structural lipids (phosphatidylcholine). However, in selected neurons, these substrates are diverted to neurotransmitter biosynthesis (acetylcholine). Similarly, many amino acids (glutamate, aspartate, glycine, tryptophan, and tyrosine) are used as neurotransmitters directly or are converted to neurotransmitters. The key point to understand, however, is that this has to be a regulated process. Neurotransmitter products represent such a small percentage of the cellular need for these molecules that it would be detrimental to divert them in an unrestricted manner. Therefore, neurotransmitter biosynthetic enzymes tend to be very heavily regulated. Tyrosine hydroxylase, for instance, is the first and rate-limiting step in norepinephrine synthesis. This one enzyme is the subject of nearly every form of enzyme regulation that has been characterized (transcriptional, translational, and posttranslational regulation; feedback inhibition; allosteric modulation; protein stability; alternative RNA splicing). Therefore, its tight regulation leads to a well-controlled diversion of tyrosine to neurotransmitter synthesis, from its larger role in protein synthesis.

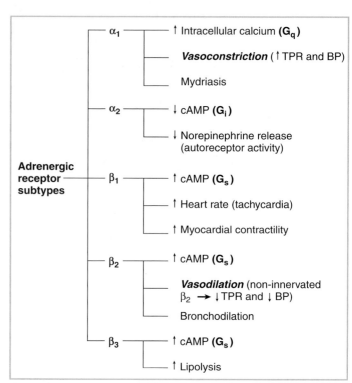

Figure 6-9. Physiology and pharmacology of adrenergic receptors.

Adrenergic β_1-receptors are found most notably on the heart, where they increase heart rate and cardiac contractility, leading to increased cardiac output. On the other hand, β_2-receptors are found on a variety of bronchial and vascular smooth muscles, where stimulation triggers muscle relaxation. In the peripheral vascular bed, β_2-receptor stimulation decreases total peripheral resistance and blood pressure.

In the case of β_2-receptors in the lungs, stimulation produces muscle relaxation and bronchodilation. For this reason, inhaled β_2 agonists are the drugs of choice for treating acute asthma. The mechanistic reasons for the seemingly opposite effects of cAMP stimulation (increased contraction in the heart vs muscle relaxation in lung and blood vessels) relate directly to the type of effector pathways engaged by specific cell types. For instance, in the case of pulmonary and vascular smooth muscle, cAMP leads to phosphorylation of myosin light chain kinase, which leads to smooth muscle relaxation; whereas in cardiac muscle, cAMP ultimately stimulates pacemaker function. Finally, β_3-receptors have been identified relatively recently. These receptors are found mainly on adipose tissue, where they seem to be involved in regulating fat metabolism.

● ● ● ADRENERGIC DRUGS

Unlike the drugs currently available to modulate the parasympathetic (ACh) nervous system, many pharmacologic agents are available that allow us to discriminately modulate

TABLE 6-6. Mechanisms of Action of Adrenergic Receptors

Receptor	G Protein (α Subunits)	Primary Effects
α_1	G_q	↑ Phospholipase C ($\Rightarrow$ ↑ Ca^{++} and bioactive lipids)
α_2	G_i/G_o	↓ Adenylyl cyclase (↓ cAMP) ↑ Potassium channel activity ↓ Calcium channel activity
$\beta_1/\beta_2/\beta_3$	G_s	↑ Adenylyl cyclase ($\Rightarrow$ ↑ cAMP)

individual adrenergic receptor subtypes. These characteristics of adrenergic receptors provide opportunities to treat certain disorders. In the following section, we broadly consider the various classes of adrenergic drugs and their uses (Table 6-7). The pharmacologic details, however, are left to chapters on specific organ systems or therapeutic needs.

Alpha Drugs

There are highly selective agonists and antagonists for α-adrenoceptor subtypes (see Table 6-7 and Fig. 6-12). Indeed, given their selectivity, these drugs are used clinically in a variety of settings.

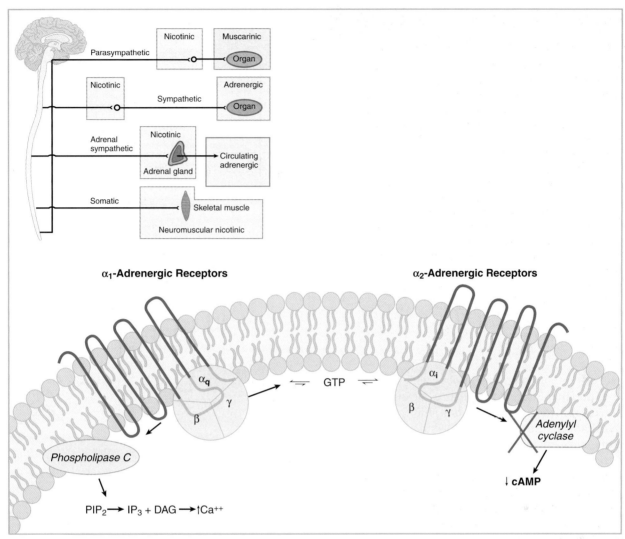

Figure 6-10. Reciprocal regulation by the α_1- and α_2-receptors. The α-receptors are 7TM-GPCRs and are coupled to lipid metabolism or inhibition of cAMP synthesis.

Alpha-Adrenergic Agonists
Norepinephrine, Methoxamine, Phenylephrine, Clonidine, and Dexmedetomidine

As shown in Figure 6-12, there are several α-selective drugs. Indeed, Table 6-7 identifies the prototypical agonists for each receptor subtype. First, let's consider the main, naturally occurring, autonomic neurotransmitters (epinephrine and norepinephrine). Epinephrine is released from the adrenal medulla and interacts, via the circulation, with all adrenergic receptors. As a result of its actions, epinephrine raises blood pressure and increases cardiac output. It is therefore used to treat anaphylactic shock. Additionally, epinephrine may be used clinically to treat mucosal congestion associated with hay fever, rhinitis, or sinusitis; status asthmaticus; symptomatic relief of serum sickness, urticaria, angioedema; glaucoma; and prolongation of local/regional anesthetics by vasoconstrictive actions.

In contrast to epinephrine, norepinephrine is released from nerves, where it interacts with receptors in the synapse. Norepinephrine is the primary mediator of β_1 tone in the heart. Moreover, norepinephrine, released in the vasculature, interacts with α_1-receptors and is responsible for the maintenance of total peripheral resistance and blood pressure (Fig. 6-13).

Methoxamine is a synthetic catecholamine with selectivity for α-receptors (with a slight preference for α_1 over α_2). Methoxamine is used clinically to maintain blood pressure during anesthesia through its ability to stimulate α_1 and raise total peripheral resistance. (Do not forget, however, that the resulting increase in blood pressure will lead to reflex activity of the baroreceptors, decreasing sympathetic outflow.)

Phenylephrine is the prototypical α_1 agonist. Because of its selectivity, phenylephrine has dramatic vasoconstrictor effects (see Fig. 6-9). It has historically been used as a nasal decongestant when topically applied to the nasal mucosa. It also has been used to overcome vascular failure in shock and supraventricular tachycardia.

On the other hand, clonidine is the prototypical α_2 agonist. This compound, which is predominantly thought of as an autoreceptor agonist, is used to lower blood pressure—through

TABLE 6-7. Examples of Selective and Nonselective Adrenergic Agonists and Antagonists

Receptor	Agonist	Antagonist
α_1	Phenylephrine	Prazosin Phentolamine (α_1/α_2) Phenoxybenzamine (α_1/α_2) Labetalol (α_1 and β)
α_2	Clonidine Dexmedetomidine	Yohimbine Phentolamine (α_1/α_2) Phenoxybenzamine (α_1/α_2)
β_1	Dobutamine Isoproteronol ($\beta_1/\beta_2/\beta_3$)	Metoprolol Acebutolol Atenolol Propranolol (β_1/β_2) Labetalol (α_1 and β)
β_2	Terbutaline Albuterol Isoproteronol ($\beta_1/\beta_2/\beta_3$)	Propranolol (β_1/β_2) Labetalol (α_1 and β)
β_3	Isoproteronol ($\beta_1/\beta_2/\beta_3$)	

agonist actions on autoreceptors located within the CNS as opposed to peripheral receptor activities. Dexmedetomidine is another α_2-agonist that has a higher affinity for CNS α_2-receptors. Although its use is associated with hypotension and bradycardia, dexmedetomidine is primarily used to provide deep intravenous sedation without causing respiratory depression.

Alpha-Adrenergic Antagonists
Phentolamine, Phenoxybenzamine, Prazosin, Doxazosin, Terazosin, and Yohimbine

Like the adrenergic agonists, there are selective antagonists for α- and β-receptors (see Fig. 6-12). Phentolamine and phenoxybenzamine are α antagonists (but do not discriminate between α_1 and α_2). The two drugs differ in that the

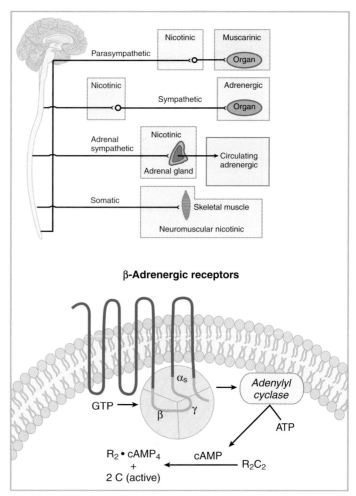

β-Adrenergic receptors

Figure 6-11. Stimulation of adenylyl cyclase by the β-receptors. All the β-receptors are coupled to a stimulatory G protein (G_s) and increase synthesis of cAMP. Stimulation of β-receptors produces widely different effects depending on downstream effectors that are present in specific cells. In this case, the cAMP triggers dissociation of the inactive PKA holoenzyme (R_2C_2) into regulatory subunit dimers ($R_2 \cdot cAMP_4$) and active catalytic subunits (C).

Figure 6-12. Pharmacologic profiles of adrenergic drugs. **A**, Adrenergic agonists. **B**, Adrenergic antagonists. Selectivity is indicated by the position of the drug on the α-to-β continuum.

α-Selective	Mixed	β-Selective
Methoxamine norepinephrine Phenylephrine (α_1) Clonidine (α_2) Dexmedetomidine (α_2)	Epinephrine	Isoproteronol Terbutaline (β_2) Albuterol (β_2) Dobutamine (β_1) Dopamine (β_1)

A

α-Selective	Mixed	β-Selective
Phenoxybenzamine Phentolamine Prazosin (α_1) Yohimbine (α_2)	Labetolol	Propranolol Timolol Atenolol (β_1) Metoprolol (β_1) Acebutolol (β_1)

B

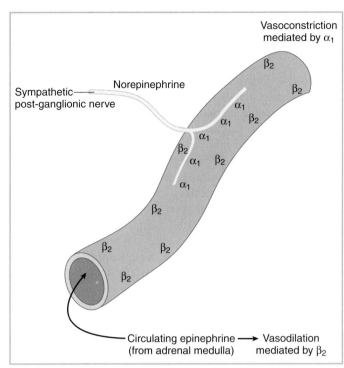

Figure 6-13. Role of noninnervated β-receptors in the regulation of blood pressure. Peripheral blood vessels are innervated by sympathetic nerves that release norepinephrine and stimulate α₁-receptors. In addition, the vessels contain noninnervated β₂-receptors that normally respond to circulating epinephrine. The former receptors produce vasoconstriction (increased BP), whereas the latter produce vasodilation (decreased BP).

former is a *reversible* antagonist, while the latter is an *irreversible* blocker. Clinically, their primary use is preoperative management of patients with pheochromocytoma (a catecholamine-secreting adrenal medullary tumor). This adrenal tumor releases high concentrations of epinephrine. These drugs prevent the effects of epinephrine on the body and "desensitize" the body to circulating catecholamines. This is particularly important during surgery because surgical manipulations of the tumor also trigger release of epinephrine.

Examples of drugs with α₁-selective antagonist actions include prazosin (and related compounds doxazosin and terazosin). These drugs have historically been used to treat hypertension, by decreasing total peripheral resistance and preventing sympathetic-mediated vasoconstriction. Recall, in the vasculature, sympathetic tone predominates because there is no parasympathetic innervation. Therefore, a major side effect of these drugs is postural hypotension (especially with the first dose).

Recently, α₁-receptor antagonists have fallen out of favor as antihypertensives because, as blood pressure falls, the kidneys secrete renin. Renin release counteracts the vasodilation induced by these drugs, and activation of the RAAS (renin-angiotensin-aldosterone system) has been associated with increased incidence of heart failure. However, these drugs are still widely used to treat benign prostatic hyper-

trophy. Adrenergic α₁ blockade in prostatic tissue causes relaxation of prostate muscle, allowing better urine flow.

Yohimbine is a selective α₂-autoreceptor antagonist (recall that the α₂-receptor is a release-modulating autoreceptor). This drug has a variety of effects and does not enjoy widespread use in the clinical setting. It has been used as a treatment for erectile dysfunction and as a mydriatic. However, numerous other drugs are effective in these applications, so yohimbine is not widely used.

Beta Drugs

Beta Adrenergic Agonists
Isoproterenol, Dobutamine, Albuterol, Salmeterol, Terbutaline, Ritodrine, and Dopamine

Isoproterenol is the prototypical β agonist. Unfortunately, because of its lack of selectivity (it is equipotent at β₁ and β₂), it does not enjoy widespread clinical use. It may be used to manage hypovolemic and septic shock. β-Selectivity comes in the form of two important classes of compounds. Dobutamine is a β₁-selective compound and is beneficial for selectively *increasing* cardiac output in patients with congestive heart failure (see Fig. 6-9). β₂-Selective agonists like albuterol are beneficial for the treatment of asthma. Indeed, inhaled β₂ agonists are drugs of choice for managing acute asthma attacks. A lipophilic version of albuterol (salmeterol) has a long duration of action, making this drug useful in asthma prophylaxis (it is the β₂ agonist component of fluticasone/salmeterol combinations). Because it has a delayed time for onset of action, it has never been used in an acute asthma attack. Additionally, β₂-selective drugs such as terbutaline and ritodrine are used as tocolytics (medications to inhibit labor), since β₂ agonist activity in the uterus causes relaxation of uterine smooth muscle.

Dopamine deserves consideration at this point. As noted in Figure 6-8, dopamine is the direct chemical precursor to norepinephrine. However, dopamine is also an important neurotransmitter in its own right and plays prominent roles in mental health, substance abuse, and motor function (loss of dopamine neurons in the CNS is the underlying cause of Parkinson's disease). At high enough doses, dopamine also binds to adrenergic receptors, with selectivity for β₁-receptors. β₁-selectivity increases cardiac output. At low doses, dopamine stimulates *bona fide* dopamine receptors (D₂) in the renal vasculature. This produces vasodilation and increases blood flow to the kidneys. These are important considerations in cases of shock. When dopamine is used to manage cardiogenic shock, activity at β-receptors increases cardiac output, while stimulation of renal dopamine receptors may prevent renal failure. At extraordinarily high doses, dopamine will act on α-receptors and cause vasoconstriction (useful in patients in hemorrhagic shock).

Beta-Adrenergic Antagonists (β-Blockers)
Propranolol, Timolol, Acebutolol, Pindolol, Labetalol, Carvedilol, and Metoprolol

Note that the names of these drugs end in "-lol."

The β-blockers have long enjoyed clinical utility because of their ability to decrease cardiac output, myocardial oxygen demand, and total peripheral resistance without leading to debilitating postural hypotension. This is because they do not affect the α_1 tone that regulates blood pressure (see Fig. 6-9). Propranolol is the prototypical β-blocker. It lacks selectivity and effectively blocks both β_1 and β_2. Clinically, β-blockers are used in a variety of settings. First and foremost, they are used to treat hypertension. They are also effective in angina (by reducing workload and the concomitant oxygen demand) and in the treatment of atrial fibrillation, where they reduce AV nodal conduction and protect the ventricles. Additionally, β-blockers are effective cardioprotectants following a myocardial infarction (and are a standard treatment modality). β-Blockers (timolol, in particular) also reduce intraocular pressure and are beneficial in long-term management of glaucoma (where they decrease aqueous humor production). Finally, certain β-blockers, such as carvedilol and metoprolol, are effective in the treatment of congestive heart failure, where there have been few classes of drugs shown to reduce mortality.

Acebutolol (as well as pindolol) represents a novel antagonist that has weak intrinsic *agonist* activity—also called partial agonist activity, or in the case of the cardiovascular system, "intrinsic sympathomimetic activity" (ISA). The best way to understand these dual effects is to remember that these compounds bind to receptors and block endogenous stimulation by epinephrine and norepinephrine, yet elicit weak stimulatory effects of their own. This minimizes the bradycardia that is usually associated with β-blockade.

Labetalol is another drug with a unique mechanism of action: it is a nonselective α_1 and β_1/β_2 blocker. Based on this spectrum of activity, labetalol decreases cardiac output *and* total peripheral resistance (see Fig. 6-9). Similarly, carvedilol has both α_1- and β_1-selective blocking properties. Orthostatic hypotension is a significant side effect of these agents.

●●● CLINICALLY IMPORTANT INDIRECT EFFECTORS OF AUTONOMIC FUNCTION

Discussions up to this point have focused primarily on direct-acting agonists and antagonists. However, there is a long list of pharmacologic compounds that act indirectly. Here, we review merely those that have an immediate and noteworthy presence in the clinical setting. Of immediate and widespread relevance is the ability to block catecholamine reuptake (dopamine, norepinephrine, and epinephrine; Table 6-8). Recall that this is the primary mechanism by which sympathetic signals are terminated. Reuptake is mediated by an Na^+-dependent symporter pump (the norepinephrine/epinephrine transporter and the dopamine transporter). As discussed in Chapter 13, the norepinephrine transporter is a target for tricyclic antidepressants (e.g., imipramine). Contrasting with this therapeutically beneficial approach, the dopamine and norepinephrine transporters (along with the serotonin transporter) are targets of an abused drug, cocaine. In all cases, the result of transporter blockade is an increased amount of time that the neurotransmitter spends in the synapse, increasing the *apparent* sympathetic activity. This leads to the designation of these compounds as *indirect-acting sympathomimetics*. Through a differing mechanism, amphetamines accomplish the same effect. In the case of amphetamines, neurotransmitters are released from synaptic vesicles and through a reversal of the symporter pump, catecholamines are released into the synapse via backward flow through the transporter.

Considering the toxicologically relevant inhibition of acetylcholinesterase (see Fig. 6-9), the toxicology profile of AChE inhibitors should be apparent. Any intervention that prevents the cell from terminating a cholinergic response will result in heightened stimulation of nearly every branch of the ANS either directly or indirectly (through ganglionic

TABLE 6-8. Clinically Important Indirect Effectors of Autonomic Function

Activity	Agents	Effects
Block catecholamine reuptake	Cocaine, tricyclic antidepressants	Increase norepinephrine in synapse; have sympathomimetic actions
Facilitate catecholamine release	Amphetamine	Stimulate sympathetic nervous system by releasing norepinephrine; have sympathomimetic actions
Block ACh breakdown	Cholinesterase inhibitors (pesticides and nerve gas agents)	Block ACh degradation; overstimulate cholinergic systems (muscarinic → SLUD syndrome)
Block catecholamine breakdown	MAO inhibitors (pargyline, selegiline) COMT inhibitors (entacapone, tolcapone)	Increase norepinephrine/epinephrine activities without direct stimulation (augment existing activities)

ACh, acetylcholine; COMT, catechol-O-methyltransferase; MAO, monoamine oxidase; SLUD, salivation, lacrimation, urination, defecation.

stimulation of the sympathetic nervous system, for example). This is what makes nerve gas agents, such as sarin, so deadly.

Finally, there are a number of new approaches that increase adrenergic function in the nervous system by modulating the degradation of catecholamines. Most signal termination is accomplished through reuptake transporters. However, a small amount of metabolic degradation occurs via MAO (monoamine oxidase) and COMT (catechol-O-methyltransferase), and these enzymes are the targets of compounds like pargyline and selegiline as well as tolcapone and entacapone. Although this approach is more common in the CNS (see Chapter 13), it is interesting to note that interfering with neurotransmitter metabolism does not interfere with tone of the system. That is, molecules will still be packaged and released in an integrated neuronal fashion. However, the effectiveness of neurotransmitter release can be enhanced by increasing catecholamine levels in the synapse.

●●● TOP FIVE LIST

1. Sympathetic and parasympathetic nerves use essentially two neurotransmitters (norepinephrine and ACh, respectively). They generate pharmacologic diversity through multiple receptor subtypes.
2. Nicotinic ACh receptors are poor choices for pharmacologic intervention because they serve too many different functions.
3. While muscarinic ACh receptors are pharmacologically suitable drug targets, we lack compounds with receptor selectivity.
4. Adrenergic receptors are strong pharmacologic targets—there is drug selectivity for numerous receptor subtypes.
5. Different adrenergic receptors on the same organ can have opposite effects. At the same time, similar adrenergic receptors on different organs can have opposite effects.

Hematology

CONTENTS

It's all about keeping the plumbing clear. Numerous arterial (e.g., myocardial infarct, stroke, and peripheral ischemia) and venous (e.g., deep vein thrombosis and pulmonary embolism) pathologies occur as a result of occlusions (stenotic lesions) within the vasculature. Under normal circumstances, blood clot formation (hemostasis) and breakdown (fibrinolysis) take place along a physiologic continuum. However, when these processes go awry, pathologic consequences such as thrombi arise, leading to potentially severe consequences. Understanding the physiologic and biochemical mechanisms underlying blood clotting offers not only a prospectus on how these processes are altered by aging and in diabetes, inflammation, cardiovascular and renal diseases, but also identifies pharmacologic targets for therapeutic interventions.

In addition to its ability to buffer extracellular pH, blood plays a number of important roles in maintaining internal equilibrium. Among these various functions is hemostasis, or the cessation of bleeding from damaged blood vessels. The process of hemostasis comprises three major interrelated steps: vessel constriction, platelet plug formation, and clotting. As a result of injury to the vessel, platelets are activated, resulting in release of vasoconstrictors, including thromboxane A_2, serotonin (5HT), and adenosine diphosphate (ADP). Vascular constriction is the initial response to blood vessel injury. Soon after vasoconstriction occurs, collagen—which underlies the vessel endothelium and is exposed as a result of the injury—allows platelet adherence and aggregation to form a platelet plug. Platelet activation and aggregation also expose glycoprotein IIb/IIIa, a receptor site for fibrinogen, the precursor molecule to formation of a fibrin clot (Fig. 7-1).

Clotting, which is the final step in hemostasis, results in a meshwork of fibrin that traps blood cells. Its main function is to reinforce the platelet plug and to provide a relatively strong seal at the site of vascular injury. Fibrin clots are the end result of the proteolytic activation of clotting factors, which make up both the intrinsic (blood trauma) and extrinsic (tissue trauma) pathways. Activation of either the intrinsic or the extrinsic pathway ends with activation of thrombin, which converts fibrinogen to fibrin to form a fibrin clot. Physicians have three major types of drugs to prevent or diminish thrombus formation: anticoagulants, platelet inhibitors, and thrombolytics (Fig. 7-2).

●●● ANTICOAGULANT DRUGS

In hypercoagulable states, the risk of thrombus formation is elevated and pharmacologic management is centered on the prevention of pathologic clot formation. It is important to remember that the liver plays a crucial role in coagulation, since it is a site that produces many clotting factors. The liver is also the site of production of bile salts that facilitate absorption of vitamin K and aid in production of clotting factors II, VII, IX, and X. The major types of anticoagulants are:
- Heparins
- Vitamin K cofactor antagonists (warfarin)
- Direct thrombin inhibitors

PATHOLOGY

Lines of Zahn

When thrombi form in the heart or aorta, they may have apparent laminations, referred to as lines of Zahn. These lines are produced by alternating pale layers of platelets and fibrin mixed with darker layers containing red blood cells. The main significance of lines of Zahn is that they imply antemortem thrombus formation at a site of blood flow.

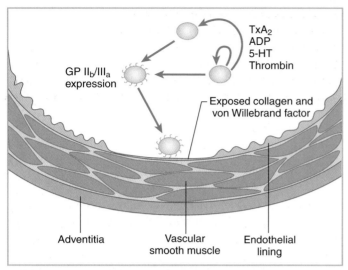

Figure 7-1. Platelet activation. Release of ADP, thromboxane, serotonin, and thrombin from adhered platelets induces additional platelet recruitment and augmented expression of glycoprotein IIb/IIIa. These glycoprotein receptors bind fibrinogen and von Willebrand factor to lead to platelet aggregation at the site of endothelial injury. The anionic phospholipid surface of the aggregated platelet mass helps localize the coagulation cascade factors that ultimately activate thrombin, the enzyme that forms fibrin from fibrinogen. ADP, adenosine diphosphate; 5HT, serotonin; TxA_2, thromboxane A_2.

Heparins

Unfractionated heparin was, for many years, the clinician's primary option when selecting a parenteral anticoagulant. However, more selective forms of heparins, known as the fractionated, low-molecular-weight heparins (LMWHs), can now be administered.

Unfractionated Heparin

Mechanism of action. Heparin is a large, endogenous, sulfated glycosaminoglycan found in mast cells. Under normal circumstances, it is rapidly destroyed and not detected in

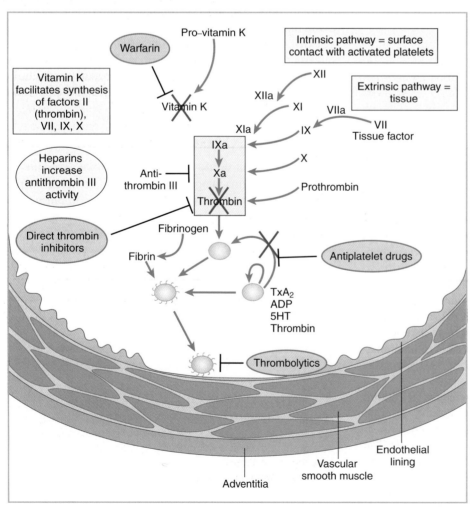

Figure 7-2. A platelet-centric view of coagulation. Both the intrinsic and extrinsic clotting pathways activate thrombin, which converts bound fibrinogen on platelet IIb/IIIa receptors into fibrin, which reinforces the clot and may lead to blood flow occlusion. The major sites of pharmacologic intervention are depicted in red. In addition, thrombolytics can be used to lyse pathologic thrombi.

plasma. The heparin used pharmacologically is extracted from bovine lung or porcine intestinal mucosa.

Heparin's anticoagulant action is derived from its binding to antithrombin III. Antithrombin III inhibits activated coagulation factors, especially thrombin (factor II), Xa, and IXa. When heparin binds to antithrombin III, a conformational change is induced that opens the reactive site of antithrombin III, increasing its ability to inhibit coagulation factors by 1000-fold.

Pharmacokinetics. The large molecular size of heparin prevents the drug from crossing membranes; thus, heparin must be given parenterally. Heparin has a short half-life and is both metabolized by heparinase in the liver and degraded in the periphery by endothelial cells. Patient response to heparin is quite variable. In part, this variability occurs because heparin binds nonspecifically to plasma proteins. Since each individual possesses differing amounts of plasma proteins to which heparin may bind, heparin's effects vary greatly between individuals. When heparin is bound to plasma proteins, it is unable to bind to antithrombin III.

Clinical uses. Heparin is a first-line agent for anticoagulation in patients with an acute deep vein thrombosis (DVT), pulmonary embolism (PE), or myocardial infarction (MI). Heparin is also used for preventing postoperative DVT and PE in high-risk patients, including pregnant women. The need for continuous intravenous infusions of heparin or repeated subcutaneous injections significantly reduces its usefulness in long-term outpatient management.

Antidote. In hemorrhagic situations, protamine sulfate can be administered. Protamine sulfate binds to heparin by virtue of positively charged protamine interacting with the sulfates on heparin and interferes with heparin's ability to bind to antithrombin III.

Adverse effects. Aside from hemorrhage, other prominent adverse effects include skin necrosis at the injection site, osteoporosis with long-term use, severe thrombocytopenia, and hypersensitivity reactions.

Contraindications. Since heparin is derived from animal sources, hypersensitivity to bovine or porcine components may cause anaphylactic reactions. Heparin should always be avoided in any situation in which a patient is likely to bleed (Box 7-1).

Monitoring. Activated partial thromboplastin time (aPTT) is used to monitor heparin's efficacy. Typically, the aPTT goal to manage a hypocoagulated patient is 1.5 to 2.5 times baseline (normal adult control values range from 28 to 42 seconds).

Low-Molecular-Weight Heparins
Enoxaparin, Dalteparin, and Ardeparin

Mechanism of action. While similar to unfractionated heparin, LMWHs are more selective in action. Like heparin, LMWHs increase the activity of antithrombin III; however, with LMWHs, factor Xa is preferentially affected over other clotting factors.

Pharmacokinetics. Unlike unfractionated heparin, there is less nonspecific binding to plasma proteins with LMWHs. This results in fewer drug interactions, a more predictable anticoagulant response, and less interpatient variability. Additional advantages of LMWHs over unfractionated heparin are listed in Box 7-2. LMWHs are eliminated renally, and dosage adjustments are needed in patients with renal insufficiency.

Clinical uses. LMWHs can be used to prevent or treat DVT and PE and to prevent ischemic complications associated with unstable angina and non-Q-wave MI. In many situations, LMWHs have replaced unfractionated heparin.

Adverse effects. Although bleeding, osteoporosis, thrombocytopenia, and skin reactions near the injection site may occur with LMWHs, the incidence and severity of these side effects are greatly reduced compared with those for unfractionated heparin.

Monitoring. Routine coagulation monitoring is not required although specific tests are available to monitor factor Xa activity periodically in patients with renal insufficiency or morbid obesity or in pregnant women.

Synthetic Heparin Alternatives

Fondaparinux is a synthetic pentasaccharide that is virtually the shortest sequence within heparin that binds to antithrombin III to inactivate factor Xa. Since this is a synthetic drug, there is less potential for hypersensitivity reactions, as compared with unfractionated heparins from bovine or porcine sources. Yet, unlike heparin, no antidote is available in the event of bleeding complications.

Direct Thrombin Inhibitors
Lepirudin, Bivalirudin, and Argatroban

Mechanism of action. These drugs directly bind to the active site of thrombin, inhibiting its effects on fibrinogen. The drug lepirudin is a recombinant form of hirudin, the irreversible thrombin inhibitor derived from leeches. Yes, the same leeches used for medicinal purposes for centuries. The FDA in 2004 approved the use of leeches for certain medical

---

Box 7-1.   CONTRAINDICATIONS TO HEPARIN DUE TO BLEEDING RISKS

- Hemophilia and all bleeding disorders
- Gastrointestinal ulcers/bleeding
- Thrombocytopenia
- Recent brain, spinal cord, or eye surgery
- During or before lumbar puncture or regional anesthetic blockade

Box 7-2.   ADVANTAGES OF LMWHS OVER UNFRACTIONATED HEPARIN

- Can be used by patients at home (SC vs IV injection)
- Routine monitoring of coagulation times is unnecessary
- Predictable dose-response relationships
- Improved bioavailability
- Longer half-life ($t_{1/2}$)
- Once or twice daily dosing

TABLE 7-1. Drugs That Increase Risk of Bleeding When Used with Warfarin

Inhibit Warfarin Metabolism	Displace Warfarin from Plasma Protein Binding Sites	Interfere with Vitamin K	Platelet Effects	Mechanism Unknown
Azole antifungals	Loop diuretics	Aminoglycosides	NSAIDs	Cephalosporins (parenteral)
HMG-CoA reductase inhibitors	Valproate	Tetracyclines	Penicillins (parenteral)	Disulfiram
Metronidazole		Vitamin E	Fish oils	Fibric acid
				Pentoxifylline
				SSRIs
				Streptokinase
				Thrombolytics
				Urokinase

purposes, such as removal of pooled blood from under a skin graft to promote healing, restoration of circulation in blocked veins, and surgical reattachment of fingers and ears. Lepirudin, bivalirudin, and argatroban are administered parenterally. Orally active thrombin inhibitors are currently being evaluated.

Clinical use. Lepirudin, bivalirudin, and argatroban are used in patients who have experienced heparin-induced thrombocytopenia. These drugs may also be administered to patients undergoing angioplasty.

Adverse effects. As with other anticoagulants, bleeding is the most common adverse event.

Vitamin K Antagonists (Orally Active Anticoagulants)

Warfarin

Note: For students who sometimes wonder how drug names are selected, warfarin is derived from the *Wisconsin Alumni Research Foundation*, the patent-holding arm of the University of Wisconsin, where warfarin was discovered.

Mechanism of action. Warfarin inhibits the synthesis of vitamin K–dependent clotting factors, which are factors II, VII, IX, and X. Specifically, synthesis of these clotting factors requires γ-carboxylation, a process that utilizes vitamin K. In the process of γ-carboxylation, vitamin K gets oxidized. Oxidized vitamin K must be reduced to regenerate active vitamin K, but warfarin interferes with the reduction step by inhibiting the actions of the enzyme, vitamin K epoxide reductase.

Pharmacokinetics. Warfarin has a slow onset of action. In fact, warfarin's therapeutic effect is delayed for 4 to 5 days, until all existing activated factors II, VII, IX, and X are depleted from the circulation.

Warfarin binds extensively and nonspecifically to plasma proteins. From 97% to 99.9% of warfarin is protein bound, with only a small percentage of the drug free in circulation to exert its biologic effects. As a result, coadministration of other highly protein-bound drugs may displace warfarin from its binding sites, leading to greater amounts of freely circulating

warfarin and increased risks of bleeding. Other drug-drug interactions with warfarin may occur as a result of the inhibition of warfarin's hepatic metabolism or pharmacodynamic actions with other drugs that also alter coagulation (e.g., aspirin, NSAIDs, salicylates). Table 7-1 lists drugs that may increase the risk of bleeding when used with warfarin, and Table 7-2 lists drugs that decrease warfarin's efficacy. Numerous foods that are rich in vitamin K also antagonize warfarin's anticoagulant effects, leading to reduced efficacy (Box 7-3). Furthermore, numerous herbal or natural products alter the effects of warfarin; these interactions can either increase or decrease the risk of bleeding (Boxes 7-4 and 7-5). Of note are the "4 Gs": garlic, ginger, *Ginkgo biloba*, and ginseng—four commonly used supplements that increase warfarin's anticoagulant actions. More food, drug, and herbal interactions occur with warfarin than with any other drug.

It is worth noting that resistance to warfarin therapy is usually due to excessive vitamin K intake from diet or supplements. However, hereditary warfarin resistance due to mutations in vitamin K epoxide reductase has been reported. Conversely, variant CYP2C9 alleles (the P-450 hepatic microsomal enzyme that typically inactivates warfarin) may enhance sensitivity to warfarin.

TABLE 7-2. Drugs That Decrease Anticoagulant Effects of Warfarin

Decreased Absorption or Increased Elimination	Induction of Hepatic Microsomal Cytochrome P-450 Enzymes	Unknown Mechanism
Spironolactone	Barbiturates	Clozapine
Sucralfate	Carbamazepine	Oral contraceptives
Thiazide diuretics	Dicloxacillin	Estrogens
Vitamin K (antagonizes warfarin)	Nafcillin	Griseofulvin
	Rifampin	Haloperidol
		Trazodone

Box 7-3. FOODS RICH IN VITAMIN K THAT CAN DIMINISH WARFARIN'S ANTICOAGULANT ACTIONS

Brussels sprouts
Broccoli
Cabbage
Chickpeas
Lettuce
Spinach
Seaweed
Turnip greens
Bok choy
Kohlrabi

Box 7-4. NATURAL PRODUCTS THAT INCREASE THE RISK OF BLEEDING WHEN USED WITH WARFARIN

Black cohosh
Fenugreek
Feverfew
Fish oils
Garlic
Ginger
Ginkgo biloba
Ginseng (Panax)
Horseradish
Licorice
Red clover
Sweet clover
Vitamin E

Box 7-5. NATURAL PRODUCTS THAT DIMINISH THE ANTICOAGULANT EFFECTS OF WARFARIN

Agrimony
Goldenseal
Mistletoe
Yarrow

Box 7-6. CONTRAINDICATIONS TO WARFARIN THERAPY

- Bleeding tendency of any type
- Severe hepatic or renal disease
- Chronic alcoholism
- Vitamin K deficiency
- Malignant hypertension

Clinical use. Warfarin is used for long-term prophylaxis and treatment of DVT and PE. Other uses for warfarin include prophylactic treatment of patients with atrial fibrillation to prevent mural thrombi (although some recent literature indicates aspirin may be a suitable alternative in appropriate patients), rheumatic heart disease, and patients with prosthetic heart valves. Warfarin may also be used as an adjunctive treatment when coronary arteries are occluded.

Adverse effects. The major factor limiting the use of warfarin is the risk of hemorrhage. Warfarin should be discontinued if skin necrosis or nonhemorrhagic purple-toe syndrome occurs. Teratogenicity (including hemorrhagic disorders and abnormal bone formation) prohibits warfarin use during pregnancy. Other contraindications to warfarin use are listed in Box 7-6. It is worth noting that while there is an increased risk of bleeding when warfarin is combined with NSAIDs or salicylates, these combinations are frequently utilized for synergistic anticoagulation.

Antidote. For minor bleeding, warfarin therapy may simply be interrupted. However, for major bleeding, vitamin K may be administered. In emergency situations, clotting factors may be replenished via administration of fresh-frozen plasma or by administration of commercially available factor IX or recombinant factor VIIa.

Monitoring. Historically, prothrombin time (PT) has been used to monitor a patient's response to warfarin therapy. However, since PT is variable depending on the type of thromboplastin used in laboratory assays, the International Normalized Ratio (INR) is currently the recognized gold standard for monitoring warfarin. The INR standardizes PT times so that they are consistent no matter which type of thromboplastin is utilized. For most indications, an INR of 2.0 to 3.0 is sufficient, although in patients with prosthetic (metallic) heart valves or patients with recurrent systemic emboli, an INR of 2.5 to 3.5 may be desired.

Summary

Table 7-3 is a summary of key points that distinguish unfractionated heparin from warfarin. Remember that heparins inhibit activated coagulation factors via activation of antithrombin III, in contrast to warfarin, which inhibits vitamin K–dependent synthesis of coagulation factors (see Fig. 7-2).

●●● ANTIPLATELET DRUGS

While interfering with clotting factors is a good approach for preventing thrombosis, the risk of hemorrhage associated with anticoagulants has necessitated the use of drugs that work through alternative mechanisms. As mentioned previously, platelet adhesion and activation occur at sites of vascular injury where factors such as thromboxane A_2, ADP, collagen, serotonin (5HT), and thrombin facilitate increased expression of glycoprotein IIb/IIIa receptors. This, in turn, leads to platelet adhesion via cross-linking reactions, which occurs following an initial fibrinogen-glycoprotein IIb/IIIa bond. Antiplatelet drugs work on one or more of these targets. Table 7-4 lists endogenous factors and drugs that affect platelet aggregation. Platelet inhibitors include (Fig. 7-3):

- salicylates
- phosphodiesterases

CLINICAL MEDICINE

INR (International Normalized Ratio)

Coagulation of whole blood can be completely prevented in vitro by adding a Ca^{++} chelator such as citrate or EDTA (calcium is required at a variety of different stages of blood clotting in both the extrinsic pathway and the intrinsic pathway). By adding a variety of factors back to citrated platelet-poor plasma, such as phospholipids, kaolin, and thromboplastin, bleeding times can be altered (see the table below).

	Clotting Time
Whole blood	4–8 min
Whole blood + EDTA or citrate	Infinite
Citrated platelet-poor plasma + Ca^{++}	2–4 min
Citrated platelet-poor plasma + phospholipids + Ca^{++}	60–85 sec
Citrated platelet-poor plasma + **kaolin** + phospholipids + Ca^{++}	21–32 sec (aPTT)
Citrated platelet-poor plasma + **thromboplastin** + Ca^{++}	11–12 sec (PT)

The aPTT is used to monitor coagulation status of the intrinsic pathway when heparin is administered, whereas the PT provides an estimate of the coagulation status of the extrinsic pathway when warfarin is given. Since numerous companies manufacture their own thromboplastin (protein + phospholipids) and concentrations of various components tend to vary between different manufacturers, a need for standardization was apparent. In fact, patients' bleeding times were variable depending on the laboratory where their blood was drawn. As a result, each batch of thromboplastin is now required to be "standardized." Today, that standardization is taken into account when the PT is measured and PTs are converted to an international normalized ratio (INR). As a result of thromboplastin standardization, a patient's INR will be consistent regardless of which laboratory is utilized.

- ADP inhibitors
- glycoprotein IIb/IIIa inhibitors

Salicylates

Aspirin

Mechanism of action. Aspirin's main effect is blockade of thromboxane A_2 production from arachidonic acid (Fig. 7-4; see also Fig. 7-3) in platelets, by irreversibly acetylating the enzyme cyclooxygenase, the rate-limiting step in thromboxane synthesis. Remember that aspirin is acetylsalicylic acid and that acetylation of cyclooxygenase leads to inactivation of this enzyme. Platelets lack nuclei, so once aspirin inactivates cyclooxygenase, additional enzyme cannot be resynthesized, which limits most of the actions of aspirin to platelets. Aspirin also inhibits production of prostacyclin from endothelial cells, a prostaglandin that inhibits platelet aggregation. However, this endothelium-specific effect is short-lived since endothelial cells, unlike platelets, can resynthesize cyclooxygenase.

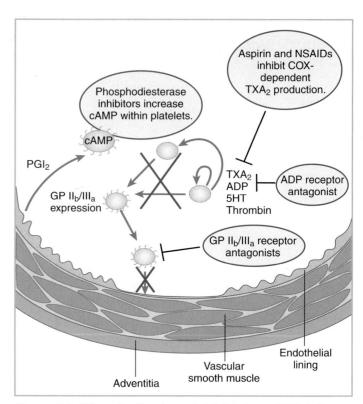

Figure 7-3. Sites of action for antiplatelet drugs. PGI_2 is the natural signal from endothelial cells for inactivating platelet responses through generation of cAMP. PGI_2, prostaglandin I_2.

Clinical use. The most common uses of aspirin are preventing and treating myocardial infarctions and cerebrovascular accidents. Aspirin may also be used in atrial fibrillation and transient ischemic attacks (TIAs). Of course, aspirin is also used for its analgesic, antipyretic, and anti-inflammatory effects as well.

Adverse effects. Children under the age of 12 may develop Reye's syndrome if given aspirin products. Aspirin is known to induce bronchospasm and gastrointestinal hemorrhage, thereby limiting its utility in patients with asthma or peptic ulcer disease.

Phosphodiesterase Inhibitors

Dipyridamole and Cilostazol

Mechanism of action. These phosphodiesterase inhibitors prevent breakdown of cAMP within platelets, and the resultant increase in intracellular cAMP levels leads to diminished platelet activity. Dipyridamole may also inhibit platelet aggregation via inhibiting adenosine uptake by red blood cells or by inhibiting thromboxane A_2 formation.

Clinical use. Dipyridamole may be used adjunctively with warfarin for preventing postoperative thromboembolic complications associated with prosthetic cardiac valves or in combination with aspirin to prevent cerebrovascular ischemia. Cilostazol is used to treat intermittent claudication (exercise-induced pain in legs due to advanced peripheral vascular disease).

Adverse effects. Side effects are mainly limited to hypotension and accompanying dizziness, abdominal distress, headache, and rash.

TABLE 7-3. Warfarin versus Heparin

Parameter	Heparin	Warfarin
Molecular structure	Large polysaccharide, water-soluble	Small molecule, lipid-soluble derivatives of vitamin K
Pharmacokinetics	Given parenterally (IV/SC), hepatic and reticuloendothelial elimination, $t_{1/2} = 2$ hr, no placental access	Given orally (PO), >98% protein bound, liver metabolism, $t_{1/2} = 30+$ hr, placental access
Mechanism of action	↑ Binding of antithrombin III to factors IIa and Xa	↓ Hepatic synthesis of vitamin K–dependent factors II, VII, IX, X → warfarin prevents γ-carboxylation. No effect on factors already present in vivo
Laboratory tests	Activated partial thromboplastin time (aPPT) for unfractionated heparin	Prothrombin time (PT)/international normalized ratio (INR)
Overdose treatment	Protamine sulfate—chemical antagonism, fast onset	Vitamin K ↑ cofactor synthesis = slow onset; fresh-frozen plasma = fast onset
Clinical utility	Rapid anticoagulation (intensive) for thromboses, emboli, unstable angina, disseminated intravascular coagulation (DIC), open-heart surgery	Longer term anticoagulation (controlled) for thromboses, emboli, post-MI, heart valve damage, atrial arrhythmias, cerebrovascular accidents
Adverse effects	Bleeding, osteoporosis, heparin-induced thrombocytopenia (HIT), hypersensitivity	Bleeding, skin necrosis (if low protein C), purple toe syndrome, drug interactions, teratogenicity (bone dysmorphogenesis)

TABLE 7-4. Endogenous Factors and Drugs Affecting Platelet Aggregation

Increased Aggregation	Decreased Aggregation
ADP	PGI_2
5HT	cAMP
Thromboxane A_2	Aspirin
Thrombin	Dipyridamole
	Ticlopidine
	Clopidogrel

PATHOLOGY

Reye's Syndrome

Although rare, Reye's syndrome occurs in childhood and is characterized by encephalitis combined with liver failure. Symptoms may develop during the apparent recovery phase of a viral infection. Treatment focuses on controlling cerebral edema and correcting metabolic abnormalities, but significant mortality occurs from brain damage. While the cause is unknown, aspirin has been implicated and should be avoided in children less than 12 years of age unless specifically indicated. It is suggested that inhibition of cyclooxygenase by aspirin in these patients results in "shuttling" of phospholipase A_2–released arachidonic acid from impaired cyclooxygenases to lipoxygenases, which drives inappropriate production of leukotrienes to initiate and maintain anaphylactoid reactions.

ADP Inhibitors

Clopidogrel and Ticlopidine

Mechanism of action. These agents irreversibly block the ADP receptor on platelets, thus reducing platelet aggregation. Antiplatelet effects persist for the life of the platelet.

Clinical use. Currently, ADP inhibitors are considered the main alternatives to aspirin for preventing thrombotic events in atherogenic patients with recent myocardial infarctions, strokes, TIAs, and unstable angina.

Adverse effects. Similar to other antiplatelet agents, ADP inhibitors increase the risk of bleeding. Clopidogrel is preferred over ticlopidine because of life-threatening hematologic reactions associated with ticlopidine, including neutropenia /agranulocytosis and thrombotic thrombocytopenic purpura.

Glycoprotein IIb/IIIa Inhibitors

Abciximab, Eptifibatide, and Tirofiban

Mechanism of action. Eptifibatide and tirofiban are small-molecule antagonists of the glycoprotein IIb/IIIa receptor on platelets, and abciximab is a monoclonal antibody that targets the same receptor. (Note that abciximab ends in "-mab," denoting that it is a monoclonal antibody.) Activation of this receptor causes fibrinogen and von Willebrand factor to bind to platelets, which subsequently leads to platelet aggregation. These drugs prevent fibrinogen from interacting with platelet glycoprotein IIb/IIIa receptors, thereby inhibiting platelet aggregation.

Clinical use. Glycoprotein IIb/IIIa receptor antagonists are primarily used to manage acute coronary syndromes and to

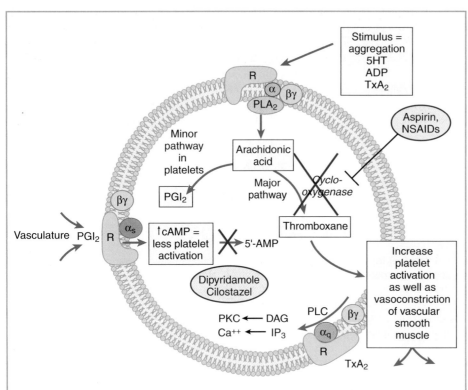

Figure 7-4. Aspirin inhibits cyclooxygenase to prevent thromboxane synthesis. The phosphodiesterase inhibitors increase cAMP, which in turn decreases platelet activation. DAG, diacylglycerol; IP_3, inositol triphosphate; NSAIDs, nonsteroidal anti-inflammatory drugs; PKC, protein kinase C; PLA_2, phospholipase A_2; PLC, phospholipase C; R, receptor; TxA_2, thromboxane A_2.

prevent acute cardiac ischemia in patients undergoing percutaneous coronary intervention.

Adverse effects. In addition to the possibility of hypersensitivity reactions with abciximab, the major adverse effect associated with glycoprotein IIb/IIIa receptor antagonists is bleeding.

●●● THROMBOLYTIC DRUGS

Thrombolytics are the only drugs that actually lyse thrombi. These drugs act by facilitating conversion of plasminogen to plasmin. Plasmin is a nonspecific protease that digests fibrin clots (as well as other clotting factors). These drugs play important roles during acute ischemic events (transmural MI, pulmonary embolism, deep vein thrombosis, and arterial thrombosis and emboli) by not only dissolving clots but also by restoring hemodynamic flow and promoting faster recovery. Notably, there may be greater than a 60% decrease in mortality if thrombolytics are used within 3 hours of an acute MI.

First-generation Thrombolytics

Streptokinase and Urokinase

Mechanism of action. Streptokinase is a protein (but, despite its name, not an enzyme) synthesized by β-hemolytic streptococci that forms a stable 1:1 complex with plasminogen, altering its conformation to facilitate its conversion to plasmin. Owing to its antigenic nature, streptokinase is quickly removed from circulation. Urokinase is an enzyme

produced by human kidney cells that directly converts plasminogen to active plasmin. Both streptokinase and urokinase act on clot-bound plasminogen and free plasminogen. Thus, these thrombolytics not only dissolve pathologic thrombi but also may digest fibrin deposits at other body sites. As such, these drugs tend to be hemorrhagic, creating a lytic state throughout the body, which can result in major bleeding events.

Clinical use. These pharmacologic agents are indicated during treatment of acute events such as evolving transmural MI, pulmonary emboli, deep vein thrombosis, and other arterial thrombosis and emboli.

Adverse effects. Owing to their biological origins, streptokinase is highly antigenic and can cause hypersensitivity reactions, including anaphylaxis. Patients with antistreptococcal antibodies can develop fever or allergic reactions and demonstrate therapeutic resistance. Of course, bleeding events are among the most frequent adverse effects and can be fatal.

Second-generation Thrombolytics: Tissue Plasminogen Activators

Alteplase, Reteplase, and Tenecteplase

Note that the drug names end in "-plase."

Mechanism of action. Recombinant plasminogen activator (t-PA) is released by endothelial cells in response to stasis produced by vascular occlusion. t-PA is co-localized to fibrin. Therefore, exogenous t-PA will preferentially activate plasminogen that is in close proximity to fibrin clots, making

TABLE 7-5. Contraindications to Thrombolytic Therapy

Major Contraindication	Relative Contraindication
Recent surgery or internal biopsy	Paracentesis
Recent cerebrovascular process or neurosurgical procedure	Thoracentesis
	Prolonged CPR
Recent needle puncture of noncompressible vessels	Septic thrombophlebitis
Active bleeding	Any other condition deemed to be a bleeding risk
Uncontrolled hypertension	
Intracranial malignancy	
Pregnancy	
Recent trauma with possible internal injury	
CPR with rib fractures	

these drugs somewhat clot-specific. However, no empiric evidence indicates that the incidence of bleeding events is actually lower with these drugs. In contrast to alteplase or reteplase, tenecteplase may offer an advantage because it is administered as a bolus rather than a 90-minute infusion.

Clinical use. Similar to streptokinase and urokinase, t-PAs are used during management of acute MI, acute ischemic strokes, and acute PE. Yet, in contrast to streptokinase, hypersensitivity reactions are not problematic with these recombinant t-PAs.

Adverse effects. Again, bleeding is the most common adverse effect, with a three-fold higher risk with these agents compared with heparin. Although relatively rare, hemorrhagic stroke is a major concern. Thrombocytopenia may also occur with t-PA. Contraindications are listed in Table 7-5.

●●● BLEEDING DISORDERS

The flip side to drugs that dissolve clots is drugs that induce clotting. The cause of bleeding disorders can generally be classified into one of three groups: genetic, acquired, or iatrogenic (treatment-associated). Hereditary bleeding disorders are rare and typically present as either hemophilia A (factor VIII deficiency), hemophilia B (factor IX deficiency), or von Willebrand's disease (abnormal bruising and mucosal bleeding as a result of a qualitative defect in platelet activity). Acquired causes primarily result from liver disease or vitamin K deficiency. The most important iatrogenic causes for bleeding disorders are the use of anticoagulant therapy and the administration of fibrinolytics. Therapeutic interventions to correct bleeding disorders include administration of clotting factors (fresh-frozen plasma [FFP; factor VIIa, factor VIII, and factor IX concentrates], cofactors [vitamin K], heparin antidotes [protamine], clotting factor agonists [desmopressin], and antifibrinolytic agents [aminocaproic acid, tranexamic acid]). Of note, vitamin K should be infused slowly to prevent

adverse reactions. In addition to its use as an antidote to reverse the effects of oral anticoagulation with warfarin, maternal therapy with vitamin K is used prophylactically to manage drug-induced hypoprothrombinemia as well as hemorrhagic diseases in newborns. Aminocaproic acid and tranexamic acid prevent activation of plasminogen and therefore prevent fibrinolysis. These drugs are especially useful in hemophiliac patients who have undergone surgical procedures or during surgical procedures where large blood losses maybe expected.

●●● ANEMIA

Anemia is a common problem worldwide. Anemia is defined as a hematocrit or hemoglobin value below a normal reference range for specific populations. It is a serious disease in its own right but frequently is a symptom of some other underlying disease. It is further histologically characterized as being microcytic hypochromic (RBCs are small in size and pale), macrocytic hyperchromic (RBCs are large in size and dark) (Fig. 7-5). The most common types of anemias usually result from either blood loss or a deficiency of vitamin B_{12}, folate, and/or iron (the most common cause worldwide) (Table 7-6). The best indicator of iron deficiency is decreased serum ferritin (a storage form of iron) in conjunction with an elevated total iron-binding capacity (TIBC). Causes of iron deficiency typically include inadequate gastrointestinal absorption, blood loss (slow gastrointestinal bleeds), and increased demands for iron (pregnancy, adolescence).

Agents to Treat Anemias

Supplementation with Iron, Vitamin B_{12}, and Folate

Mechanism of action. Dietary supplementation with iron increases serum iron as well as amount of iron stored in liver and bone. Iron is crucial for normal erythropoiesis as well as for the formation of numerous iron-containing proteins (such as hemoglobin). Both vitamin B_{12} and folate are crucial for DNA synthesis and vital for effective erythropoiesis (generation of new RBCs). Megaloblastic anemias result when folic acid– or vitamin B_{12}–dependent nucleic acid synthesis is impaired in immature erythrocytes, since a series of reactions catalyzed by vitamin B_{12} and folate are necessary for both DNA and RNA synthesis. With inadequate amounts of these vitamins, DNA and RNA synthesis is slowed and mitotic divisions are skipped, thus producing abnormally large cells.

Pharmacokinetics. The preferred method of iron supplementation is via the oral route. However, only about 40% to 60% of orally administered iron is absorbed. Foods that are rich in iron, as well as foods that aid gastrointestinal iron absorption or inhibit iron absorption, are listed in Box 7-7. As a general rule, iron is best absorbed on an empty stomach, but gastrointestinal intolerance may render this impossible. Doses of iron should be based on the elemental dose of iron. Table 7-7 shows the amount of elemental iron obtained from different ferrous salts. Parenteral iron is an option for patients

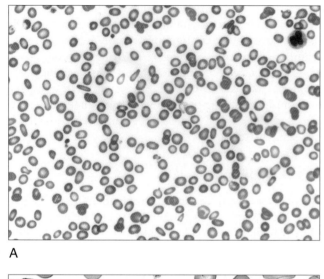

A

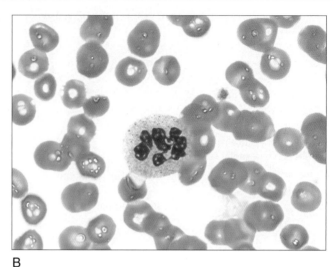

B

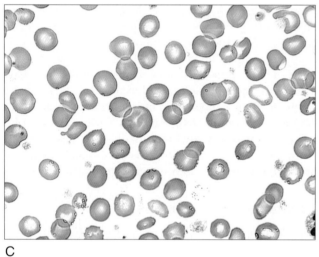

C

Figure 7-5. Red blood cells. **A**, Normal RBCs. **B**, Hypochromic microcytes. **C**, Oval macrocytes. (Courtesy of Alvin Telser, PhD, Northwestern University.)

who are intolerant of or noncompliant with oral iron therapy; who continue to experience blood loss, perhaps via gastrointestinal bleeding; and who have malabsorptive disorders, perhaps due to bowel removal. Iron can form complexes with other medications, impairing the absorption of both iron and the target drug. Drugs that interfere with iron absorption include tetracyclines and fluoroquinolone antibiotics.

Oral vitamin B_{12} may be used for nutritional deficiencies; however, parenteral B_{12} (cyanocobalamin or hydroxycobalamin) should be used if a lack of transcobalamin is causing inadequate B_{12} absorption.

Clinical use. Iron is helpful for treating certain types of microcytic anemias. Hematologic responses begin within 3 days of initiation of iron replacement therapy. Vitamin B_{12} and folate are used to treat macrocytic anemias that are caused by B_{12} and folate deficiency, respectively (Box 7-8). It is also recommended that all women of childbearing age take folate to prevent neural tube defects in their offspring. While recent data show that folate lowers homocysteine levels, it may not offer protection against atherosclerosis.

Adverse effects. Iron causes GI upset including nausea, vomiting, constipation, a metallic taste, and darkened stools.

Patients who experience constipation may be supplied with a stool softener. Iron may also discolor the urine. Iron tablets are the most common cause of accidental overdose (and death) for children under 6 years of age. Parenterally administered iron may cause anaphylactic hypersensitivity reactions, serum sickness, and pain at the site of injection. Parenterally administered vitamin B_{12} may be associated with anaphylaxis. Hyperuricemia, hypokalemia, and Na retention may also occur, and these laboratory parameters should be monitored.

Hemapoietic Stimulating Factors

Erythropoietins (epoetin α, darbepoetin α), Granulocyte Colony-stimulating Factor (G-CSF; filgrastim, pegfilgrastim), Granulocyte-macrophage Colony-stimulating Factor (GM-CSF; sargramostim)

Note: The drugs in parentheses are recombining forms of natural hormones.

Mechanism of action. Erythropoietin is normally produced in the kidneys in response to a decrease in blood O_2 tension.

TABLE 7-6. Comparing Three Common Anemias

Anemia	Microscopic Appearance	Clinical Features	Laboratory Findings
Iron deficiency	Microcytic	Pallor	Decreased hematocrit
		Tachycardia	Decreased hemoglobin
		Lightheadedness	Low or normal reticulocyte count
		Breathlessness	Decreased serum iron
		Fatigue	Decreased serum ferritin
		Headache	Elevated TIBC
		Sensitivity to cold	Decreased transferrin saturation ratio
		Loss of skin tone	
Vitamin B_{12} deficiency	Macrocytic	Weakness	Low or normal reticulocyte count
		Painful, enlarged tongue	Decreased vitamin B_{12}
		Paresthesias	Mean corpuscular volume typically elevated
		Nausea	
		Anorexia	
		Ataxia	
		Dementia	
Folate deficiency	Macrocytic	Pallor	Low or normal reticulocyte count
		Fatigued	Decreased serum folate
		Cardiac symptoms	Decreased hematocrit
			Decreased hemoglobin

Box 7-7. FOODS THAT AFFECT IRON ABSORPTION

Good dietary sources of iron

Red meats
Raisins
Fish
Eggs
Legumes
Potatoes
Rice

Foods that aid iron absorption

Vitamin C
Meat
Orange juice

Foods/drugs that impair iron absorption

Milk
Tea
Phytates
Antacids
Tetracyclines
Fluoroquinolones

TABLE 7-7. Elemental Iron in Various Iron Salts

Iron Salt	Amount of Elmental Iron
Ferrous sulfate 300 mg	60 mg
Ferrous gluconate 300 mg	35 mg
Ferrous fumarate 100 mg	33 mg

Box 7-8. RISK FACTORS FOR FOLATE DEFICIENCY

Decreased absorption caused by

Celiac disease
Crohn's disease

Inadequate intake caused by

Alcoholism
Advanced age
Malnutrition/poverty

Hyperutilization caused by

Pregnancy
Growth spurts

Vitamin B$_{12}$ and Folate Demand

Since all animal products contain vitamin B$_{12}$, only strict vegetarians are at risk of B$_{12}$ dietary deficiencies. Other risk factors for vitamin B$_{12}$ deficiencies include decreased gastrointestinal absorption (possibly due to removal of the bowel) and inadequate utilization due to transcobalamin (a transport protein) deficiency in the gastrointestinal tract. Folate deficiency is more common than vitamin B$_{12}$ deficiency. Humans must obtain folate through their diet, and the most common cause of folate deficiency is lack of dietary green vegetables. In addition to inadequate intake, other risk factors include decreased absorption and hyperutilization. Folate demand increases during pregnancy. Evidence now shows that periconceptional folate supplementation in normal women reduces the incidence of fetal neuronal tube defects (spina bifida, meningocoele, anencephaly). Folate is absolutely necessary for the developing fetal nervous system. Newborns with congenital folate malabsorption syndrome are born with mental retardation, cerebral calcifications, seizures, and peripheral neuropathies.

Erythropoietin stimulates erythropoiesis (RBC production) and increases the hematocrit. Recombinant erythropoietin is the predominant form available for use in patients. Filgrastim and pegfilgrastim stimulate proliferation, differentiation, migration, and functional activity of neutrophils. Sargramostim stimulates proliferation, differentiation, and functional activity of neutrophils, monocytes, and macrophages. Unlike the filgrastims, sargramostim inhibits neutrophil migration.

Pharmacokinetics. Compared with epoetin α, darbepoetin α has a three-fold longer $t_{1/2}$, thus requiring fewer infusions per month. Pegfilgrastim (administered subcutaneously) has the advantage of a longer duration of activity over filgrastim (administered intravenously); thus, it can be administered once per chemotherapy cycle.

Clinical use. Erythropoietin has demonstrated clear benefits in patients with anemia as a result of chronic renal failure and in patients following chemotherapy. It can also be helpful before allogenic blood transfusions. Filgrastims are used to decrease the duration and extent of neutropenia. Sargramostim also decreases the duration and extent of neutropenia and is used for myeloid reconstitution after bone marrow transplantation and after chemotherapy (see Chapter 5 for review). These types of drugs can be misused by athletes for performance enhancement.

Adverse effects. With erythropoietin, there have been reports of dose-dependent increases in blood pressure and platelet counts. Some people experience influenza-like symptoms and hypersensitivities. Leukocytosis, accompanied by risk of splenic rupture, may occur if the neutrophil count rises too high with the filgrastims or sargramostims. Sargramostim may cause local reactions at the injection site (50%). This is minimized when the drug is given intravenously or very slowly by the subcutaneous route. Bone pain and anaphylaxis may occur with filgrastims or sargramostim.

TOP FIVE LIST

1. Heparin inhibits coagulation by combining with and activating antithrombin III, resulting in more efficient inactivation of clotting factors IIa, IXa, and Xa. aPTT is used to monitor the effects of heparin on the intrinsic coagulation pathway, and protamine is an antidote if excessive bleeding occurs.
2. Low-molecular-weight heparins (LMWHs) inhibit coagulation by combining with and activating antithrombin III, resulting in efficient inactivation primarily of factor Xa. LMWHs have a predictable dose-response; routine anticoagulation monitoring is not usually necessary.
3. Warfarin derives its anticoagulant actions through inhibition of hepatic carboxylation of vitamin K–dependent clotting factors, i.e., clotting factors II, VII, IX, and X. Warfarin's effects are monitored by PT (or more reliably INR). In the event of excessive bleeding, vitamin K, fresh-frozen plasma, or concentrated clotting factors may be administered. More food, drug, and herb interactions occur with warfarin than any other drug.
4. A variety of drugs—COX inhibitors, phosphodiesterase inhibitors, ADP inhibitors, and glycoprotein IIb/IIIa inhibitors—inhibit coagulation by inhibiting platelets through different signal transduction mechanisms.
5. Unlike other drugs used in anticoagulation, thrombolytics actually lyse existing clots rather than simply preventing additional clot formation.

Keep in mind that bleeding events are common with all anticoagulants.

Cardiovascular System 8

CONTENTS

It's more than just the curve, that is, the Frank-Starling curve—left ventricular end diastolic pressure is proportional to stroke volume. In more clinical terms, pathologies that result in altered cardiac output, due to changes in stroke volume or heart rate, can be treated with drugs that affect hemodynamic parameters that control left ventricular end diastolic pressure, such as preload and afterload. However, drugs that regulate hemodynamic parameters are often ineffective and do not prolong life in patients with failing hearts. In reality, it's all about making the failing heart more effective (i.e., moving the Frank-Starling curve upward and to the left). This can be accomplished pharmacologically by increasing myocardial contractility through positive inotropes, as well as by reducing inefficient cardiac hypertrophy via angiotensin-converting enzyme (ACE) inhibitors and angiotensin receptor blockers (ARBs).

Pathologies that compromise cardiac output include hypertension, coronary artery disease, heart failure, cardiac arrhythmias, and hypercholesterolemia. Since these conditions affect multiple parameters associated with cardiac output and total peripheral resistance, it should not be surprising that there is considerable overlap in the drugs used to treat these five medical conditions and the drugs frequently are used in combination.

In many ways, cardiovascular pharmacology fits hand-in-hand with autonomic pharmacology. Many drugs used for treatment of cardiovascular disease act as agonists or antagonists of the α- or β-adrenergic receptors in the heart and the vasculature. Regulation of these receptors modulates preload and afterload pressures, total peripheral resistance, and myocardial contractility, culminating in control of cardiac output.

●●● PHARMACOLOGIC MANAGEMENT OF HYPERTENSION

Regulation of blood pressure is all about communication, exquisite wireless communication between organ systems. Receptors that assess pressure and solute concentrations

PHYSIOLOGY

Defining Blood Pressure
Blood pressure is the product of cardiac output × total peripheral resistance (BP = CO × TPR). Cardiac output is a product of heart rate × stroke volume (CO = HR × SV). Stroke volume is a function of preload (the amount of blood returning to the heart), afterload (the pressure that the heart must pump against), and contractility. Antihypertensives either lower cardiac output or lower total peripheral resistance.

regulate interconnected neuronal, cardiovascular, and renal networks. The interplay between the renal, neuronal, and cardiovascular systems ultimately controls blood pressure (*total peripheral resistance* and *cardiac output*) through tight control of fluid and solute load as well as endogenous regulators of vasoconstriction. Disturbances in these feed-forward and feed-back pathways lead to exacerbations of cardiovascular disease and identify targets for pharmacologic intervention.

Identifiable causes of hypertension (and methods for controlling it) are summarized in Box 8-1 and Figure 8-1. In patients with hypertension, baroreceptors acquire a new set point that is higher than normal, resulting in central stimulation of the sympathetic nervous system. This heightened sympathetic tone increases norepinephrine release.

In the heart, norepinephrine increases myocardial contractility and heart rate via actions at β_1-receptors, thereby increasing cardiac output. Increased noradrenergic activity in the vasculature directly stimulates vasoconstriction via actions at α_1-receptors, which increases total peripheral resistance.

Norepinephrine also stimulates renal β_1 receptor–mediated release of renin, which activates the renin-angiotensin-aldosterone pathway. Renin is the enzyme that cleaves angiotensinogen to form angiotensin I, which is then hydrolyzed by ACE into angiotensin II. Angiotensin II is a potent vasoconstrictor. Angiotensin II also stimulates the release of aldosterone from the adrenal gland, which leads to sodium reabsorption. Ultimately, activation of the renin-angiotensin-aldosterone (RAA) system increases total peripheral resistance via vasoconstriction and increases cardiac output via sodium (and water) retention.

Box 8-1. IDENTIFIABLE CAUSES OF HYPERTENSION

Sleep apnea
Illicit drug use (cocaine, amphetamines)
Chronic kidney disease
Primary aldosteronism
Renovascular disease
Chronic steroid therapy
Cushing syndrome
Pheochromocytoma
Coarctation of the aorta
Thyroid disease
Parathyroid disease

CLINICAL MEDICINE

Controlling Blood Pressure

As blood pressure rises, there is a greater risk of coronary artery disease, stroke, and kidney disease. Therefore, it is imperative to get blood pressure under control to reduce related cardiovascular morbidity and mortality. When hypertension is first noted, an identifiable cause should be considered, but 95% of the time an obvious cause cannot be found.

Figure 8-1. Network control of blood pressure.

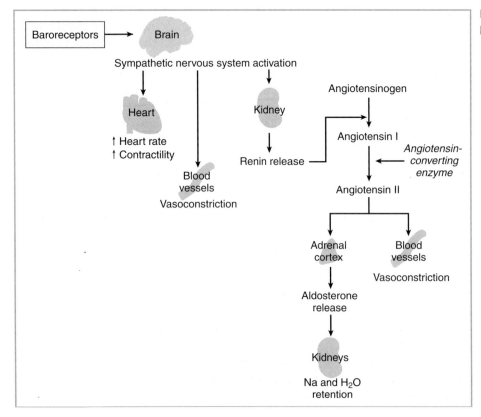

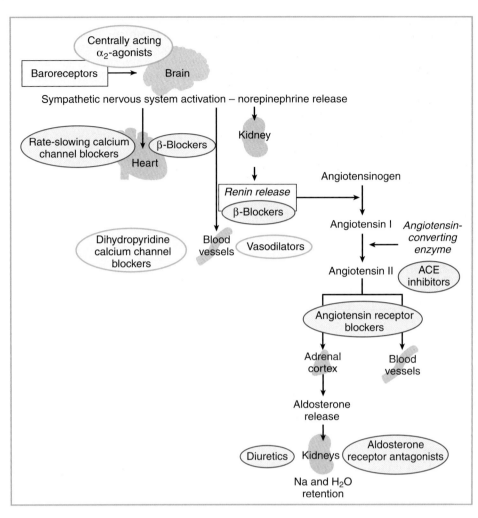

Figure 8-2. Site of action for antihypertensive drugs.

Identifying the mechanisms that underlie hypertension helps define targets or pathways suitable for pharmacologic intervention (Fig. 8-2). Briefly, centrally acting α_2-agonists inhibit norepinephrine release. β-Blockers decrease cardiac output by slowing heart rate and decreasing myocardial contractility. β-Blockers also antagonize renal β_1-receptors to block renin release, thereby preventing activation of the renin-angiotensin-aldosterone system. ACE inhibitors, ARBs, and aldosterone receptor antagonists block various steps within the RAA pathway. Diuretics reduce cardiac output by increasing excretion of Na^+ and H_2O. Direct-acting vasodilators may be used to directly vasodilate the vasculature to reduce total peripheral resistance. Additionally, calcium channel blockers, which inhibit the actions of Ca^{++} in the myocardium or the periphery, may also be used to decrease myocardial contractility and heart rate and reduce total peripheral resistance.

The Joint National Committee on Prevention, Detection, Evaluation, and Treatment of High Blood Pressure published its seventh set of guidelines for managing hypertension in 2003 (JNC-VII). These guidelines are summarized in Figure 8-3. Although these guidelines are currently the gold standard for hypertension management, some hypertension specialists prefer to treat patients according to whether they exhibit high

plasma renin activity or have a volumetric (sodium) excess. Drug choices for each of these types of hypertension are listed in Table 8-1.

The following classes of drugs are used to treat hypertension:

- Diuretics
- β-Blockers
- ACE inhibitors
- ARBs
- Aldosterone-receptor antagonists
- α_1-Blockers
- Ca^{++} channel blockers
- Centrally acting α_2-blockers
- Vasodilators

TABLE 8-1. Antihypertensive Treatment Options*

Volumetric Excess	High Renin Activity
Thiazide or loop diuretics	ACE inhibitors
Spironolactone	ARBs
Ca^{++} channel blockers	β-Blockers
α-Blockers	

*Based on volumetric excess or high renin activity.

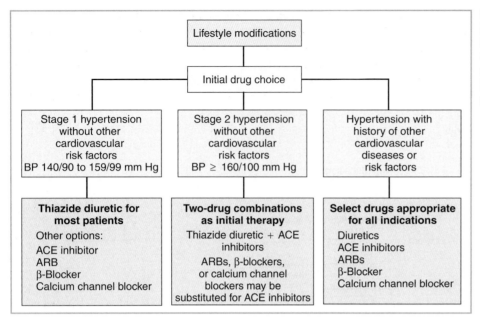

Figure 8-3. Algorithm for initial hypertension treatment. (Data from the Seventh Report of the Joint National Committee on Prevention, Evaluation, and Treatment of High Blood Pressure, Dec. 2003. www.nhlbi.nih.gov/guidelines/hypertension/index.htm.)

Diuretics

Thiazides, Loop Diuretics, and K⁺-sparing Drugs

Thiazides include hydrochlorothiazide, chlorthalidone, metolazone, indapamide. Examples of loop diuretics are furosemide and bumetanide. K^+-sparing drugs are spironolactone, triamterene, and amiloride.

An initial strategy for managing hypertension is often to alter volumetric excess through dietary restriction of Na^+. Diuretics (see Chapter 9) essentially capitalize on sodium restriction, since these drugs facilitate sodium excretion. Diuretics are often included in antihypertensive treatment regimens.

In hypertension management, diuretics initially decrease blood volume by facilitating Na^+ excretion, hence reducing extracellular fluid volume; however, antihypertensive effects are maintained even after excess Na^+ has been diuresed. It has been speculated that high plasma sodium increases vessel rigidity; thus, antihypertensive effects are maintained because low plasma sodium indirectly induces vasodilation.

According to JNC-VII, thiazide diuretics are the first-line antihypertensive for most patients. These drugs are particularly effective antihypertensives for patients of African ancestry and the elderly. Note, however, that with the exception of metolazone, thiazides are not effective at low glomerular filtration rates; therefore, loop diuretics are preferred when kidney function is compromised. In addition, thiazides are often not first-line choices for diabetic patients or patients with hyperlipidemias, since the drugs may exacerbate these conditions. Often, K^+-sparing diuretics (amiloride and triamterene) are used in combination with thiazides to offset K^+ loss.

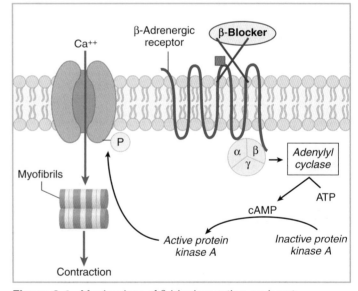

Figure 8-4. Mechanism of β-blocker action on heart.

Beta-Blockers

Beta-1 Selective: Acebutolol, Atenolol, Betaxolol, and Bisoprolol

Nonselective: Carteolol, Esmolol, Labetolol, Metoprolol, Nadolol, Penbutolol, Pindolol, Propranolol, Sotolol and Timolol

Note that the drug names all end in "-olol."

Mechanism of action. β-Blockers are antagonists of β-adrenergic receptors. Figure 8-4 illustrates how β-blockade *prevents* accumulation of cAMP and activation of protein kinase A, thereby reducing Ca^{++} entry into myocardial cells, decreasing heart rate, and reducing myocardial contractility.

These combined effects reduce cardiac output and are responsible for initial antihypertensive effects. In addition, β-blockers exert sustained antihypertensive actions by antagonizing β$_1$-receptors in the kidneys, an effect that reduces renin release and decreases total peripheral resistance.

β-Blockers are not all created equal. For the most part, selective β$_1$-receptor blockers, such as metoprolol and atenolol, are the preferred β-blockers to treat hypertension, especially for patients with peripheral vascular disease or airway diseases such as asthma or chronic obstructive pulmonary disease (COPD). Remember that nonselective blockade of β$_2$-receptors in the lung can aggravate pulmonary bronco-constriction and airway resistance. Therefore, propranolol may aggravate these conditions, since it blocks both β$_1$- and β$_2$-receptor subtypes.

Other nonselective β-antagonists, such as pindolol, possess intrinsic sympathomimetic activity (ISA) because they exhibit partial agonist activity. A partial agonist *weakly* stimulates the receptor to which it is bound but simultaneously blocks the activity of stronger endogenous agonists (epinephrine or nonepinephrine). It is difficult to define pindolol as a β-antagonist when, in fact, it is really a poor agonist. This partial β-agonist activity decreases blood pressure, but it does not induce bradycardia. β-Blockers that possess intrinsic sympathomimetic activity should not be used in patients with angina or those who are post–myocardial infarction.

β-Blockers such as labetalol and carvedilol also are not selective β$_1$-blockers, but these drugs antagonize both α- and β-adrenergic receptors. By antagonizing α-adrenergic receptors in the vasculature, these drugs preferentially reduce total peripheral resistance in the periphery without causing significant effects on heart rate or cardiac output. Thus, these drugs are especially useful to manage special hypertensive situations such as pheochromocytoma (an epinephrine-secreting tumor of the adrenal medulla) and hypertensive crisis. Clinically relevant pharmacologic differences among various β-blockers are highlighted in Table 8-2.

Clinical use. In addition to their use as antihypertensives, β-blockers are used as antiarrhythmics and for management of angina and treatment of heart failure, and they should be included in most post–myocardial infarction therapeutic regimens. β-Blockers also are used prophylactically to prevent migraine headaches and may be administered ocularly to reduce intraocular pressure (IOP). Timolol decreases IOP by preventing production of aqueous humor. Some unique indications for β-blockers are listed in Table 8-3.

Adverse effects. Since β-blockers depress myocardial contractility and excitability, they may cause hypotension, may precipitate cardiac conduction abnormalities (second- or third-degree AV block), may worsen acutely decompensated congestive heart failure, and may cause bradycardia. β-Blockers are *absolutely contraindicated* in patients who have profound sinus bradycardia and greater than first-degree heart block or signs of bronchoconstriction. Therapy with β-blockers should not be stopped abruptly, because rebound hypertension may occur. β-Blockers commonly cause fatigue, malaise, sedation, depression, and sexual dysfunction. These drugs may also impair the ability to exercise, since they lower the maximal exercise-induced heart rate. Additionally, β-blockers inhibit sympathetically stimulated lipolysis, inhibit hepatic glycogenolysis, mask symptoms of hypoglycemia (e.g., tremor, cardiac palpitations), mask symptoms of hyperthyroidism, and adversely affect cholesterol levels. Overall, relative contraindications for β-blockers are listed in Box 8-2.

Angiotensin-converting Enzyme (ACE) Inhibitors

Enalapril, Lisinopril, Captopril, Benazepril, Fosinopril, Quinapril, Ramipril, Moexipril, and Perindopril

TABLE 8-2. Pharmacologic Differences Among β-Blockers (Commonly Used Drugs)

β$_1$/β$_2$ Non-selective Antagonists	β$_1$-Selective Antagonists	Nonselective Agents with Intrinsic Sympatho-mimetic Activity (ISA)	α- and β-Antagonists
Carteolol	Acebutolol	Acebutolol	Carvedilol
Nadolol	Atenolol	Carteolol	Labetalol
Penbutolol	Betaxolol	Pindolol	
Pindolol	Bisoprolol		
Propranolol	Esmolol		
Sotalol	Metoprolol		
Timolol			

TABLE 8-3. Unique Uses for Commonly Used β-Blockers

β-Blocker	Use
Esmolol	Hypertensive emergencies (IV)
Timolol	Ocular hypotensive effects in glaucoma
Labetalol	Hypertensive crisis
Propranolol	Migraine prophylaxis
Carvedilol	Congestive heart failure

Box 8-2. RELATIVE CONTRAINDICATIONS FOR USE OF β-BLOCKERS

- Asthma
- AV block
- Bradycardia
- Chronic obstructive pulmonary disease (COPD)
- Uncontrolled diabetes mellitus

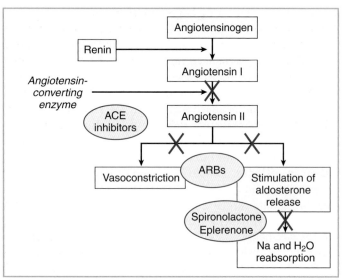

Figure 8-5. Hypertension can be controlled by pharmacologically regulating the renin-angiotensin-aldosterone (RAA) system.

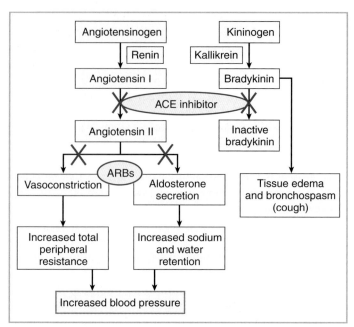

Figure 8-6. ACE inhibitors cause bradykinin accumulation.

Note that the drug names all end in "-pril."

Mechanism of action. ACE inhibitors reduce total peripheral resistance by blocking the actions of angiotensin-converting enzyme, the enzyme that converts angiotensin I to angiotensin II (Fig. 8-5). Recall that angiotensin II is a potent vasoconstrictor and stimulates release of aldosterone from the adrenal cortex, which causes sodium and water retention. ACE inhibitors are balanced vasodilators, meaning that they cause vasodilation of both arteries and veins. Unlike other vasodilators, this class of drugs does not exert reflex actions on the sympathetic nervous system (tachycardia, increased cardiac output, fluid retention). Finally, as angiotensin II also possesses mitogenic activity in the myocardium, inhibition of angiotensin II may lead to diminished myocardial hypertrophy or remodeling, situations often seen in patients with hypertension or heart failure.

Clinical use. ACE inhibitors are especially useful antihypertensives in young and middle-aged Caucasians. Elderly and black patients are relatively resistant to the antihypertensive effects of ACE inhibitors, but resistance can be overcome by adding diuretics to the regimen. Some of this resistance has been linked to a high-salt diet, which induces hypertension despite a low renin state. ACE inhibitors have beneficial actions in heart failure and reduce the risk of strokes, even in patients with well-controlled blood pressure. ACE inhibitors also slow progression of kidney disease in patients with diabetic nephropathies. Renal benefits are probably due to improved renal hemodynamics from decreased glomerular arteriolar resistance.

Adverse effects. As many as 40% of patients cannot tolerate ACE inhibitors due to induction of a dry cough. This cough is thought to occur as a result of accumulation of bradykinin. Normally, ACE converts bradykinin to inactive metabolites. However, when ACE is inhibited, bradykinin concentration rises. Bradykinin causes tissue edema and bronchospasm, so

PHYSIOLOGY

Sodium and Water Retention

Diminished afferent arteriolar pressure causes the kidney to release renin, which then converts angiotensinogen to angiotensin I. Angiotensin-converting enzyme removes two terminal amino acids from angiotensin I to form angiotensin II. Angiotensin II stimulates aldosterone secretion from the adrenal cortex. Aldosterone release increases expression of renal Na^+ channels, facilitating sodium reabsorption and water retention.

bradykinin accumulation is thought to be responsible for causing the cough (Fig. 8-6). Bradykinin accumulation may also induce angioedema of the lips and tongue, even after patients have used ACE inhibitors for many years. Dysgeusia (unpleasant taste in the mouth) and rashes are possible. Severe hypotension may occur in patients who are volume-depleted. Hyperkalemia may also occur, due to inhibition of aldosterone, especially in patients using potassium supplements and potassium-sparing diuretics. ACE inhibitors are contraindicated during the second and third trimesters of pregnancy because of adverse effects on the fetus (fetal hypotension, anuria, renal failure, fetal malformation). ACE inhibitors are also contraindicated in patients with bilateral renal artery stenosis, in whom they can cause acute renal failure.

Angiotensin Receptor Blockers

Losartan, Candesartan, Eprosartan, Irbesartan, Olmesartan, Telmisartan, and Valsartan

Note that all end in "-sartan."

Mechanism of action. In contrast to ACE inhibitors, which inhibit production of angiotensin II, ARBs block the effects of angiotensin II by acting as antagonists at angiotensin II receptors. This action results in decreased vasoconstriction and decreased release of aldosterone and antidiuretic hormone.

Clinical use. ARBs are used for treating the same conditions as ACE inhibitors. However, ARBs may be better tolerated than ACE inhibitors because of the lack of bradykinin-induced bronchospasm.

Adverse effects. ARBs are less likely than ACE inhibitors to cause angioedema or cough. However, like ACE inhibitors, ARBs can cause hyperkalemia and are contraindicated during pregnancy.

Aldosterone Receptor Antagonists

Spironolactone and Eplerenone

Mechanism of action. These drugs bind to cytosolic mineralocorticoid receptors and block aldosterone from binding its receptors and inducing nuclear localization. Thus, the action of aldosterone to increase blood pressure, by reabsorbing Na^+, is inhibited. When aldosterone receptors are blocked, Na^+ is excreted but K^+ is retained. Thus, as discussed in Chapter 9, spironolactone is known as a K^+-sparing diuretic. Spironolactone also antagonizes other steroid receptor subtypes, explaining its adverse endocrine effects. Eplerenone is a specific antagonist of aldosterone receptors.

Adverse effects. Spironolactone and eplerenone can cause hyperkalemia. Eplerenone is contraindicated in patients with poor renal function or patients using potent P-450 3A4 inhibitors (e.g., "azole" antifungals, clarithromycin, ritonavir), since eplerenone is metabolized by hepatic P-450 enzymes.

Alpha-1 Receptor Blockers

Prazosin, Doxazosin, and Terazosin

Note that all end in "-zosin."

Mechanism of action. These drugs antagonize α_1-receptors in the periphery, leading to vasodilation. However, patients compensate through reflex tachycardia (due to baroreceptor-induced sympathetic neuronal activity) and increased release of renin.

Clinical use. Unfortunately, these compensatory mechanisms have been shown to contribute to heart failure. As a result, α_1-receptor blockers are not routinely recommended for treating hypertension and are reserved as last-line agents. Another use for these drugs is in management of benign prostatic hypertrophy. In the prostate and the neck of the bladder, α_1-antagonists reduce smooth muscle tone, thus relieving urinary symptoms.

Calcium Channel Blockers

Myocardial Specific: Verapamil and Diltiazem
Vascular-acting Dihydropyridines: Amlodipine, Felodipine, Isradipine, Nicardine, Nifedipine, Nimodipine, and Nisoldipine

Note that the dihydropyridines all end in "-dipine."

Mechanism of action. All calcium channel blockers prevent Ca^{++} from entering either cardiac or vascular smooth muscle cells. Verapamil and diltiazem preferentially block calcium entry into myocardial cells. In myocytes, Ca^{++} binds to troponin, which relieves troponin's inhibitory effects, thus allowing actin and myosin to interact. The actions of verapamil or diltiazem result in bradycardia, reduced contractility, and slowed AV conduction. Antihypertensive effects occur as a result of decreased cardiac output.

Dihydropyridines interfere with vasoconstriction by blocking Ca^{++} entry into vascular smooth muscle cells. In vascular smooth muscle cells, Ca^{++} binds to calmodulin. This calcium-calmodulin complex activates calmodulin kinase, which phosphorylates myosin, thus stimulating contraction. Antihypertensive effects occur as a result of diminished vascular smooth muscle contraction and reduced total peripheral resistance.

Nifedipine is unique in that it blocks Ca^{++} influx in both myocardial tissues and the vasculature, exhibiting properties of both verapamil and the dihydropyridines; however, the effects on the myocardium are much less than those in the periphery.

Clinical use. Calcium channel blockers are especially useful antihypertensives in patients who have low-renin hypertension. Heart rate–slowing Ca^{++} channel blockers, like verapamil and diltiazem, are also used as antiarrhythmics. Additional uses for Ca^{++} channel blockers include angina, migraine prophylaxis, and preterm labor.

Adverse effects. Calcium channel blockers that cause bradycardia (verapamil and diltiazem) should be avoided in patients with heart failure or cardiac conduction defects, especially if patients are also prescribed β-blockers. Dihydropyridines cause peripheral edema, hypotension, dizziness, flushing, and headaches, due to their vasodilatory effects. All Ca^{++} channel blockers may cause or worsen gastroesophageal reflux disease (GERD), by lowering lower esophageal sphincter tone. Many Ca^{++} channel blockers are highly protein-bound, so drug interactions are likely when other highly bound drugs are given concurrently.

Centrally Acting Alpha-2 Agonists

Methyldopa and Clonidine

Mechanism of action. These drugs act as agonists of synaptic α_2-receptors in the central nervous system (Fig. 8-7). Essentially, these receptors are autoreceptors; when stimulated, they feed-back to negatively inhibit adrenergic tone and decrease norepinephrine release in the periphery. Ultimately, antihypertensive effects result from (1) decreased total peripheral resistance, (2) blunted baroreceptor reflexes (these drugs cause very little tachycardia), (3) decreased heart rate, and (4) reduced renin activity.

Pharmacokinetics. Clonidine exerts its actions directly on α_2-receptors. In contrast, methyldopa acts indirectly. Methyldopa is converted to α-methylnorepinephrine by the same enzymes involved in the biosynthesis of dopamine and is released as a false neurotransmitter (Fig. 8-8). Methylnor-

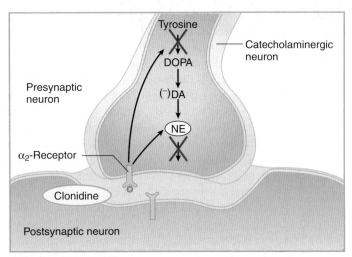

Figure 8-7. Mechanism of centrally acting α_2-agonists. Clonidine binds to α_2-autoreceptors and via feedback inhibition, prevents neurotransmitter synthesis and release. DA, dopamine; NE, norepinephrine.

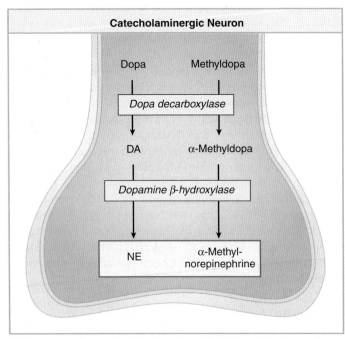

Figure 8-8. Central activation of methyldopa. DA, dopamine; DOPA, dihydroxyphenylalanine; NE, norepinephrine.

epinephrine is the "active" drug that stimulates presynaptic α_2-receptors centrally. Clonidine is available as an oral tablet and as a transdermal patch that is applied once weekly.

Clinical use. Methyldopa is often used to manage eclampsia during pregnancy. In addition to its antihypertensive actions, clonidine is used off-label to manage numerous conditions including alcohol withdrawal, attention deficit hyperactivity disorder, mania, psychosis, and restless leg syndrome. Clonidine is useful in combination with vasodilators, to blunt reflex tachycardia.

Adverse effects. The adverse effects associated with these two drugs are quite different from each other. Prolonged use of methyldopa causes sodium and water retention; therefore, it is best used in combination with diuretics. Orthostatic hypotension may occur and is more likely in patients who are volume-depleted. Methyldopa can cause hepatitis, so liver function tests should be monitored regularly during therapy, and methyldopa may also cause hemolytic anemia. Because of structural similarities with dopamine, Parkinson symptoms, hyperprolactinemia, galactorrhea, gynecomastia, and decreased libido may also occur.

Clonidine is associated with central side effects including sedation, sleep disturbances, nightmares, and restlessness. These effects are worsened when the drug is used simultaneously with other central nervous system depressants. Clonidine should never be discontinued abruptly, because severe rebound hypertension occurs from massive release of catecholamines from the adrenal gland.

Vasodilators

Sodium Nitroprusside, Hydralazine, and Minoxidil

Mechanism of action. These drugs directly relax vascular smooth muscle, decreasing total peripheral resistance. Nitroprusside is metabolized in vascular endothelial cells to nitric oxide. Nitric oxide activates guanylyl cyclase to form cGMP. cGMP exerts vasodilatory actions in both arteries and veins, thus making nitroprusside a useful intravenous option for managing hypertensive crisis. (Additional nitric oxide–producing drugs are discussed later in more detail as treatments for stable angina.) The mechanism of hydralazine is unknown, but it directly relaxes smooth muscle only in the arteries. Minoxidil stimulates ATP-activated potassium channels in smooth muscle. Increased intracellular potassium stabilizes the membrane at resting potential and makes vasoconstriction less likely. Like hydralazine, minoxidil vasodilates only arteries.

Pharmacokinetics. Metabolism of hydralazine is by acetylation and is genetically determined. Roughly half the population are rapid acetylators, and half slow acetylators. Hydralazine has a plasma half-life of only 1 hour, yet its hypotensive effects persist for 12 hours—a phenomenon for which there is no explanation, in part because the mechanism of this drug is unknown.

Nitroprusside has a rapid onset of action and a short half-life. Typically, the effects of this drug subside within 1 to 2 minutes of discontinuing infusions. The drug is metabolized to cyanide and nitrite ions, both of which are responsible for adverse effects.

Clinical use. Typically hydralazine and minoxidil are reserved for treatment-resistant hypertension. Since compensatory mechanisms tend to counteract the actions of vasodilators, these drugs are most effective when combined with a diuretic (to counteract sodium retention) and a β-blocker (to counteract reflex sympathetic activation that causes reflex tachycardia and renin release). As mentioned, nitroprusside is usually reserved for hypertensive crisis (Box 8-3 lists other drugs that are also used to manage hypertensive crisis.)

Box 8-3. EXAMPLES OF INTRAVENOUS DRUGS USED TO MANAGE HYPERTENSIVE CRISIS

Enalaprilat
Esmolol
Hydralazine
Labetalol
Nicardipine
Nitroglycerin
Nitroprusside

Topically, minoxidil is used to treat male-pattern baldness.
Adverse effects. Tachycardia and fluid retention occur to compensate for drug-induced vasodilation. In addition, flushing, headache, and hypotension occur because of vasodilation. Since arterial vasodilators cause reflex tachycardia, these drugs can exacerbate angina or myocardial ischemia.

Hydralazine can cause lupus-like syndromes; therefore, arthralgias, myalgias, rash, fever, anemia, antinuclear antibodies, and complete blood counts should be monitored regularly.

Hypertrichosis, or hair growth, may be an unwanted adverse effect associated with oral minoxidil.

Cyanide toxicity may occur when sodium nitroprusside is administered rapidly or for longer than 2 days. Methemoglobinemia may also occur as a result of nitroprusside metabolism to nitrite ions. Nitrite ions complex with hemoglobin, forming methemoglobin, and methemoglobin has a low affinity for binding to O_2.

Summary

The bottom line in the approach to hypertension management is to make sure it is treated! Guidelines are in place to select appropriate therapy. Patients with comorbidities may respond better to one class of medications than to another. Table 8-4, a special-populations pocket guide, lists drugs that are preferred, as well as those to avoid, in some special situations.

●●● PHARMACOLOGIC MANAGEMENT OF STABLE ANGINA

Angina is a symptom of ischemic heart disease. Angina pectoris (pain in the chest) is an example of poor oxygen economics—there is an imbalance of O_2 supply and O_2 demand. The goal of therapy is to (1) increase blood flow to ischemic tissues and/or (2) reduce the O_2 demand of the heart.

To reduce myocardial O_2 demand, treatments include reducing heart rate/contractility, reducing afterload/arterial pressure, and reducing preload/cardiac filling. Treatment strategies for managing stable angina are listed in Box 8-4. For the most part, β-blockers are the primary agents to prophylactically manage chronic stable angina (Table 8-5), although Ca^{++} channel blockers may also be used in patients with stable angina or patients with spasmodic, non-exercise-

TABLE 8-4. Drug Considerations for Special Populations and Comorbidities with Hypertension

Population or Comorbidity	Comment
Blacks	Tend to respond well to diuretics. Diuretics improve responsiveness to ACE inhibitors.
Children	Respond well to β-blockers and clonidine. Children with hypertension tend to have increased cardiac output rather than increased total peripheral resistance.
Elderly	Tend to respond well to diuretics. The elderly are especially sensitive to volume-depletion.
Angina	β-blockers and rate-slowing Ca^{++} channel blockers are good choices. Dihydropyridine Ca^{++} channel blockers may cause reflex tachycardia because of their vasodilatory effects, which will worsen angina.
Post–myocardial infarction	Good choices are β-blockers that lack intrinsic sympathomimetic activity (because sympathetic stimulation is unwanted post-MI) and ACE inhibitors or ARBs. Optimally, every patient post-MI will receive a β-blocker and an ACE inhibitor or ARB.
Diabetes mellitus	Good choices are ACE inhibitors, Ca^{++} channel blockers, and $α_2$-agonists. Use β-blockers with caution, since they can mask hypoglycemia.
Gout	Avoid diuretics, since thiazides and loops can worsen uric acid control.
Bilateral renal artery stenosis	Avoid ACE inhibitors and ARBs, since these drugs can precipitate acute renal failure in this population.
Advanced renal insufficiency	Select a loop diuretic over a thiazide diuretic. Select other antihypertensives on the basis of which ones are *not* excreted renally.
Heart failure	Good choices are loop diuretics (which will also reduce edema and congestive symptoms), β-blockers, ACE inhibitors, ARBs, and aldosterone antagonists.
Asthma/COPD	Do not use β-blockers in patients who are actively wheezing.

Box 8-4. TREATMENT OF STABLE ANGINA

Reduction of risk factors through life-style modifications
    Smoking cessation
    LDL cholesterol reduction
    Weight loss
β-Blockers
Nitrates
Low-dose aspirin
Ca^{++} channel blockers

Box 8-5. BENEFITS OF NITRATES

- Reduce myocardial oxygen demand by dilating veins and increase venous pooling of blood
- Increase systemic arteriolar vasodilation (intravenous forms only)
- Directly dilate undiseased coronary arteries, helping restore blood flow deep within myocardial tissues
- Decrease ventricular wall tension due to increased venous pooling
- Improve exercise tolerance

TABLE 8-5. Rationale for Use of β-Blockers in Angina Management

Antagonize actions of norepinephrine in cardiac tissue

Decrease heart rate

Increase diastolic perfusion

Decrease contractility

Decrease blood pressure

Decrease total peripheral resistance by preventing renin release

Reduce oxygen demand and increase oxygen supply

Box 8-6. CLINICAL UTILITY OF NITRATES

- Termination of acute anginal attacks
- Long-term prophylaxis of anginal attacks
- Prophylaxis of stress- or effort-induced attacks
- For patients with frequent symptoms
- For patients who are nonresponsive to or intolerant of β-blockers or Ca^{++} channel blockers

TABLE 8-6. Rationale for Use of Ca^{++} Channel Blockers in Angina

Type of Ca^{++} Channel Blocker	Rationale
Verapamil and diltiazem	Reduce myocardial contractility and conduction velocity
Dihydropyridines	Vasodilate systemic arterioles and coronary arteries Decrease arterial pressure Decrease coronary artery vasculature resistance Prevent coronary artery vasospasm

induced Prinzmetal's angina (Table 8-6). Since these agents were previously reviewed for hypertension control, we will focus on another class of drugs, the nitrates, that reduce myocardial oxygen demand by reducing preload via venous vasodilation. See Chapter 7 for treatments for unstable angina (e.g., thrombus-causing myocardial infarction).

Nitrates

Nitroglycerin, Isosorbide Mononitrate, and Isosorbide Dinitrate

Mechanism of action. As discussed earlier, nitrates induce vasodilation via direct activation of guanylyl cyclase by nitric oxide and the resultant increase in cGMP. All nonintravenous forms of nitrates predominantly vasodilate veins, thereby reducing preload. In contrast, intravenous nitrates are balanced vasodilators, with vasodilatory actions in both veins and arteries.

Pharmacokinetics. Nitrates are available as oral tablets, transdermal patches, sublingual tablets, translingual sprays, topical ointments, and intravenous infusions. The onset of action of sublingual forms of nitroglycerin occurs within 1 to 3 minutes, but effects are terminated in less than an hour because of rapid metabolism. Nitroglycerin sublingual tablets must be kept in their original glass container because the medication adsorbs onto standard plastic prescription vials. The benefits provided by nitrates for patients with angina are featured in Box 8-5.

Clinical use. Nitrates are used to treat acute anginal attacks and as prophylaxis against recurrent attacks. They may also be used during a myocardial infarction, as well as to manage perioperative hypertension. Box 8-6 lists additional situations in which nitrates may be useful.

Adverse effects. Tolerance, termed *tachyphylaxis*, develops quickly to the effects of nitrates. To prevent tolerance from occurring there should be a nitrate-free interval (at least 12 hours) during each 24-hour period (typically overnight). Headaches, flushing, and postural hypotension accompanied by reflex tachycardia may occur as a result of vasodilation. Nitrates are contraindicated with phosphodiesterase-5 inhibitors, which are used for erectile dysfunction (e.g., sildenafil, vardenafil, and tadalafil), since these drugs inhibit the breakdown of cGMP. Fatal hypotension has occurred when phosphodiesterase-5 inhibitors have been combined with nitrates.

Summary

Often combinations of drugs are used to manage stable

TABLE 8-7. Rationale for Use of Drug Combinations in Angina

Drug Combination	Rationale
Nitrates and β-blockers	Nitrates decrease preload and cause venous pooling β-Blockers prevent nitrate-induced reflex tachycardia
Nitrates and Ca++ channel blockers	Nitrates reduce preload Dihydropyridines decrease afterload or rate-slowing Ca++ channel blockers reduce heart rate
Ca++ channel blockers and β-blockers	β-Blockers prevent reflex tachycardia associated with dihydropyridine-induced blood pressure decrease
Nitrates, Ca++ channel blockers, and β-blockers	Dihydropyridines reduce afterload Nitrates reduce preload β-Blockers decrease heart rate and contractility to blunt nitrate-induced and dihydropyridine-induced reflex tachycardia

TABLE 8-8. Factors That May Precipitate Heart Failure

Factor	Drug Examples
Uncontrolled hypertension Cardiac arrhythmias Myocardial infarction Negative inotropes	Antiarrhythmics β-Blockers
Heart-rate-slowing Ca++ channel blockers	Verapamil Diltiazem
Cardiotoxic chemotherapies	Daunorubicin Doxorubicin
Drugs that cause sodium/water retention	Carbenicillin/ticarcillin Glucocorticoids NSAIDs

angina. Nitrates are frequently given in concert with β-blockers and calcium channel inhibitors. Rationales for these combinations are given in Table 8-7. Because some unstable angina symptoms may be caused by acute coronary syndrome (see Chapter 7), a review of the drugs used to restore coronary flow (antiplatelet agents, anticoagulants, antithrombin agents) is suggested.

●●● PHARMACOLOGIC MANAGEMENT OF HEART FAILURE

Essentially, congestive heart failure (CHF) occurs when myocardial dysfunction (myocardial hypertrophy and fibrosis) is so severe that the cardiac output is no longer adequate to provide oxygen for the tissues. Signs and symptoms of heart failure include decreased exercise tolerance, shortness of breath, tachycardia, cardiomegaly, fatigue, as well as peripheral and pulmonary edema. Precipitating factors are listed in Table 8-8.

Using the Frank-Starling curve (Fig. 8-9), note that patients with heart failure have reduced cardiac output for any end-diastolic pressure on the curve. As myocardial activity worsens, congestive symptoms such as pulmonary edema occur, as do low-output symptoms like fatigue and oliguria (producing abnormally small volumes of urine). Initially, the baroreceptors attempt to compensate for reduced cardiac output through activation of compensatory reflexes like heightened sympathetic tone and activation of the RAA system. However, these compensatory mechanisms only worsen myocardial function by increasing total peripheral resistance and increasing afterload (Fig. 8-10). This only makes the failing heart work more inefficiently, leading to further maladaptive myocardial hypertrophy and remodeling

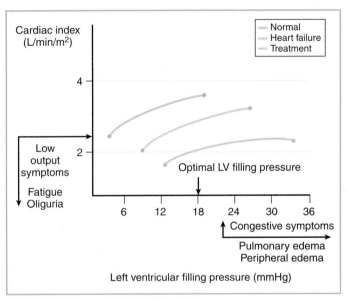

Figure 8-9. Frank-Starling curve.

(an example of a deadly feed-forward mechanism, "vicious cycle").

The primary goal of pharmacotherapeutic management of life-threatening heart failure is to slow ventricular remodeling and the maladaptive ventricular changes (e.g., apoptosis, abnormal gene expression) associated with it. Diuretics move the depressed Frank-Starling cardiac output curve only to the left, providing symptomatic relief from edema, but diuretics do not increase cardiac output. In contrast, vasodilators, ACE inhibitors, ARBs, spironolactone, eplerenone, β-blockers, and positive inotropes (e.g., digoxin) shift the depressed cardiac output curve upward. As with most cardiovascular diseases, a combination of therapies is used to manage CHF symptoms. Rationale for each of the pharmacotherapies is listed in Table 8-9. The "ABCDs" for managing patients with worsening heart failure are listed in Table 8-10. Note that pharmacologic interventions can be beneficial in high-risk patients even before symptoms begin.

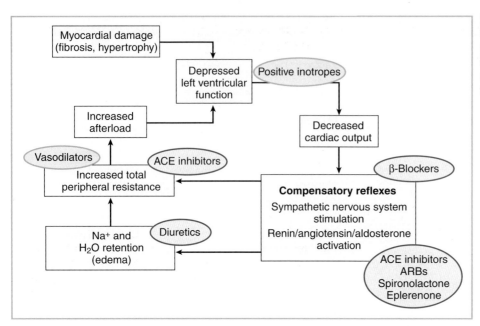

Figure 8-10. Drug therapies to break the vicious cycle of heart failure. The primary pharmacologic goal in heart failure treatment is to reduce symptoms. The secondary goal is to reduce myocardial fibrosis and hypertrophy in the failing heart.

TABLE 8-9. Rationale for Pharmacotherapies Utilized in Managing Heart Failure

Goal	Rationale and Pharmacotherapy

Improve heart function	Decrease myocardial remodeling and fibrosis (by blocking effects of aldosterone)
	    ACE inhibitors
	    ARBs
	    Spironolactone
	    Eplerenone
	Enhance contractility
	    Positive inotropes
	Improve ventricular function
	    β-Blockers

Decrease preload	Loop diuretics
Decrease afterload	Vasodilators ACE inhibitors, ARBs
Other	Correct arrhythmias Warfarin anticoagulation

TABLE 8-10. ABCDs of Managing Heart Failure

Symptoms	Management
A. Patient does not have heart failure but is at high risk owing to uncontrolled hypertension, coronary artery disease, diabetes	Encourage blood pressure control Encourage lipid control ACE inhibitors or ARBs are recommended
B. Patient does not have symptoms of heart failure but has structural damage or recently had a myocardial infarction	ACE inhibitors or ARBs *and* β-blockers are recommended
C. Patient has structural disease *and* symptoms of heart failure (These are the patients usually thought of as *having* heart failure)	Diuretics are recommended for fluid retention ACE inhibitors or ARBs are recommended unless contraindicated β-Blockers are recommended if patient is stable Digoxin is recommended if patient is symptomatic
D. Patient has refractory symptoms even at rest	Ventricular assistance devices Continuous inotropic infusions Heart transplantation

For the most part, the first-line therapeutics are the previously described drugs that blunt the RAA system. Drugs that block the formation (ACE inhibitors) or the actions (ARBs) of angiotensin II are balanced vasodilators and will reduce preload and afterload (Box 8-7). In addition, since angiotensin II is a potent stimulus for myocardial hypertrophy, inhibiting its actions with either ACE inhibitors or ARBs will diminish or reverse myocardial remodeling and disease progression. Spironolactone and the selective aldosterone receptor antagonist eplerenone can decrease heart failure mortality by 30% by blocking the effects of elevated aldosterone in CHF patients (Box 8-8). It is also believed that aldosterone receptor blockers diminish the

maladaptive cardiofibrosis associated with CHF. In clinical trials, spironolactone improved survival in patients with heart failure. Yet, life-threatening complications due to hyperkalemia are common. Patients using spironolactone need to have their K^+ levels monitored closely. When congestive symptoms of CHF are evident, loop diuretics are used to manage fluid retention.

In patients with CHF, β-blockers are often prescribed. This should appear counter-intuitive. In fact, β-blockers are

Box 8-7. ADVANTAGES OF ACE INHIBITORS AND ARBS IN HEART FAILURE MANAGEMENT

- Provide balanced vasodilation (arteries and veins)
- Improve myocardial function
- Improve cardiac workload and stroke volume
- Reduce blood pressure
- Improve exercise tolerance
- Slow disease progression (decrease myocardial fibrosis and hypertrophy)
- Improve survival

Box 8-9. ADVANTAGES OF β-BLOCKERS IN COMPENSATED HEART FAILURE MANAGEMENT

- Prevent adverse effects of norepinephrine on the heart
- Prevent myocardial remodeling (fibrosis and hypertrophy)
- Improve ventricular function
- Improve exercise tolerance
- Decrease renin release
- Decrease oxidative damage
- Prolong survival
- Slow progression of heart failure

Box 8-8. ADVANTAGES OF SPIRONOLACTONE IN HEART FAILURE

- Assist in sodium/fluid excretion
- Prevent myocardial remodeling, which improves heart function
- Prevent myocardial fibrosis, which reduces the likelihood of arrhythmias
- Reduce vascular fibrosis

contraindicated in patients with acutely decompensated CHF owing to diminished myocardial contractility. Yet, surprisingly, three β-blockers—metoprolol XL, bisoprolol, and carvedilol—are approved for managing heart failure. As summarized in Box 8-9, these β-blockers slow progression of heart failure by diminishing oxidative damage and myocardial remodeling or hypertrophy by blocking the adverse effects of norepinephrine on myocardial tissues.

Another class of drugs used to manage symptomatic CHF is the positive inotropes (digoxin, milrinone, dobutamine, dopamine, and nesiritide), which improve myocardial contractility. These drugs are introduced below.

Positive Inotropes

Digoxin

Mechanism of action. Digoxin inhibits Na^+/K^+-ATPase pumps by binding to the potassium-binding site. The resulting increase in intracellular Na^+ drives the Na^+/Ca^{++} exchanger which increases intracellular Ca^{++}. Digoxin may also facilitate Ca^{++} release from the sarcoplasmic reticulum. Excess intracellular Ca^{++} facilitates interactions between actin and myosin; therefore, digoxin increases the force of myocardial contractility to improve the efficiency of the failing heart (Fig. 8-11).

As digoxin increases cardiac stroke volume and cardiac output, baroreceptor-regulated compensatory sympathetic neuronal pathways are diminished. This leads to predominance of parasympathetic tone, which slows heart rate and vasodilates the vasculature. Improved renal hemodynamics also allows edematous fluid to be excreted, which reduces preload. However, despite all the beneficial contractile and hemodynamic effects of digoxin, the drug has never been shown to improve survival. For this reason, digoxin is usually not a first-line drug for the treatment of heart failure. However, digoxin also possesses antiarrhythmic activity, and it is sometimes a first-line choice for patients with both congestive heart failure and atrial fibrillation.

Pharmacokinetics. Digoxin has a narrow therapeutic index of 1 to 2 ng/mL. In general, clinicians should aim for plasma levels of 1.0 ng/mL because greater than 2.0 ng/mL is always toxic.

Figure 8-11. Mechanism of digoxin.

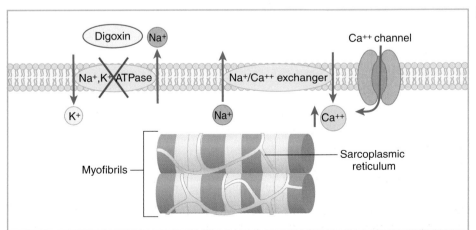

Bioavailability of digoxin varies among various formulations (tablet, gel cap, oral elixir, intravenous injection) and differs between patients. One reason for this interpatient variability is altered metabolism within the gut. Roughly 10% of the population carries *Eubacterium* as a part of their normal gastrointestinal flora. This microorganism inactivates digoxin. In these patients, treatment with antibiotics (which eliminates *Eubacterium*) may suddenly increase digoxin's toxicologic potential. Digoxin is about 90% nonspecifically bound to plasma proteins, which makes drug interactions possible when administered with other highly protein-bound drugs. About 70% of digoxin is excreted renally, so renal function should be monitored.

Adverse effects. Diogin toxicity, if untreated, can be fatal. The first symptoms of digoxin toxicity are gastrointestinal (abdominal cramps, vomiting, diarrhea) and visual disturbances (green or yellow halos, "fuzzy shadows"—like driving at night with dirty glasses). Confusion and yellow vision may occur with chronic toxicity, followed by AV blockade, bradycardia, and ventricular arrhythmias. Digoxin toxicity is managed according to Box 8-10. Digoxin toxicity is worsened by hypokalemia, renal insufficiency, and hypothyroidism.

Milrinone

Mechanism of action. Milrinone is a phosphodiesterase inhibitor. Phosphodiesterases degrade cyclic nucleotides, such as cAMP. Inhibiting phosphodiesterase in myocardial cells increases cAMP concentration, so milrinone acts as a positive inotrope (Fig. 8-12).

Pharmacokinetics. Milrinone is given as a continuous intravenous infusion.

Adverse effects. Since milrinone is a positive inotrope, it can also be proarrhythmogenic. It is used only in cases of acute heart failure because prolonged usage results in increased mortality.

Dobutamine

Mechanism of action. Dobutamine is a β_1-adrenergic receptor agonist. Exactly opposite to β-blockers, dobutamine increases stroke volume in the failing heart. At low doses, cardiac output increases with little change in heart rate.

Pharmacokinetics. Dobutamine is administered as a continuous intravenous infusion. As such, it is used only in cases of acute heart failure.

Adverse effects. As a positive inotrope, dobutamine may cause hypertension, tachycardia, arrhythmias, or angina.

Dopamine

Mechanism of action. Dopamine is primarily a dopamine receptor agonist; however, at higher doses, dopamine activates α- and β-adrenergic receptors too. Dopamine is administered as a continuous intravenous infusion. At low doses, dopamine preferentially stimulates D1 and D2 receptors in the renal vasculature, which leads to vasodilation and promotes renal blood flow to preserve the glomerular filtration rate. At intermediate doses, dopamine also stimulates β_1-receptors on the heart. At high doses, dopamine stimulates α-adrenergic receptors in the vasculature, which exacerbates heart failure by increasing afterload. (However, this may be a desired effect in patients who are in hemorrhagic shock.)

Clinical use. Dopamine is especially useful in situations of cardiogenic shock, in which there is inadequate perfusion of vital organs.

Adverse effects. Same as for dobutamine.

Nesiritide

Box 8-10. MANAGING DIGOXIN TOXICITY

1. Discontinue digoxin.
2. Discontinue K⁺-depleting drugs (remember that digoxin and K⁺ compete for the same binding site on Na⁺/K⁺-ATPase) .
3. Give K⁺ if needed.
4. Administer an antiarrhythmic (only if needed).
5. Administer Digibind, a digoxin-specific antibody.

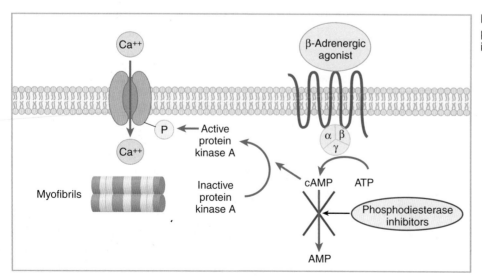

Figure 8-12. Mechanism of phosphodiesterase inhibitors (milrinone) in heart failure.

Mechanism of action. Nesiritide is a B-type natriuretic peptide. Like endogenous atrial natriuretic factor produced by the heart, this drug activates guanylyl cyclase to form the potent vasodilator cGMP. Administration of the drug leads to balanced vasodilation in the arteries and veins, diuretic effects (via enhanced Na^+ excretion), suppression of the RAA system, and suppression of the sympathetic nervous system. As a result, not only does circulation improve, but symptoms of heart failure improve as well.

Pharmacokinetics. Nesiritide is administered as a continuous intravenous infusion.

Adverse effects. Although less likely than dobutamine to cause tachycardia or arrhythmias and better tolerated than intravenous nitroglycerin, nesiritide has been associated with prolonged hypotension. Additionally, there is new concern with respect to the potential of this drug to increase the risk of renal impairment and mortality. Even though nesiritide has been shown to be hemodynamically beneficial in the short term, it may not be beneficial in the long term.

Summary

The bottom line for heart failure management is that it is best to prevent it from happening in the first place. However, once the heart begins to fail, drug combinations may be indicated, including diuretics to decrease congestive symptoms; ACE inhibitors, ARBs, or aldosterone receptor antagonists to decrease myocardial fibrosis and remodeling; β-blockers to block effects of sympathetic nervous stimulation; and positive inotropes to improve myocardial contractility.

●●● PHARMACOTHERAPY OF ANTIARRHYTHMICS

Box 8-11. CONDITIONS THAT PROVOKE ARRHYTHMIAS

- Ischemic damage
- Heart failure
- Hypovolemia
- Hypercapnia
- Hypotension
- Electrolyte disturbances (K^+, Mg^{++}, Ca^{++})
- Drug toxicities (digoxin, antiarrhythmics, caffeine, alcohol)

Box 8-12. MECHANISMS OF ANTIARRHYTHMIC DRUGS

- Decrease the slope of phase 4 depolarization
- Elevate the threshold potential for phase 0 upward shoot
- Shorten refractoriness in area of unidirectional block to allow anterograde conduction to proceed
- Prolong refractoriness in area of unidirectional block to cause bidirectional block so that the impulse cannot proceed in a retrograde fashion

One of the most serious complications of CHF and other cardiovascular diseases is cardiac arrhythmia (Box 8-11). Whether due to an ectopic focus or a reentrant circus rhythm, abnormal electrical conductance pathways can be life-threatening. Antiarrhythmic drugs work by several different mechanisms (Box 8-12). Since these drugs alter electrical conduction, all antiarrhythmics can potentially worsen conduction. There is a narrow margin of safety between obtaining the desired antiarrhythmic effect and provoking a new arrhythmia.

Antiarrhythmics are classified according to their predominant pharmacologic effects into classes I, II, III, and IV agents (Table 8-11).

Although a given drug may fall into a particular *class*, many of the antiarrhythmics used today have activities that fall into more than one class.

Class I: Sodium Channel Blockers

Class IA, IB, and IC Drugs

Class IA: Quinidine, Procainamide, and Disopyramide

Class IB: Lidocaine, Tocainide, and Mexiletine

Class IC: Propafenone and Flecainide

Mechanism of action. All class I antiarrhythmics block Na^+ channels, but the pharmacokinetics of this blockade differs among individual drugs, producing action potential differences (Table 8-12 and Fig. 8-13). Class IA drugs increase the refractory period (see Fig. 8-13A), whereas class IB antiarrhythmics decrease the refractory period (see Fig. 8-13B).

ANATOMY

Normal Conduction Pathway of the Heart

The electrical activity in the heart is generated by the sinoatrial (SA) node. Normally, the SA node has the highest degree of spontaneous firing. The impulse produced by the SA node spreads throughout the atria and then is slightly delayed at the atrioventricular (AV) node. This delay allows time for the atria to contract. The electrical impulse propagates to the bundle of His and then bifurcates to travel down the Purkinje fibers, exciting the cardiac muscle of both ventricles.

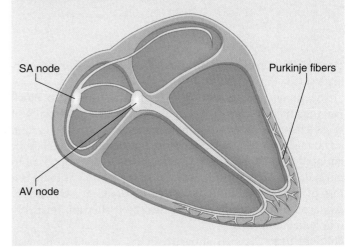

PHYSIOLOGY

Phases of Ventricular Membrane Depolarization

The electrical properties of the heart are often described as ventricular membrane depolarizations. Ventricular action potentials have four phases. Prior to excitation, an electrical gradient exists in which the inside of the myocytes are −80 to −90 mV more negative with respect to the outside of the cell. Electrical stimulation (or depolarization) occurs when ions begin entering the cell. Phase 4 is unique to pacemaker cells. Other cell types lack this slow, inward, positive current that is seen during diastole. During phase 4, there is a slow leak of Na^+ ions into the cell and a slow K^+ efflux. Over time, K^+ efflux diminishes but Na^+ influx continues. Once a critical threshold potential is reached, voltage-gated Na^+ channels open and Na ions rapidly rush into the cell. This is known as phase 0 or "depolarization." During phase 1, there is passive chloride ion influx and potassium efflux. The hallmark features of phase 2, or the "plateau" phase, are calcium influx and potassium efflux. During phase 3, the cell repolarizes as potassium efflux continues. Recall that depolarization cannot occur again until the cell has completely repolarized. Note: the Na^+/K^+-ATPase is constantly working to reestablish Na^+ and K^+ homeostasis.

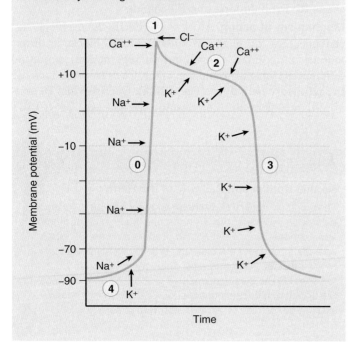

Drugs falling into class IC markedly slow phase 0 depolarization (see Fig. 8-13C).

The unique ability of class IB antiarrhythmics to block Na^+ channels when activated or inactivated (especially if those channels remain in a polarized state) provides certain advantages. For example, lidocaine (an example of a class IB antiarrhythmic) preferentially affects diseased, as opposed to normal, tissue. As a result, with lidocaine treatment there is a loss of excitability and conduction blockade in ischemically damaged tissues, while normal, healthy tissues are relatively unaffected by the drug.

Clinical use. Class IB antiarrhythmics are used to manage

TABLE 8-11. Predominant Pharmacologic Effects of Antiarrhythmics

Class	Conduction Velocity	Refractory Period	Automaticity	Ion Block
IA	↓	↑	↓	Na^+
IB	−/↓	↓	↓	Na^+
IC	↓↓	−	↓	Na^+
II	↓	↑	↓	Ca^{++} (indirectly)
III	−	↑↑	−	K^+
IV	↓	↑	↓	Ca^{++}

Note: Most antiarrhythmics decrease automaticity and conduction velocity by altering movement of specific ions (Na^+, Ca^{++}, K^+).

TABLE 8-12. Class I Na^+ Channel Blockers

Antiarrhythmic Drug	Kinetics with Na^+ Channel	Effect
Class IA	Intermediate rate of association	Slows rate of rise (phase 0) of action potential. Prolongs action potential (increases refractory period)
Class IB	Rapid rate of association	Shortens refractory period (phase 3 repolarization). Decreases duration of action potential
Class IC	Slow rate of association	Markedly slows phase 0 depolarization. No effect on refractory period

ventricular arrhythmias, especially during cardiac procedures or following myocardial infarction. Drugs in this class shorten phase 3 repolarization and decrease the duration of the action potential (see Fig. 8-13B). Class IB antiarrhythmics have accentuated effects for turning areas of unidirectional block into "no block at all." With these drugs, anterograde conduction is allowed to proceed because the refractory period of damaged tissue has been reduced.

Class IA and IC drugs are not first-line agents because therapeutic approaches currently focus on heart *rate* control rather than *rhythm* control. Quinidine and procainamide (class IA drugs) were historically used to chemically convert atrial fibrillation back to a normal sinus rhythm and to maintain normal sinus rhythms after direct current conversions. Class IA antiarrhythmics prolong the refractory period and turn areas of unidirectional block into bidirectional block (see Fig. 8-13). Similarly, class IC antiarrhythmics are not usually first-choice antiarrhythmics because they are quite proarrhythmogenic and increase mortality.

PATHOLOGY

Ectopic Foci and Reentrant Circus Rhythms

Ectopic foci occur when myocardial cells located outside the SA node take over the normal pacemaker function of the SA node by becoming unusually "automatic." Reentrant circus rhythms occur when an impulse is propagated indefinitely. When a premature impulse encounters refractory tissue (tissue that has not yet repolarized), the impulse is simply terminated. If, however, the impulse proceeds in a different direction and "reenters" the area, which has now repolarized, the impulse may proceed in a retrograde (i.e., backward) manner. Thus, the impulse may continue to propagate itself indefinitely in a circular fashion.

Pharmacokinetics. Numerous drug interactions are likely with many of the class I antiarrhythmics owing to interactions that result from hepatic metabolism by the P-450 microsomal enzymes and nonspecific binding to plasma proteins. Lidocaine (a class IB drug) is administered parenterally to avoid first-pass hepatic metabolism. Tocainide and mexiletine can be thought of as "oral lidocaine."

Adverse effects. As a class, these drugs have an extremely narrow therapeutic window. Many are proarrhythmogenic or possess negative inotropic properties.

Class IA antiarrhythmics are proarrhythmogenic because they cause QT prolongation, which can lead to potentially fatal torsades de pointes, a life-threatening ventricular arrhythmia. Quinidine is also associated with a conglomeration of symptoms termed *cinchonism*, in which patients may experience tinnitus, blurred vision, headache, nausea, delirium, and psychosis. Additionally, quinidine and disopyramide possess severe anticholinergic adverse effects.

Due to lipid solubility, central nervous system adverse effects are likely with lidocaine. Tocainide is associated with adverse hematologic effects and pulmonary fibrosis.

Although class IC drugs do not prolong the QT interval, these drugs are also quite prone to inducing new arrhythmias.

Class II: Beta-Blockers

Propranolol and Esmolol

Mechanism of action. Yes, β-blockers (class II antiarrhythmics) also have antiarrhythmic actions. β-Blockers indirectly prevent calcium entry into myocardial cells; therefore, β-blockers slow conduction velocity, slow automaticity, and prolong the refractory period.

Clinical use. Because certain exercise-induced arrhythmias are produced by heightened sympathetic tone, β-blockers are often effective therapies. As another example, the sinoatrial (SA) and atrioventricular (AV) nodes are heavily innervated by the adrenergic system, making β-blockers useful for managing tachyarrhythmias in which these nodes are abnormally automatic or involved in a reentrant circus rhythm. β-Blockers should be included in the therapeutic regimens of all patients following myocardial infarction to prevent ventricular tachycardia and to slow the ventricular rate in response to atrial fibrillation or atrial flutter. β-Blockers have been shown to reduce arrhythmia-related mortality, making them a common first choice for treatment of atrial tachyarrhythmias.

Class III: Potassium Channel Blockers

Bretylium, Amiodarone, Sotalol, Dofetilide, and Ibutilide

Mechanism of action. As a generalization, class III antiarrhythmics prolong cardiac action potentials, resulting in an increase in the effective refractory period. With the exception of ibutilide, which slows outward Na^+ currents during repolarization, the class III drugs block potassium channels. However, properties of individual drugs in this class vary considerably. What is consistent among class III anti-

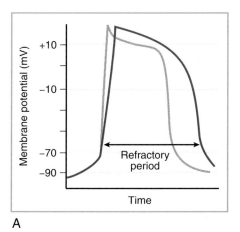

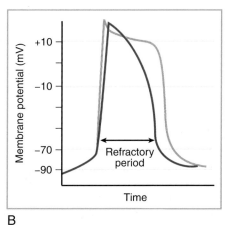

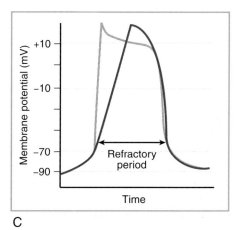

A   B   C

Figure 8-13. Actions of class I antiarrhythmics on ventricular action potential. **A,** Class IA drugs. **B,** Class IB drugs. **C,** Class IC drugs. The gray line represents a normal action potential. The red line represents the pharmacologic effect of the antiarrhythmic. Note that the refractory period is lengthened by class 1A agents, shortened for class 1B drugs, and relatively unchanged for class 1C therapies.

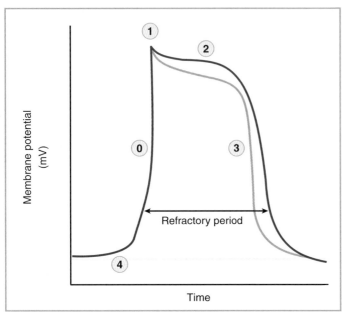

Figure 8-14. Actions of class III antiarrhythmics on ventricular action potential.

arrhythmics is that they prolong phase III repolarization without changing phase 0 depolarization (Fig. 8-14). This reduces myocardial automaticity, prolongs action potentials, increases the refractory period, and increases the QT interval. Prolongation of the QT interval is one mechanism by which class III antiarrhythmics can induce secondary arrhythmias (these drugs are proarrhythmogenic).

Pharmacokinetics. Bretylium and ibutilide are poorly absorbed from the gastrointestinal tract and are administered only intravenously. Amiodarone has a long $t_{1/2}$, roughly 40 to 60 days; therefore, it takes a long time for the drug to reach steady state. Additionally, when adverse effects occur, they are slow to resolve, since it takes a long time for the drug to be eliminated from the body. More than 96% of amiodarone is nonspecifically bound to plasma proteins. Amiodarone is metabolized by hepatic P-450 microsomal enzymes and inhibits these metabolic enzymes. As a result, numerous drug interactions occur, since amiodarone increases plasma drug concentrations of digoxin, quinidine, phenytoin, flecainide, and warfarin.

Clinical use. Bretylium is reserved primarily for treating life-threatening ventricular arrhythmias and for attempts to resuscitate patients from ventricular fibrillation. Amiodarone is used to manage recurrent ventricular fibrillation or ventricular tachycardia. Its use has been shown to decrease mortality following myocardial infarction and in heart failure patients. Sotalol decreases the fibrillation threshold and is used to prevent atrial and ventricular fibrillation. Dofetilide is used to convert atrial fibrillation or flutter to normal sinus rhythm and to maintain normal sinus rhythm after cardioversion. Ibutilide is used for rapid conversion of atrial fibrillation or atrial flutter of recent onset (<90 days) to sinus rhythm. Patients with atrial arrhythmias of a longer duration are less likely to respond to ibutilide.

Box 8-13. ADVERSE EFFECTS OF AMIODARONE

Serious pulmonary toxicity (interstitial lung disease)
Liver damage
Heart block
Bradycardia
Hypotension
Corneal deposits
Optic neuritis
"Smurfism"
Hypo- or hyperthyroidism
Photosensitivity
Neuropathy
Muscle weakness

Adverse effects. For the most part, class III agents can induce life-threatening QT prolongation. Patients require close monitoring for life-threatening ventricular arrhythmias. In fact, amiodarone should be prescribed only by physicians who are thoroughly familiar with its risks. A substantial number of patients experience adverse effects with high doses of amiodarone, often necessitating that the drug be discontinued, since adverse effects are sometimes fatal. A partial listing of adverse effects is located in Box 8-13. The chemical structure of amiodarone contains iodine and is structurally related to thyroid hormone. This accounts for amiodarone's adverse effects on the thyroid gland and for "smurfism," which is an iodine-induced blue-gray skin discoloration. Because of the numerous adverse effects, patients should regularly have their visual function, cardiac function (electrocardiogram), thyroid function, pulmonary function, and liver function checked. Owing to the risk for QT prolongation, prescriptions for dofetilide may only be written by physicians who have completed specialized training.

Class IV: Calcium Channel Blockers

Rate-slowing Calcium Channel Blockers
Verapamil and Diltiazem

Mechanism of action. Yes, some Ca^{++} channel blockers are also antiarrhythmics. Rate-slowing Ca^{++} channel blockers directly block slow inward Ca^{++} currents from entering myocardial cells. This action decreases and prolongs phase 4 spontaneous depolarization. These effects are most prominent in tissues that (1) fire frequently, (2) are less polarized at rest, and (3) depend upon Ca^{++} for activation.

Clinical use. Like β-blockers, rate-slowing Ca^{++} channel blockers are most useful for managing tachyarrhythmias in which the SA node or the AV node are abnormally automatic or involved in a reentrant circus rhythm. These Ca^{++} channel blockers slow AV conductance in atrial fibrillation, thus protecting the ventricles.

Other Antiarrhythmics

Adenosine

Mechanism of action. Adenosine is a naturally occurring nucleoside that slows conduction through the AV node by opening K^+ channels.

Pharmacokinetics. Because the drug has an extremely short $t_{1/2}$ (15 seconds), it is administered only intravenously.

Clinical use. Adenosine may be used to convert acute reentrant supraventricular tachycardias at the AV node back to normal sinus rhythm.

Adverse effects. Adverse effects associated with adenosine include bronchospasm, flushing, sweating, chest pain, and hypotension.

Summary

Because all antiarrhythmics alter ionic conductances in myocardial tissue—thereby slowing automaticity and conduction velocity—caution must be utilized when prescribing these drugs due to their ability to induce new arrhythmias.

●●● HYPERLIPIDEMIAS

Hyperlipidemia is defined as an elevation of cholesterol or triglycerides. Cholesterol is, of course, essential for synthesis of plasma membranes, steroid hormones, and bile acids. Likewise, triglycerides play essential roles in transporting and storing fatty acids for energy. However, these lipids may contribute to disease processes. Elevated levels of cholesterol can lead to atherosclerosis and coronary artery disease; elevated triglycerides can lead to pancreatitis. Classical therapy is directed at lowering low-density lipoproteins (LDLs), lowering triglycerides, or raising high-density lipoproteins (HDLs).

Cholesterol and triglycerides are synthesized by the liver or obtained from dietary sources (Fig. 8-15). As lipids, cholesterol and triglycerides are insoluble in blood; therefore, they must be transported within lipoproteins, which differ from each other in composition and mission. Key points about the drugs used to manage hypercholesterolemia are summarized in Table 8-13.

Statins

Lovastatin, Pravastatin, Simvastatin, Atorvastatin, Fluvastatin, and Rosuvastatin

Note that all these drug names end in "-statin."

Mechanism of action. Statins inhibit 3-hydroxy-3-methyl-glutaryl-coenzyme A (HMG-CoA) reductase. This enzyme catalyzes the rate-limiting step in hepatic cholesterol

TABLE 8-13. Pharmacotherapy of Hyperlipidemia in a Nutshell

Drugs	Clinical Utility	Clinical Drawbacks
Statins	Effective for lowering LDL and increasing HDL	Only mildly effective for lowering triglycerides
Fibrates	Effective for lowering triglycerides	Only minimally effective for lowering LDL or increasing HDL
Niacin	Effective for lowering triglycerides, lowering LDL, and increasing HDL	Adverse effects may limit utility
Bile acid resins	Moderately effective for lowering LDL	Increase triglycerides
Ezetimibe	Moderately effective for lowering LDL	Only minimally effective for increasing HDL

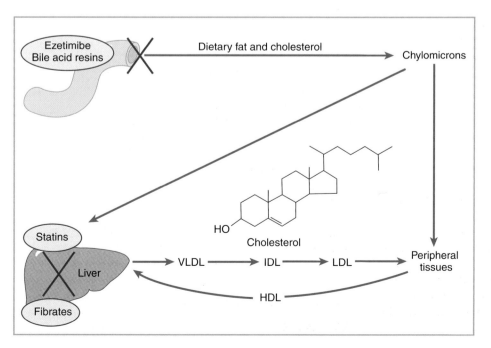

Figure 8-15. Cholesterol transport. In contrast to statins and fibrates (which work at the level of the liver), ezetimibe and bile acid resins work by blocking absorption. VLDL, very low density lipoprotein; IDL, intermediate-density lipoprotein; LDL, low-density lipoprotein; HDL, high-density lipoprotein.

PHYSIOLOGY

Lipoproteins: It's All about Density

Chylomicrons are rich in triglycerides. They are formed from dietary fat, and they transport lipids from the gastrointestinal tract to the liver.

Very low density lipoproteins (VLDLs) contain triglycerides that are synthesized in the liver but are converted to low-density lipoproteins (LDLs) in the bloodstream. The role of VLDL is to transport triglycerides and cholesterol synthesized hepatically to the tissues.

LDL is formed once VLDL has donated triglycerides and fatty acids to the tissues. LDL is the major cholesterol transport mechanism, but cholesterol is loosely bound and can be deposited in the vasculature. Receptors for LDL exist in the liver, the adrenal gland, and cells of peripheral tissues. When LDL binds to its receptors, it undergoes endocytosis and is broken down intracellularly. (LDL is the "bad" cholesterol.)

High-density lipoproteins (HDLs) are synthesized in the liver and gut. The role of HDL is to scavenge excess cholesterol from peripheral tissues and transport it back to the liver, where it may be secreted into bile and excreted, a process known as *reverse cholesterol transport*. (HDL is the "good" cholesterol.)

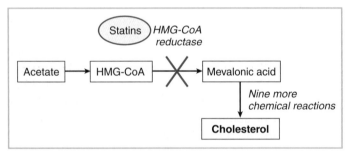

Figure 8-16. Statins inhibit HMG-CoA reductase, the rate-limiting step in cholesterol synthesis.

synthesis (Fig. 8-16). Reduced hepatic cholesterol synthesis decreases hepatocyte cholesterol concentration, leading to increased hepatic expression of LDL receptors, which is the primary mechanism by which LDL is internalized and degraded.

Pharmacokinetics. With the exceptions of pravastatin and rosuvastatin, most statins are metabolized by the hepatic P-450 microsomal enzymes and are contraindicated with drugs that inhibit the P-450s. Grapefruit juice also decreases P-450 activity and is contraindicated with most statins. Lovastatin should be taken with food to increase its bioavailability; other statins may be taken without regard to meals.

Clinical use. Statins lower LDL cholesterol by 15% to 60%, lower triglycerides by 25% to 40%, and raise HDL by 6% to 10%.

Adverse effects. Statins are usually well tolerated. Predictable side effects associated with statins are listed in Box 8-14. Major adverse side effects are myopathy and hepatotoxicity. Baseline liver transaminase levels should be obtained prior to beginning therapy. Rosuvastatin is the only statin that may

PATHOLOGY

Atherosclerotic Lesions

Atherosclerotic lesions may occur after injury to the endothelium. If LDL cholesterol is retained in arterial walls, it may get oxidized, which recruits monocytes and macrophages (foam cells) to the area, provoking an inflammatory response. This process is exacerbated by high levels of cholesterol. Hypercholesterolemia may occur because of genetic disturbances in cholesterol synthesis, transport, or catabolism. Secondary causes of hypercholesterolemia include the use of certain drugs (progestins, glucocorticoids, or anabolic steroids) as well as the nephrotic syndrome, diabetes, systemic lupus erythematosus, and hypothyroidism. Pharmacotherapy is useful to lower cholesterol and triglyceride levels when dietary changes are not successful.

Box 8-14. ADVERSE EFFECTS ASSOCIATED WITH STATINS

Muscle aches, myopathy, muscle inflammation, rhabdomyolysis
Peripheral neuropathies
Hepatotoxicity (increase in transaminase)
Gastrointestinal upset
Headache
Rash
Itching

cause renal toxicity, and this is more likely to occur when the drug is administered at high doses. The risk of myopathy or rhabdomyolysis increases when statins are administered with P-450 inhibitors, gemfibrozil, or niacin. (Note: rhabdomyolysis involves breakdown of muscle fibers and release of myoglobin into the circulation; myoglobin and its metabolites may be toxic to the kidneys and can result in kidney failure. Creatinine kinase levels may be checked to monitor for muscle breakdown.)

Fibrates

Gemfibrozil and Fenofibrate

Mechanism of action. Fibrates reduce hepatic triglyceride levels by inhibiting hepatic extraction of free fatty acids and thus hepatic triglyceride production. These drugs may also lower cholesterol by increasing endothelial lipoprotein lipase activity.

Clinical use. Fibrates are most commonly prescribed to reduce triglyceride levels. Fibrates lower triglyceride levels by approximately 40%, have only a marginal effect on LDL, and increase HDL by approximately 5%.

Adverse effects. Patients should be monitored for elevated liver enzymes. A decrease in WBCs may also occur. Adverse effects associated with fibrates are listed in Box 8-15. Patients should be warned to report unusual muscle pain, tenderness, or weakness, especially if accompanied by malaise or fever.

Box 8-15. ADVERSE EFFECTS ASSOCIATED WITH FIBRATES

Myopathy/rhabdomyolysis
Elevated liver function tests
Fatigue
Infections/influenza
Pain
Headache

Box 8-16. EXAMPLES OF DRUGS WITH REDUCED BIOAVAILABILITY WHEN ADMINISTERED CONCURRENTLY WITH BILE ACID RESINS

Aspirin (NSAIDs)	Glipizide
Clindamycin	Hydrochlorothiazide
Digoxin	Hydrocortisone
Fat soluble vitamins (A, D, E, K)	Phenytoin
Furosemide	Thyroxine

Fenofibrate is contraindicated in patients with liver disease, gallbladder disease, or severe renal disease. Fibrates may cause cholelithiasis (gallstones) resulting from increased cholesterol excretion into bile. Several severe drug interactions may occur with fibrates, including increased risk of bleeding when fenofibrate is given with warfarin, myopathy or rhabdomyolysis when it is administered with HMG-CoA reductase inhibitors (statins), and hypoglycemia when it is given with sulfonylureas.

Ezetimibe

Mechanism of action. Ezetimibe inhibits intestinal absorption of cholesterol originating from dietary or biliary sources. This decreases the amount of cholesterol that is transported to the liver; thus, hepatic stores of cholesterol are decreased and clearance of plasma cholesterol increases.

Clinical use. Ezetimibe lowers LDL cholesterol by 20% and triglycerides by 10%. It is often combined with statins.

Adverse effects. Generally, ezetimibe is well tolerated. It has been associated with allergic responses, respiratory infections, back pain, arthralgias, and gastrointestinal upset. Rarely, liver function tests may be elevated, but this resolves when the drug is discontinued.

Bile Acid Sequestrants (Resins)

Cholestyramine, Colestipol, and Colesevelam

Mechanism of action. Bile acid resins are positively charged, nonabsorbable resins that bind to negatively charged bile acids in the intestinal tract and prevent their reabsorption. This results in fecal elimination of bile acids. As the bile acid pool is depleted, hepatic enzymes increase conversion of cholesterol to bile acids. This increased hepatic demand for cholesterol causes increased synthesis of hepatic LDL receptors and ultimately lowers LDL cholesterol in the plasma.

Pharmacokinetics. These positively charged resins are not bile-specific and therefore bind to all negatively charged materials in the gut. As a result, drug interactions occur when acidic drugs are given concurrently. Absorption of fat-soluble vitamins (vitamins A, D, E, and K) may be impaired with bile acid resins, and bioavailability of acidic drugs is reduced (Box 8-16).

Clinical use. Bile acid resins decrease total cholesterol by 15% to 25%. These drugs are also used off-label to reduce diarrhea.

Adverse effects. Bile acid resins may actually increase triglyceride levels by 15%; therefore, they are best used in combination with drugs that lower triglyceride levels. Frequently, bile acid resins cause constipation, bloating, and flatulence, which can be managed by increasing fluid intake or using stool softeners.

Niacin

Mechanism of action. The mechanisms of niacin are not completely understood but may involve inhibition of a putative lipid translocase that normally liberates free fatty acids from adipose tissue to the liver. Ultimately, synthesis of triglycerides is reduced, which translates to reduced synthesis of very low density lipoprotein (VLDL), which subsequently reduces LDL levels as well. Niacin also increases HDL levels.

Clinical use. Niacin reduces LDL and triglycerides by 15%. Niacin also decreases uptake of HDL by the liver, resulting in a 25% increase in HDL at relatively low doses. Niacin is frequently combined with bile acid resins for additive effects.

Adverse effects. Niacin often causes flushing and itching due to release of prostaglandins. These adverse effects may be prevented by preadministration of aspirin. Hepatitis may occur, and as dosages are increased, liver function tests must be monitored. Immediate-release formulations are associated with substantial flushing. Sustained-release niacin formulations are associated with less flushing but a higher incidence of hepatotoxicity. Intermediate-acting formulations are a compromise between the adverse effects. Niacin is teratogenic in pregnancy. Additional adverse effects associated with niacin are listed in Box 8-17.

Summary

In essence, drugs that reduce cholesterol synthesis (by the liver) or block cholesterol or bile acid absorption through the gastrointestinal tract are effective therapies. Many patients who consume low-fat diets still require pharmacotherapy due to genetic predispositions for hyperlipidemia ("It's not just the frank you eat, but also your Uncle Frank").

●●● COMPLEMENTARY AND ALTERNATIVE MEDICINE

CLINICAL MEDICINE

Lowering "Bad" Cholesterol

Statins are usually the best choice for initial therapy to lower LDL. Patients typically get the most benefits at low- to mid-range doses. Doubling the statin dose usually provides only a modest additional reduction in LDL cholesterol and makes adverse effects more likely. It is often more effective to add a second drug. Adding a bile acid sequestrant provides an additional 10% to 20% reduction in LDL, adding ezetimibe lowers LDL an additional 15%, and adding niacin lowers LDL 10% to 15% (and can increase HDL and lower triglycerides also).

Box 8-17. ADVERSE EFFECTS ASSOCIATED WITH NIACIN

Flushing
Itching
Hyperuricemia (elevated uric acid; can precipitate gout)
Hyperglycemia
Gastrointestinal disturbances
Myopathy
Hepatitis
Peptic ulcer reactivation

Patients use a variety of natural products to lower their cholesterol. Some of these alternatives are probably safe and effective; others, however, may not be.

Plant sterols and stanols are being added to foods like orange juice and margarine. They prevent cholesterol from being absorbed. Regular use of these health foods may decrease LDL by 5% to 17%.

Fibrous foods that contain at least 51% whole grains (e.g., whole wheat, whole oats, corn, barley) may help reduce cholesterol. It is the fiber content in whole grains that seems to reduce cholesterol and the risk of heart disease. Oat bran can reduce LDL cholesterol by as much as 26% by increasing the viscosity of food in the stomach and delaying absorption. Psyllium, another source of fiber, can decrease cholesterol by absorbing dietary fats in the gastrointestinal tract, preventing cholesterol absorption, and increasing cholesterol elimination in fecal bile acids.

Fish oil contains omega-3 fatty acids that have been shown to reduce triglycerides by 20% to 50%, but supplements containing these fatty acids should be used cautiously in patients who are using anticoagulants, since fish oil may increase the risk of bleeding.

Products that contain red yeast rice are extracts of rice that has been fermented with red yeast. The natural fermentation process yields several different HMG-CoA reductase inhibitors (including lovastatin). These natural products are essentially statins in disguise. Because the natural substances produced via the fermentation process are statins, hepatotoxicity and myopathy can occur as adverse effects. The fact that these natural products are unregulated means that they may contain too much or too little of the active ingredients.

TOP FIVE LIST

1. Antihypertensives lower blood pressure by reducing cardiac output (β-blockers) or lowering total peripheral resistance (the rest of the drugs).
2. Drugs used to manage angina reduce myocardial oxygen demand or increase oxygen supply.
3. Heart failure therapies focus on preventing additional hypertrophy or remodeling damage; positive inotropes should be reserved for patients who are symptomatic after other therapies have been tried.
4. Antiarrhythmics possess a variety of different mechanisms that target ion channels; however, these drugs may also induce secondary arrhythmias by perturbing these ion channels (proarrhythmogenic).
5. Antihyperlipidemics lower cholesterol or triglyceride levels, but many are associated with muscle aches and elevations of liver function tests.

Renal System

9

CONTENTS

It's all about osmotic balance. Essentially, renal physiology can be reduced to one simple equation: what goes in must equal what comes out. Despite a variable load of solute and solvent ingestion, the kidney is capable of finely regulating osmotic balance. Multiple Na^+ cotransporters, antiporters, and channels serve to reabsorb Na^+ along the nephron to create the osmotic gradient necessary for water reabsorption. Physicians have at their disposal a vast arsenal of drugs to circumvent Na^+ and water retention, especially in diseases such as congestive heart failure where retained fluid must be eliminated. The administration of these drugs (diuretics) leads to both diuresis (water loss) as well as natriuresis (Na^+ loss). Diuretics increase the rate of urine formation. By increasing urine volume, there is a net loss of water and accompanying solute. The net loss of electrolytes varies among diuretic agents depending upon the drug's site of action. Figure 9-1 provides an overview of the site of action for six classes of diuretic agents.

Given their role in the regulation of water and salts, diuretics are used to manage diseases such as hypertension, congestive heart failure, edema, hypercalciuria, and historically glaucoma.

●●● ELIMINATION

Renal elimination refers to the process by which the kidney removes substances from the body and is the net result of three inter-related processes: namely, glomerular filtration, secretion, and reabsorption (Box 9-1). Filtration is a passive, nonsaturable, linear process by which small ionized and unionized molecules are filtered from the plasma via the glomerulus. It is important to remember that only free, unbound drug is filtered. Protein-bound drugs do not enter the filtrate as long as renal function is normal.

ANATOMY

Structure Defines Function

To fully understand the actions of diuretics, practitioners must appreciate the exquisite anatomy of the nephron that underlies renal physiology. In other words, structure (anatomy) drives function (physiology), which can be exploited (pharmacology). The nephron, the functional unit of the kidney, is composed of the glomerulus (the filtration unit) and a series of downstream tubules (proximal, loop of Henle, distal and collecting ducts) that serve to reabsorb solutes and fluid into the peritubular capillary network. Three examples of structure-function relationships within the nephron are described below.

1. The process of selective filtering or sieving within a glomerulus is mediated by the fenestrated endothelial cells of the capillary lumen in juxtaposition to the foot processes of the epithelial cells of the tubule network. The mesenchymal cells within the capillary network of the glomerulus, known as mesangial cells, provide the mechanical constrictive force to regulate GFR by changing the surface area available for filtration.

2. The distal tubule of the nephron winds its way between both the afferent and efferent arterioles as well as the glomerulus. This anatomic feature, known as the macula densa, allows for cross-talk between nephron elements. Cells within the afferent arteriole (juxtaglomerular cells) release renin, the enzyme that converts angiotensinogen to angiotensin I, by integrating signals from the afferent arteriole (perfusion pressure), renal sympathetic nerves, and distal tubule (solute load). In a similar scenario, the process of tubuloglomerular feedback is mediated by sensing solute load within the distal tubule and turning that information into intracellular signals that modify glomerular filtration rate via mesangial cell contractility.

3. Based on the anatomic hairpin loop of Henle as well as the discrete localization of $Na^+/K^+/2Cl^-$ cotransporters in the thick ascending loop of Henle, an osmotic gradient is generated in the renal medulla that provides the driving force to reabsorb greater than 99% of filtered water.

Box 9-1. CALCULATING RENAL CLEARANCE

Any discussion of renal elimination warrants a review of the concept of clearance (see Chapter 1). Clearance is defined as the volume of blood cleared of drug per unit time. Although this chapter is primarily about renal elimination, recall that there are other routes of elimination as well, including hepatic, fecal, pulmonary, and through lactation. In such cases, total body clearance (CL_T) may be represented as

$$CL_T = CL_R \text{ (renal clearance)} + CL_{NR} \text{ (nonrenal clearance)}$$

Drugs that undergo first-order elimination have a constant clearance, since their rate of elimination is directly proportional to plasma levels. Also, when no active secretion or reabsorption occurs, renal clearance is the same as glomerular filtration rate (GFR). Since only "free" drugs are filtered at the glomerulus, when a drug is protein bound, the renal clearance is represented as follows:

$$CL_{Renal} = GFR \times \text{free fraction of drug}$$

Kidney function is most commonly quantified in terms of creatinine clearance (CrCl). Creatine clearance is a direct measure of renal function. This value is estimated using what is known as the Cockcroft-Gault method. The formula for males is

$$CrCl \text{ (mL/min)} = \frac{(140 - age)(body\ weight\ [kg])}{(Serum\ creatinine\ [mg/dL])(72)}$$

The formula for females is

$$CrCl \text{ (mL/min)} = \frac{(140 - age)(body\ weight\ [kg])}{(Serum\ creatinine\ [mg/dL])(72)} \times 0.85$$

These equations are useful unless the patient's weight is excessive. If patients weigh more than 30% over their ideal body weight (IBW), this is accounted for by using the following equation for weight, where TBW stands for total body weight (kg) and IBW is ideal body weight (kg).

$$\text{Corrected body weight} = IBW + [0.4(TBW - IBW)]$$

Ideal body weight is calculated as follows:
For men,

$$IBW = 50\ kg + 2.3(\text{number of inches} > 60)$$

For women,

$$IBW = 45\ kg + 2.3(\text{number of inches} > 60)$$

Knowledge of a patient's kidney function is imperative when prescribing any medications that are eliminated renally. For a healthy young adult, creatinine clearance should be approximately 100 to 120 mL/min or 20 mg/kg/day. Since creatinine clearance declines with declining renal function, doses of medication handled by the kidneys will need to be decreased accordingly to prevent adverse effects resulting from drug accumulation. While not a 1:1 correlation, drug doses are decreased proportionately to diminished creatinine clearance.

PHYSIOLOGY

Role of the Glomerulus

During glomerular filtration, the plasma is filtered through the capillary endothelium, a basement membrane, and the epithelium of Bowman's capsule. The most important barriers to prevent substances from freely leaking through the glomerulus are negatively charged heparin sulfates in the basement membrane and the podocytes, which are specialized epithelial cells that stabilize the glomerulus.

Unlike filtration, secretion, is an active, saturable process (Fig. 9-2). The kidney has evolved multiple mechanisms to actively secrete both unionized and charged substances by way of energy-dependent transporters.

Not all drugs that are passively filtered at the glomerulus or actively secreted into the renal filtrate are immediately eliminated from the body. Drugs that are nonpolar and un-ionized may be reabsorbed from the renal filtrate and reenter the bloodstream. On the other hand, drugs that are polar or ionized become "trapped" in the filtrate and are eliminated from the body in the urine. As should be remembered, the

CLINICAL MEDICINE

Competition for Renal Secretion

Sometimes drugs compete for the renal active transport protein system. For example, under normal circumstances, penicillins are actively secreted into the renal tubules from the peritubular capillary network. In certain situations, it is desirable to slow penicillin's elimination from the body and increase the drug's concentration in the plasma. The drug probenecid, an anti-inflammatory typically prescribed for gout, can compete with penicillin for the same active transport protein carrier in the renal tubules. When probenecid competes with penicillin for the active transport carrier protein, elimination of penicillin from the body is slowed.

ultimate consequence of drug metabolism is to generate polar hydrophilic metabolites that are not reabsorbed in the tubule network and remain in the urine.

●●● OSMOTIC DIURETICS

Mannitol and Urea

Osmotic diuretics are freely filtered at the glomerulus, undergo minimal reabsorption by the renal tubules, and are rela-

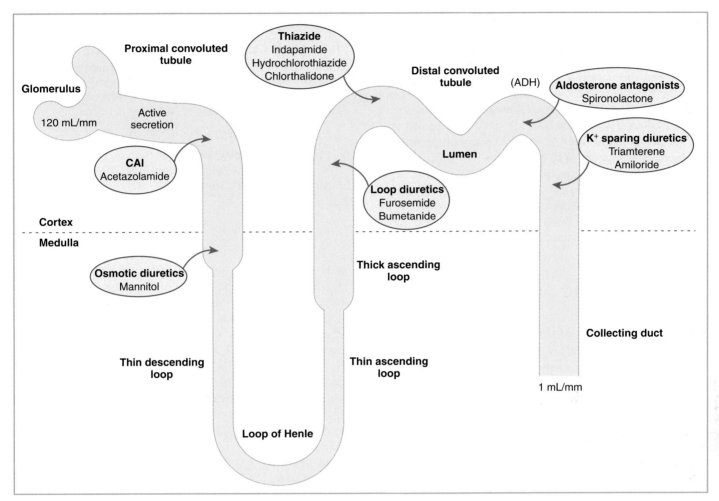

Figure 9-1. Overview of site of action for diuretic drugs. CAI, carbonic anhydrase inhibitor.

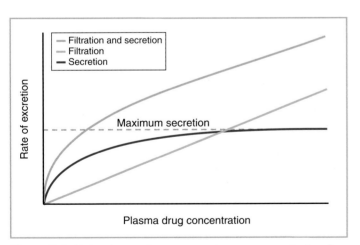

Figure 9-2. Rate of excretion versus plasma concentration for drugs. Excretion is a combination of filtration and active secretion.

tively pharmacologically and metabolically inert. Examples of osmotic diuretics are intravenous mannitol and urea.

Mechanism of action. Osmotic diuretics primarily inhibit water reabsorption in the proximal convoluted tubule (PCT) and the thin descending loop of Henle and collecting duct,

PATHOLOGY

Detoxification of Weak Acids and Weak Bases

Use NH_4Cl, vitamin C, or cranberry juice to acidify the urine. This increases ionization of weak bases, which increases renal elimination.

Use $NaHCO_3$ or acetazolamide to alkalinize the urine. This increases ionization of weak acids, which increases renal elimination.

regions of the kidney that are highly permeable to water. As Na^+ is reabsorbed in the proximal tubule, water normally follows and is reabsorbed by passive diffusion. In the presence of an osmotic diuretic, reabsorption of water is reduced relative to Na^+. In other words, despite the actions of transporters to generate an Na^+ concentration gradient favorable for osmosis, mannitol and urea negate this driving force. Osmotic diuretics also extract water from intracellular compartments, increasing extracellular fluid volume. Overall, urine flow increases with a relatively small loss of Na^+. In fact, urine osmolarity actually decreases.

Clinical uses. Osmotic diuretics are used to increase water excretion in preference to Na^+ excretion. Urine volume can be maintained even when the glomerular filtration rate is low. Osmotic diuretics are particularly effective in preventing anuria (cessation of urine production) accompanying presentation of large pigment loads to the kidney such as in hemolysis as well as rhabdomyolysis. Osmotic diuretics are used to lower intracranial pressure and for short-term reduction of intraocular pressure. These drugs also promote excretion of nephrotoxic substances such as cisplatin.

Adverse effects. Acutely, extracellular fluid volume expansion may occur, which is particularly undesirable for patients with cardiac decompensation. As mannitol is cleared by the kidneys, water follows, leading to dehydration and hypernatremia; nausea and vomiting, chest pain, and chills may occur.

●●● CARBONIC ANHYDRASE INHIBITORS

Acetazolamide and Methazolamide (Oral) and Dorzolamide (Ocular)

Mechanism of action. Carbonic anhydrase (CA) inhibitors block carbonic anhydrase on the luminal membrane and inside proximal tubule cells (Fig. 9-3). Inhibition of CA in the cytoplasm of proximal tubule cells causes a decrease in secretion of H^+ through the Na^+/H^+ antiporter. In this way, the driving force to reabsorb Na^+ in the proximal tubule is dissipated, necessitating natriuresis and diuresis. With CA on the luminal membrane also inhibited, the formation of bicarbonate from carbonic acid in the lumen is slowed,

as is the diffusion of CO_2 into the tubular cells. Overall, bicarbonate reabsorption in the proximal tubule decreases by 80%, leading to the possibility of acidosis. As a consequence of less Na^+ reabsorption via Na^+/H^+ exchange in the proximal tubule, more Na^+ is delivered to distal segments of the nephron. Sodium reabsorption in the distal tubule provides the electrogenic driving force to facilitate K^+ secretion into the tubule lumen. This is the mechanism by which most diuretics cause hypokalemia (loss of K^+). To counteract this loss of K^+, patients are often given K^+ supplements or encouraged to eat bananas or drink orange juice. Overall, the enhanced urinary excretion of Na^+ and K^+ leads to increased urine flow.

Clinical uses. As diuretics, these agents have limited utility due to rapid depletion of body bicarbonate stores and metabolic acidosis. Since CA inhibitors rapidly reduce total body bicarbonate stores, they are useful to treat chronic metabolic alkalosis. The lack of proton secretion into the tubules as a consequence of CA inhibition may be used to alkalinize the urine to enhance elimination of weak acids, such as uric acid and cystine. CA inhibitors are also useful in treatment of acute mountain sickness (they rapidly reduce pulmonary and cerebral edema). There is also a role for these agents in treating glaucoma, since CA inhibitors reduce intraocular pressure by inhibiting the formation of aqueous humor.

Adverse effects. Acetazolamide is a nonbacteriostatic sulfonamide. Sulfonamide-type adverse reactions may occur including urticaria, pruritus, rash, Stevens-Johnson syndrome, photosensitivity, bone marrow depression, and blood dyscrasias. The drug is contraindicated in those with sulfonamide hypersensitivity. Other adverse effects include hyperchloremic metabolic acidosis, renal calculi (calcium is insoluble at alkaline pH), hypokalemia, and paresthesias.

Ocular use of dorzolamide is associated with adverse ocular reactions, dysgeusia (an unpleasant taste in the mouth), and superficial punctate keratitis (corneal disease).

Drug interactions. Concurrent use of CA inhibitors and salicylates may result in accumulation and toxicity of CA inhibitors, leading to central nervous system toxicity as well as severe metabolic acidosis.

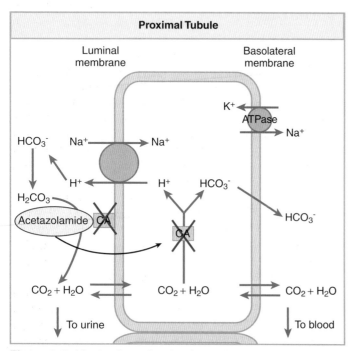

Figure 9-3. Mechanism of action for carbonic anhydrase (CA) inhibitors.

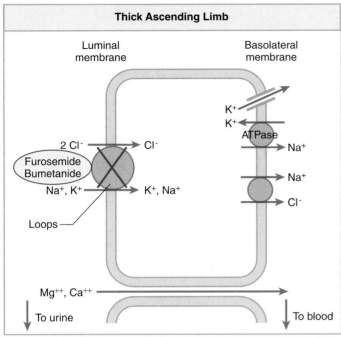

Figure 9-4. The $Na^+/K^+/Cl^-$ symporter is the site of action of loop diuretics.

●●● LOOP DIURETICS

Furosemide, Bumetanide, Ethacrynic Acid, and Torsemide

Mechanism of action. The primary mode of action of loop diuretics is inhibition of the $Na^+/K^+/2Cl^-$ cotransporter on the luminal membrane of the thick ascending limb (TAL) of the loop of Henle (Fig. 9-4). Inhibition of the $Na^+/K^+/2Cl^-$ cotransporter dissipates the Na^+ gradient generated in the renal medulla, which drives water reabsorption in the water-permeable descending limb of the loop of Henle. Inhibition of $Na^+/K^+/2Cl^-$ cotransport decreases intracellular K^+, which decreases the positive electrogenic potential and hence decreases reabsorption of Ca^{++} and Mg^{++}. Uric acid excretion is also reduced. In a nutshell, loop diuretics decrease reabsorption of Na^+, K^+, Ca^{++}, Mg^{++}, and Cl^-. Because of the large NaCl absorptive capacity of the loop of Henle, loop diuretics cause a large Na^+ load to remain in the tubule system and exert a powerful diuretic action.

Loop diuretics such as ethacrynic acid, furosemide, and bumetanide are both passively filtered at the glomerulus and actively secreted by cells of the proximal tubule. Acidic drugs like probenecid compete for this secretory transport process and can thus reduce the diuretic action of loop diuretics by reducing their concentration at the loop of Henle.

Clinical uses. Loop diuretics are useful to reduce edema associated with cardiac, hepatic, or renal disease. They are also helpful in managing acute pulmonary edema and congestive heart failure. In acute renal failure, loop diuretics may be used in an attempt to convert oliguric (small volume of urine) failure to nonoliguric failure. Loop diuretics have also been used to manage hypercalcemia and hyperkalemia.

Adverse effects. The most common adverse effects associated with loop diuretics are related to renal effects of the drugs: volume depletion, hypokalemic metabolic alkalosis, hypomagnesemia, and hypocalcemia. Furosemide and bumetanide are sulfonamide derivatives and may be contraindicated in patients with hypersensitivity to sulfa drugs. Ototoxicity may occur with loop diuretics, particularly when used intravenously, at high doses, or in combination with aminoglycosides (ethacrynic acid is more ototoxic than furosemide is). Ethacrynic acid also causes gastrointestinal disturbances.

Drug interactions. Loop diuretics may decrease lithium clearance, resulting in lithium toxicity. Use with angiotensin-converting enzyme (ACE) inhibitors may result in a precipitous fall in blood pressure, especially in the presence of Na^+ depletion. Diuretic-induced hypokalemia may increase the risk of digoxin toxicity; this occurs because digoxin binds to the K^+-site of the Na^+/K^+-ATPase. Under conditions of hypokalemia, there is less K^+ competing with digoxin, thus digoxin toxicity may occur. Concomitant use with nonsteroidal anti-inflammatory drugs (NSAIDs) reduces the blood pressuring–lowering effects of diuretics owing to the Na^+ reabsorption associated with NSAIDs.

●●● THIAZIDES

Hydrochlorothiazide, Indapamide, Metolazone, and Chlorthalidone

Mechanism of action. Thiazides increase urine output by inhibiting the NaCl cotransporter on the luminal membrane of the earliest portion of the distal convoluted tubule (DCT), often called the cortical diluting segment (Fig. 9-5). Inhibition of the NaCl cotransporter increases luminal concentrations of Na^+ and Cl^- ions in the late distal tubule; the large Na^+ load downstream promotes K^+ excretion in the late distal tubule and the collecting duct. Thiazides also lead to increased reabsorption of Ca^{++} into the blood and may lead to hypercalcemia. Thus, thiazides increase urinary levels of Na^+, K^+, and Cl^- and decrease levels of Ca^{++} in the urine.

Thiazides, as organic acids, are readily filtered and secreted but are less effective at mobilizing fluid than loop diuretics are, especially at low glomerular filtration rates (GFRs). (Loop diuretics are preferred when creatine clearance is less than 40–50 mL/min.) In fact, hydrochlorothiazide decreases GFR without altering renal blood flow.

Clinical uses. Thiazide diuretics are first-line treatment for hypertension, according to the Seventh Report of the Joint National Committee on Prevention, Detection, Evaluation, and Treatment of High Blood Pressure (JNC-VII). Initially, antihypertensive effects are due to diuresis and volume depletion. Surprisingly, as renal compensation occurs via the renin-angiotensin-aldosterone system, the antihypertensive actions of thiazides continue. It is thought that mobilization of Na^+ makes vessels more pliable and less rigid, producing a decrease in total peripheral resistance. Additionally, indapamide has vasodilating properties, which accounts for a portion of its antihypertensive effects. Because thiazides

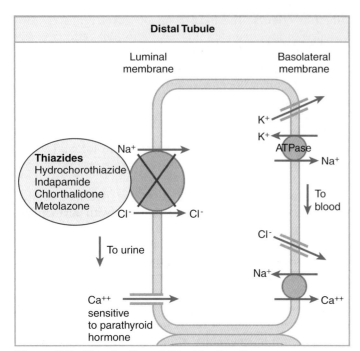

Figure 9-5. Site of action of thiazide diuretics.

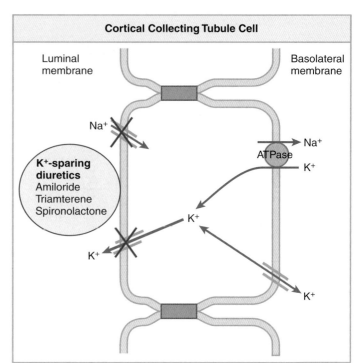

Figure 9-6. Site of action of K⁺-sparing diuretics.

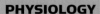

PHYSIOLOGY

Parathyroid Hormone

Parathyroid hormone (PTH), synthesized and released by the parathyroid glands, controls the distribution of Ca^{++} and $H_2PO_4^-$ in the body. High levels of PTH cause Ca^{++} transfer from bone to blood. Specifically, PTH enhances Ca^{++} reabsorption within the distal convoluted tubule through G protein–coupled regulated Ca^{++} channels as well as inhibits tubular reabsorption of phosphate. Finally, PTH also stimulates production of 1,25-dihydroxyvitamin D3 (calcitriol) within the kidney, which enhances Ca^{++} reabsorption in the gastrointestinal tract.

reabsorb calcium, they are a first-line choice for treating idiopathic hypercalciuria to reduce calcium stone formation. **Adverse effects.** Hypokalemia, hyponatremia, hypomagnesemia, and hypercalcemia may occur. Preexisting diabetes mellitus may be aggravated by thiazides. Hyperuricemia that precipitates gout can occur. Triglycerides and LDL cholesterol levels may increase initially but appear to return to pretreatment levels with long-term therapy (indapamide is an exception; it does not appear to increase serum cholesterol). Photosensitivity, decreased libido, and gastrointestinal disturbances may also occur.
Drug interactions. Same as for loop diuretics.

⬤⬤⬤ POTASSIUM-SPARING AGENTS

Spironolactone, Amiloride, and Triamterene

Mechanism of action. With their effect at the level of the collecting tubules (CT), these agents are generally considered

weak diuretics, since most of the filtered Na^+ is reabsorbed upstream (Fig. 9-6). The CT does, however, determine final urinary Na^+ concentration and is a major site of regulated K^+ and H^+ secretion.

Spironolactone is a steroid analog of the mineralocorticoid aldosterone. As an aldosterone receptor antagonist, spironolactone competitively competes with aldosterone for binding to its cytoplasmic receptor. This antagonism indirectly halts expression of new (spare or silent) Na^+ channels on the luminal membrane, decreases Na^+ conductance, and decreases Na^+/K^+-ATPase pump activity, which is the driving force behind K^+ secretion.

Remember that as Na^+ diffuses through its channels in the CT, it causes an increase in intracellular positive charge, which leads to extrusion of K^+ into the lumen. Since Na^+ is usually reabsorbed in exchange for K^+ in the CT, urinary K^+ excretion decreases with the use of spironolactone. Thus, inhibition of aldosterone via spirolactone retards K^+ secretion and is thus K^+-sparing. Since aldosterone, through undefined mechanisms, leads to proton extrusion across the luminal membrane of intercalated cells, spirolactone often alkalinizes the urine.

In contrast to spirolactone, amiloride and triamterene have slightly different mechanisms in the CT. These drugs directly block Na^+ channels on the luminal membrane in the CT, resulting in hyperkalemia and acidosis. Again, as these drugs block Na^+ channels at the site of Na^+-dependent K^+ excretion, K^+ is retained in the body (i.e., K^+ is spared). Together, all K^+-sparing diuretics produce small increases in urinary Na^+ and marked decreases in urinary K^+ and H^+.

Clinical uses. Spironolactone is helpful as an adjunct to other diuretics because of its K^+-retaining properties. As an aldosterone receptor antagonist, spironolactone is used to treat primary or secondary hyperaldosteronism. Spironolactone has also been shown to increase survival in advanced stages of heart failure and reduce edema and ascites associated with hepatic cirrhosis or nephrotic syndrome.

Triamterene is frequently used in combination with hydrochlorothiazide. This combination not only enhances the diuretic effect of the thiazide, but also counteracts the loss of K^+ normally associated with hydrochlorothiazide. Like triamterene, amiloride is used in combination with hydrochlorothiazide. Additionally, amiloride has an off-label use for preventing K^+ loss in lithium-induced diabetes insipidus.

Adverse effects. As a group, K^+-sparing diuretics may cause hyperkalemic metabolic acidosis or azotemia (excessive amounts of urea and other nitrogenous wastes in the blood). Spironolactone is usually not recommended in males owing

---

Box 9-2. NATURAL PRODUCTS HAVING DIURETIC EFFECTS

Caffeine	Foxglove
Chicory	Licorice
Corn silk	Stinging nettle
Dandelion	St. John's wort
Elderberry	

---

to the drug's antiandrogenic effects, which lead to gynecomastia and lowered libido. Nephrolithiasis (kidney stones) has been reported with triamterene.

COMPLEMENTARY AND ALTERNATIVE MEDICINE

In addition to prescription diuretics, natural diuretics are used by patients to self-treat problems such as menstrual disorders, edema, and hypertension. Although more than 90 natural products are reported to have diuretic activity, only caffeine is routinely included in over-the-counter medications for this purpose, since adequate scientific data supporting the safety and efficacy of other products are lacking. However, patients may self-medicate with dandelion, stinging nettle, corn silk, and other natural therapies. A partial listing of the most common natural products with diuretic activity is given in Box 9-2.

TOP FIVE LIST

1. Diuretics that block Na^+ reabsorption at segments proximal to the collecting duct increase Na^+ load in the late proximal tubule and collecting ducts.
2. An increase in Na^+ load leads to urinary excretion of K^+.
3. Urinary loss of K^+ may cause hypokalemia.
4. Blockade of Na^+ reabsorption by loop diuretics and thiazides drives water excretion (diuresis) and is associated with loss of H^+, resulting in alkalosis.
5. Loss of K^+ can be avoided through use of drugs that act primarily at collecting ducts (i.e., K^+-sparing diuretics)—the final site for K^+ secretion.

The major effects of diuretics on urine and blood chemistries are reviewed in Table 9-1. Choosing a diuretic in clinical practice requires a complete patient history (Table 9-2) and will vary according to underlying disease.

PHYSIOLOGY

Role of the Renin-Angiotensin-Aldosterone (RAA) Pathway During Congestive Heart Failure

For patients with congestive heart failure, cardiac output eventually becomes inadequate to provide the necessary O_2 for all the body's tissues. The body attempts to compensate in several ways. One of these compensatory mechanisms involves activation of the RAA pathway, which leads to widespread vasoconstriction and Na^+ reabsorption in an attempt to compensate for the body's perceived "lack of blood flow." Unfortunately, these compensatory mechanisms simply end up placing more stress (i.e., preload and afterload) on an already failing heart. As an antagonist of aldosterone, spironolactone inhibits one of the end-results of RAA activation, that of aldosterone secretion, and thus prevents further sodium and water retention.

CLINICAL MEDICINE

Spironolactone Is More Than Just a Diuretic.

Hirsutism and polycystic ovary syndrome (PCOS) occur in females when androgen levels are too high. Having a steroid structure, spironolactone possesses nonspecific antiandrogenic effects. Spironolactone has been used by women to treat excessive hair growth and PCOS.

TABLE 9-1. Review of Major Diuretic Classes

Drug	Mechanism	Urine Levels	Blood Chemistry
Carbonic anhydrase inhibitors	Inhibit carbonic anhydrase in PCT	Elevated Na^+, K^+, Ca^{++}, HCO_3^-, and PO_4	Hypokalemia, acidosis, hyperchloremia
Loop diuretics	Inhibit $Na^+/K^+/2Cl^-$ in TAL	Elevated Na^+, K^+, Ca^+, Mg^{++}, and Cl^- Decreased HCO_3^-	Hypokalemia, alkalosis, hypomagnesemia, hypocalcemia
Thiazides	Inhibit NaCl in PCT	Elevated Na^+, K^+, and Cl^- Decreased Ca^{++}	Hypokalemia, alkalosis, hypercalcemia, hyperuricemia
K^+-sparing agents	Inhibit Na^+ channels or antagonize aldosterone receptors in CT	Elevated Na^+ Decreased K^+	Hyperkalemia, acidosis

CT, collecting tubule; PCT, proximal convoluted tubule; TAL, thick ascending limb of the loop of Henle.

TABLE 9-2. Choice of Diuretics in Clinical Practice

Condition	Diuretic of Choice
Congestive heart failure	Furosemide
Acute pulmonary edema	Furosemide
Hypertension	Hydrochlorothiazide
Hepatic cirrhosis	Spironolactone
Lithium-induced diabetes insipidus	Amiloride
Ca^{++} stones	Hydrochlorothiazide
Idiopathic hypercalciuria	Hydrochlorothiazide
Hirsutism	Spironolactone
Polycystic ovary syndrome (PCOS)	Spironolactone
Idiopathic hypercalcemia	Furosemide
Nephrogenic diabetes insipidus	Hydrochlorothiazide

Inflammatory Disorders 10

CONTENTS

Tissue damage causes dilation of local blood vessels as well as other characteristic changes, such as increased capillary permeability and accumulation of inflammatory cells at the site of injury. Leukocytes play a central role in initiation of the inflammatory process. Yet, it is the interaction between a wide range of mediators (e.g., histamine, kinins, neuropeptides, cytokines, and arachidonic acid derivatives) that is needed to *maintain* an inflammatory response. Acute and nonspecific inflammation are primarily mediated by neutrophils and macrophages, while lymphocytes, basophils, and eosinophils are generally associated with specific, more chronic types of inflammatory responses. Under normal circumstances, inflammation is localized, is short-lived, and resolves spontaneously. However, persistent inflammation indicates an ongoing pathologic state.

●●● INTRODUCTION TO ANTI-INFLAMMATORY DRUGS

It's all a fine line. A little inflammation restores homeostatic balance, fights disease, and drives wound-healing responses. A lot of inflammation results in pathologic conditions, such as asthma, rheumatoid arthritis, inflammatory bowel diseases, gout, atherosclerosis, and quite possibly cancer. Understanding the mechanisms by which inflammatory mediators regulate tissue damage has identified pharmaceutical targets for the development of drugs that combat unchecked inflammation. Histamine blockers, cyclooxygenase (COX) inhibitors, and glucocorticoids are all examples of drug classes that put the brakes on inflammatory processes.

IMMUNOLOGY

Hypersensitivity Reactions

Hypersensitivity reactions result from antigen interactions with humoral antibodies or sensitized lymphocytes. Type I reactions occur when allergens bind to specific IgE antibodies immobilized on FcεR1 high-affinity IgE receptors, mast cells, or basophils. Activated mast cells release histamine, prostacyclin D2, and leukotrienes. Type I allergic immediate reactions are associated with allergic rhinitis, bronchial asthma, atopic dermatitis, and systemic anaphylaxis. Type II reactions are cytotoxic and typically involve IgG and IgM antibodies reacting with a tissue antigen and triggering cytotoxicity. An example of a type II reaction is hemolytic anemia, in which certain drugs cause hemolysis of red blood cells. Type III reactions are immunocomplex-mediated, in which preformed antigen-antibody complexes are deposited in tissues or blood vessels. This type of hypersensitivity reaction can lead to vasculitis. Finally, type IV hypersensitivity reactions are delayed reactions between sensitized CD^{4+} or CD^{8+} T cells and antigens expressed in the proper cellular context. Activation of these CD^{4+} T cells releases cytokines, which further recruit and activate macrophages, granulocytes, and NK cells. Activation of CD^{8+} T cells can lead to direct cellular cytotoxicity.

Drugs used to treat inflammatory disorders fall into one of the following categories:

1. Antihistamines
2. Broad-spectrum agents, which include nonsteroidal anti-inflammatory drugs (NSAIDs) and steroidal anti-inflammatory drugs (glucocorticoids)
3. Disease-specific drugs that have uses in conditions such as asthma, gout, and skin disorders.

● ● ● ANTIHISTAMINE DRUGS

Histamine is typically found at pathologic levels in the lungs, skin, and the gastrointestinal (GI) tract. It is also released from mast cells and basophils during type I hypersensitivity reactions and in response to certain drugs, venoms, and even trauma.

Histamine receptors belong to the 7-transmembrane G protein–coupled family of receptors (7TM-GPCR; Fig. 10-1). There are two main histamine receptors—H_1 and H_2—and activation leads to selective effects (Table 10-1). In clinical practice, antagonists of both histamine receptors subtypes are used. Traditionally, H_1-selective antagonists are known as antihistamines, while H_2 antagonists are known as H_2 blockers.

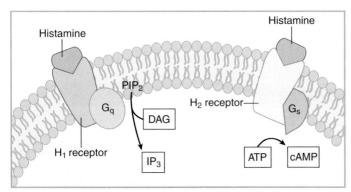

Figure 10-1. Histamine receptor signaling. H_1 receptors are G_q-coupled, while H_2 receptors are G_s-coupled.

TABLE 10-1. Characteristics of Histamine Receptor Activation

H_1 Activation	H_2 Activation
↑ Capillary dilation → ↓ blood pressure	↑ Gastric acid secretion → ↑ GI ulcers
↑ Capillary permeability → ↑ edema	↑ SA nodal rate
↑ Bronchiolar smooth muscle contraction	Positive cardiac inotrope
↑ Peripheral nociceptive receptors	↑ Cardiac automaticity
↓ AV nodal conduction	

H_1 Antagonists

Sedating Drugs: Diphenhydramine, Promethazine, and Meclizine

Low to Moderately Sedating Drugs: Cetirizine, Chlorpheniramine, Clemastine, and Cyproheptadine

Nonsedating Drugs: Loratadine, Fexofenadine, Desloratadine, and Phenindamine

Topical Nonsedating Drugs: Ketotifen, Levocabastine, Olopatadine, and Azelastine

Mechanism of action. These agents exert their pharmacologic effects through selective competitive antagonism of H_1 receptors and therefore may be ineffective in the presence of high histamine levels.

Clinical use. This class of drugs is most commonly recognized for its effectiveness in relieving allergic symptoms in hay fever, urticaria, rhinitis. They are also helpful in treating vertigo, motion sickness, and nausea, and many have sedating effects that allow them to be used as sleep aids. It should be noted that drugs like loratadine and fexofenadine are second-generation H_1 blockers and, unlike first-generation drugs, do not penetrate the central nervous system. As a result, these drugs do not cause drowsiness or provide relief from motion sickness. The sedating antihistamines impair performance, and in most states in the United States, drivers using these drugs would be considered impaired.

Some antihistamines have been developed specifically for treatment of seasonal allergies (Box 10-1).

Adverse effects. H_1 blockers are associated with muscarinic receptor blockade and accompanying "anticholinergic" side effects, sedation, and GI distress (less with second-generation drugs). On rare occasions, allergies to H_1 blockers have been reported.

H_2 Antagonists

Cimetidine, Ranitidine, Nizatidine, and Famotidine

Mechanism of action. These drugs will be discussed in detail in Chapter 11. H_2 blockers indirectly suppress activity of proton pumps in the gastric mucosa and partially antagonize HCl secretion.

Box 10-1. TOPICAL ANTIHISTAMINE TREATMENTS FOR SEASONAL ALLERGIES

Ocular Antihistamines

Ketotifen
Levocabastine
Olopatadine

Nasal Antihistamines

Azelastine

Clinical use. H_2 blockers are used in peptic ulcer disease, gastroesophageal reflux disease, as well as Zollinger-Ellison syndrome.

Adverse effects. Effects range from GI distress, dizziness, and somnolence to slurred speech and delirium (typically only in the elderly). In particular, cimetidine is a potent inhibitor of cytochrome P-450 isoenzymes and interferes with metabolism of common medications (Table 10-2).

●●● NONSTEROIDAL AND STEROIDAL ANTI-INFLAMMATORY DRUGS

It's all about the lipids, that is, the bioactive, lipid-derived second messengers that contribute to inflammation. Oxygenated metabolites of arachidonic acid, known as eicosanoids, play a central role in the majority of inflammatory reactions, and manipulation of their biosynthesis provides the basis of modern anti-inflammatory therapy (Table 10-3). Arachidonic acid itself is a 20-carbon fatty acid with four double bonds that is released from cell membrane phospholipids by the enzyme phospholipase A_2 (Fig. 10-2). Through further metabolism, arachidonic acid is converted by cyclooxygenases to prostanoids (thromboxane and prostacyclin), by lipoxygenases to leukotrienes, or by epoxygenases to hydroxyeicosatrienoic (HETEs) acids. As shown in Figure 10-3, 5-lipoxygenase products can be converted to leukotrienes, which are important mediators of inflammation and chemoattraction.

TABLE 10-2. Drug Interactions Caused by H_2 Antagonists That Inhibit Hepatic Microsomal P-450s

H_2 antagonists *increase the effects* of these drugs by decreasing their metabolism	H_2 antagonists *decrease the effect* of these pro-drugs (block activation by P-450s)
Amphetamines	"Azole" antifungals
Some β-blockers	Codeine
Some benzodiazepines	Hydrocodone
Calcium channel blockers	Oxycodone
Cyclosporine	Tramadol
Mexiletine	
Nateglinide	
Quinidine	
Phenytoin	
Risperidone	
Some selective serotonin reuptake inhibitors	
Sildenafil (and other phosphodiesterase-5 inhibitors)	
Tacrolimus	
Theophylline	
Tricyclic antidepressants	
Warfarin	

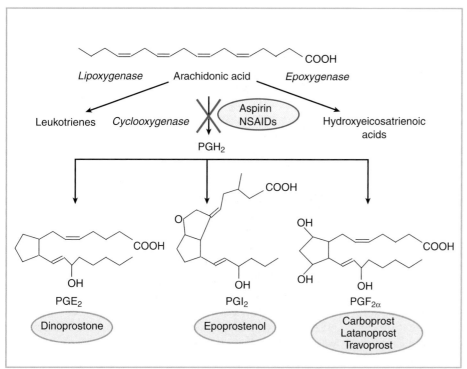

Figure 10-2. Arachidonic acid metabolites. Drugs that inhibit prostaglandin production *(burgundy)* or mimic prostaglandin action *(green)*. In rare circumstances, inhibition of cyclooxygenase with aspirin and NSAIDs may shunt arachidonic acid to leukotrienes and lead to bronchoconstriction. This is why aspirin/NSAIDs are contraindicated in asthmatics.

TABLE 10-3. Major Actions of Specific Eicosanoids and Therapeutic Uses of Several Eicosanoid Derivatives (the therapeutic eicosanoid is highlighted in color)

Eicosanoids	Actions and Uses
Leukotrienes LTA_4, LTC_4, LTD_4	Increased vascular permeability Anaphylaxis Bronchoconstriction (central role in asthma)
LTB_4	Neutrophil chemoattractant Activation of PMNs Increased free radicals, leading to cell damage
Prostaglandins PGE_1	Protection of gastric mucosa (misoprostol) Maintenance of patency of ductus arteriosus in neonates (alprostadil) Vasodilation (used in male impotence to treat erectile dysfunction) (alprostadil) Inhibition of platelet aggregation
PGE_2	Uterine smooth muscle contraction (dinoprostone) Cervical ripening and abortifacient Vasodilation and increased vascular permeability Sensitization of nociceptive fibers
$PGF_{2\alpha}$	Uterine smooth muscle contraction to terminate pregnancy/postpartum uterine bleeding (carboprost) Bronchiolar smooth muscle contraction Decreased intraocular pressure (latanoprost or travoprost) Used primarily as abortifactant and in glaucoma Vasodilation and increased vascular permeability Sensitization of nociceptive fibers
PGI_2 (prostacyclin)	Inhibition of platelet aggregation Vasodilation Used to treat pulmonary arterial hypertension (epoprostenol)
Thromboxanes TXA_2 (thromboxane)	Platelet aggregation Potent bronchoconstriction Potent vasoconstriction

Nonsteroidal Anti-inflammatory Drugs (NSAIDs)

Nonselective Cyclooxygenase (COX) Inhibitors

Examples of COX inhibitors are aspirin, ibuprofen, indomethacin, ketorolac, ketoprofen, naproxen, piroxicam, and sulindac. Somewhat selective COX-2 inhibitors include meloxicam and etodolac. Celecoxib is a selective COX-2 inhibitor.

Mechanism of action. Irreversible inhibition of cyclooxygenase is a unique property of aspirin. Aspirin (acetylsalicylic acid) was the first NSAID to be used in clinical practice (it was initially extracted from the bark of the willow tree). Aspirin covalently and irreversibly acetylates serine-520 of cyclooxygenase to inhibit its activity. All other NSAIDs work through noncovalent mechanisms.

Today, NSAIDs comprise a chemically diverse group of drugs, all of which possess the ability to competitively inhibit the enzyme cyclooxygenase to decrease formation of prostaglandins and thromboxane. Cyclooxygenase exists in two isoforms: COX-1, which is expressed in most tissues (especially in platelets, gastric mucosa, and kidneys), and COX-2, which is induced at sites of inflammation. Most NSAIDs work by indiscriminately inhibiting both cyclooxygenase isoforms and thus exhibit analgesic, antipyretic, anti-inflammatory, and antiplatelet effects. COX-2 specific inhibitors were developed to, theoretically, capitalize on the anti-inflammatory and analgesic properties of NSAIDs while simultaneously bypassing the risk of gastric bleeding associated with COX-1 inhibition. However, recent reports linking COX-2 inhibitors with cardiovascular mortality have lead to removal of rofecoxib (Vioxx) from the market. Some suggest that COX-2 specific inhibitors exert prothrombotic effects via inhibition of endothelial cell function and wound healing. Additional research will elucidate the safety issues surrounding the use of COX-2 specific inhibitors, and for now, celecoxib is the only selective COX-2 agent available. Additionally, the FDA mandated in February 2005 that all NSAIDs must carry warnings (the so-called black-box warning) that include the possibility of increased adverse cardiovascular events.

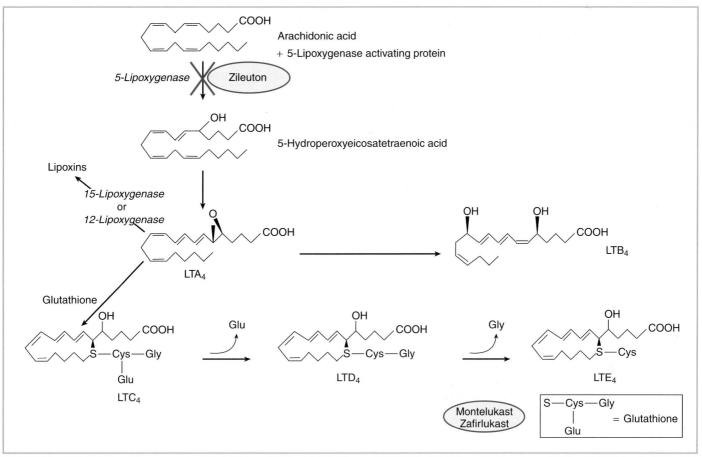

Figure 10-3. Drugs that inhibit leukotriene biosynthesis (zileuton) or antagonize the leukotriene receptors directly (montelukast and zafirlukast).

Clinical use. In general, NSAIDs are used as anti-inflammatory agents, antipyretics, and analgesics, although not all agents possess these three actions to the same extent. Depending on the desired effect, specific NSAIDs are used to treat rheumatoid arthritis, osteoarthritis, musculoskeletal pain or inflammation, postoperative pain, headaches, dental pain, and dysmenorrhea, and to provide symptomatic febrile relief. For pain, the analgesic strength profile is ketorolac > naproxen > ibuprofen > aspirin. Ketorolac, available as both oral tablets and an intramuscular injection, was developed specifically for postoperative analgesia. Even though high doses of NSAIDs may alleviate symptoms of rheumatoid arthritis, these drugs do not reduce progression of joint disease.

Acetaminophen (e.g., Tylenol), through unknown mechanisms, has antipyretic and analgesic actions similar to aspirin. However, since it is a very weak COX inhibitor, its anti-inflammatory actions are negligible. Acetaminophen is particularly useful in patients with aspirin allergies, peptic ulcer disease, and bleeding disorders and in those taking anticoagulant therapies.

Indomethacin is used in neonatal settings to encourage closure of a patent ductus arteriosus. The ductus arteriosus remains patent (open) as a result of enhanced prostanoid production. In fact, one reason NSAIDs should be avoided during pregnancy is that they may cause premature closure of the ductus arteriosus, leading to pulmonary hypertension in the fetus.

Adverse effects. Patients with GI ulcers and/or bleeding should avoid NSAIDs, since these conditions might be exacerbated. Taking NSAIDs with food lessens the risk of adverse GI effects. Ketorolac is especially problematic for the GI tract, and this drug should never be used for more than 5 days in a row to avoid GI bleeding. Hypersensitivity to NSAIDs is possible, particularly among patients with a history of nasal polyps or asthma. Cross-reactivity between agents is possible. Caution should be exercised when these drugs are used in patients with asthma, since the drugs can lead to unopposed accumulation of leukotrienes, thereby predisposing patients to bronchoconstriction (shunting of arachidonic acid to lipoxygenases; refer to Fig. 10-2).

NSAIDs are highly protein bound and can displace other drugs from plasma protein binding sites (with the exception of acetaminophen, ibuprofen, and indomethacin). This may increase the toxicity of sulfonylureas, sulfonamides, and phenytoin. Plasma levels of methotrexate and lithium may also be elevated with NSAIDs. Furthermore, chronic use of NSAIDs may lead to nephritis, nephritic syndrome, or acute renal failure, (i.e., via reduction of PGE_2 and PGI_2, which normally maintain glomerular filtration rate [GFR] and renal blood flow [RBF]). Because of the sodium retention induced by NSAIDs, antihypertensive therapies (e.g., ACE inhibitors, β-blockers, and loop diuretics) are often rendered less effective, and sodium retention may also aggravate symptoms of congestive heart failure. Renal complications are not seen with chronic use of sulindac; however, this drug can lead to pancreatitis. Indomethacin has been associated with thrombocytopenia, agranulocytosis, and CNS effects. Chronic diclofenac use is associated with hepatotoxicity. Celecoxib causes hypersensitivity reactions in patients with allergies to sulfonamides. Acetaminophen overdoses can cause hepatotoxicity, a situation that is managed by administering intravenous acetylcysteine (see Chapter 3).

Aspirin's unique mechanism (irreversible inhibition of COX) allows it to be a potent inhibitor of platelet aggregation (through reduction of TXA_2), and this has led to its successful use in primary and secondary prevention of cardiovascular and cerebrovascular events (Table 10-4). Recall that the actions of other NSAIDs are not irreversible but are competitive in nature. These disparate properties can be problematic for patients who take aspirin for cardiovascular protection, while simultaneously using chronic NSAID therapy for anti-inflammatory effects. If the NSAID reaches the COX active site first, it blocks aspirin's ability to bind, thus preventing the antiplatelet actions of aspirin. In fact, patients taking both ibuprofen and aspirin have a 73% increased risk of death due to cardiovascular events compared with patients taking aspirin alone. The bottom line is, if patients need both types of therapy, it is best to administer the "antiplatelet" aspirin first and delay other NSAID therapy for several hours.

Steroidal Anti-inflammatory Drugs (Glucocorticoids)

Oral Drugs: Methylprednisolone, Dexamethasone, Prednisolone, Prednisone, and Budesonide

Inhaled (Pulmonary, Nasal) Drugs: Triamcinolone, Mometasone, Beclomethasone, Flunisolide, Fluticasone, and Budesonide

Topical Drugs: Betamethasone, Mometasone, Triamcinolone, and Hydrocortisone

Mechanism of action. Unlike NSAIDs, which directly inhibit enzymes that generate pro-inflammatory lipid-derived second messengers, steroids are lipophilic, binding to cytosolic steroid receptors, which translocate into cell nuclei to exert their effects on glucocorticoid-responsive genes. Of particular importance to this chapter on inflammation-

---

TABLE 10-4. Unique Properties of Aspirin

Property	Description
Molecular mechanism	Irreversible covalent bond via acetylation of a serine hydroxyl group near the active site of COX enzymes.
Antiplatelet aggregation	Even a low dose (81-mg baby aspirin vs 325-mg full dose) exerts irreversible inhibition of TXA_2 synthesis; an elevation in prothrombin time is noted at high doses.
Analgesia	Moderate doses inhibit formation of prostaglandins, which in turn blunts peripheral pain receptor responses to pain mediators such as bradykinin and histamine.
Antipyresis	Pyrogens typically release IL-1, leading to increased PGE_2 in the hypothalamus and increasing the body's "set-point" temperature.
	At moderate doses, aspirin causes sufficient inhibition of PGE_2 and lowers the "set-point" to normal.
Anti-inflammatory	At moderate-to-high doses, strong inhibition of COX-2 is noted.
	Aspirin also interferes with cell surface selectins and integrins, thereby inhibiting leukocyte adhesion.
Uric acid excretion	At low-to-moderate doses, a decrease in renal tubular secretion is noted that leads to hyperuricemia; however, at high doses, a reduction of tubular reabsorption is noted, which leads to uricosuria.
Acid-base balance	At high therapeutic doses, a mild uncoupling of the oxidative phosphorylation chain leads to respiratory alkalosis and a compensatory metabolic acidosis.
	At toxic doses, inhibition of the respiratory center leads to respiratory acidosis, and severe uncoupling of the oxidative phosphorylation chain leads to metabolic acidosis, hyperthermia, and hypokalemia.
Gastrointestinal irritation	Inhibition of PGE_2 leads to gastritis, ulcers, and bleeding.
Salicylism	First signs of toxicity are often tinnitus (ringing in ears), vertigo, and decreased hearing.
Hypersensitivity	Seen most often among those with the triad of asthma, nasal polyps, and rhinitis.
Reye's syndrome	Potentially lethal condition in children that results in hepatotoxicity and/or encephalopathy due to use of aspirin during a viral illness; may be due to shunting of arachidonic acid to leukotrienes and lipoxin metabolites.

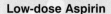

Low-dose Aspirin

Low-dose aspirin treatment (81 mg) is particularly effective to prevent additional cardiovascular and cerebrovascular accidents in patients who have suffered myocardial infarctions and strokes. This may be a reflection of the enucleated state of platelets. Platelets do not have nuclei; therefore, irreversible inactivation of platelet cyclooxygenase requires synthesis of new platelets (>24 hours) to produce vasoconstrictive and prothrombogenic thromboxanes. This is in contrast to endothelial cells, which can transcriptionally synthesize cyclooxygenase (<8 hours) to primarily generate vasodilatory and antithrombotic prostacyclins.

Putting It All Together: Anaphylactic Shock

Anaphylactic shock is a life-threatening, type I IgE-mediated systemic reaction in patients who have been previously sensitized to the antigen in question. Typical antigens that can generate anaphylaxis include insect stings, blood products, penicillin, cephalosporins, and food allergens (e.g., egg, peanut).

Activated mast cells and basophils release histamine and leukotrienes that induce bronchial constriction, vasodilatation, and vascular permeability. Bronchial constriction induced by leukotrienes leads to airway obstruction, laryngeal edema, bronchospasms and possible asphyxia and hypoxia. Vasodilation and plasma leakage into tissues, mediated by H_1 receptors, leads to hypovolemic shock, hypotension, and angioedema. First-line treatment for anaphylactic shock is intramuscular administration of epinephrine, to increase total peripheral resistance (raising blood pressure and reducing edema). In addition, antihistamines and glucocorticoids may be administered.

mediated lipid-derived second messengers, a major effect of glucocorticoids is the enhanced transcription or translation of a peptide called lipocortin that inhibits phospholipase A_2. This enzyme is responsible for mobilizing arachidonic acid from phospholipids in cell membranes. As a result of phospholipase A_2 inhibition, both prostanoids and leukotrienes are inhibited. As discussed in Chapter 5, glucocorticoids also induce immunosuppression by reducing the number and activity of immunocompetent cells in the circulation.

Clinical use. Glucocorticoids cause profound inhibition of inflammatory responses and are used to treat rheumatoid arthritis, inflammatory bowel diseases, asthma, and eczema, to name only a few uses. Various glucocorticoids have been formulated that can be delivered via nasal and oral inhalation for more local, nonsystemic, nontoxic control of asthma or allergic rhinitis.

Adverse effects. Prolonged use of systemic glucocorticoids leads to a cushingoid state, characterized by central obesity, moon face, hyperglycemia (which may lead to clinically significant diabetes mellitus), osteoporosis, and loss of skin structural integrity (seen as thin skin, easy bruising, and purple striae) as well as muscle weakness and wasting. Growth is often suppressed in children requiring systemic steroids. Adrenal suppression is also a major consideration in long-term corticosteroid users, and therefore a slow, tapered withdrawal must be employed. Immunosuppression increases susceptibility to pathogenic and opportunistic infections. Thus, a high index of suspicion for infection must be maintained in patients on long-term corticosteroids, since normal indicators of infection (such as inflammation) are suppressed. Other adverse effects include oral or nasal thrush (typically with inhaled corticosteroids), perforation of the nasal septum (with nasally administered corticosteroids), mood changes (euphoria or psychosis), peptic ulceration, and eye disorders (cataracts or glaucoma). With the exception of growth suppression and osteoporosis, inhaled glucocorticoids do not manifest systemic adverse effects, and the inhaled steroids do not have to be tapered. However, they cannot be used as substitutes for systemic formulations.

As specific examples, we will look at four specific inflammatory conditions (acne, asthma, gout, and rheumatoid arthritis) for which additional disease-specific anti-inflammatory agents are also used.

●●● INFLAMMATORY DISORDERS OF THE SKIN

Drug Classes: Corticosteroids, T-Cell Immunomodulators (Eczema) and Retinoids (Acne)

Two common skin disorders, eczema and acne, also have inflammatory components. In the case of eczema, topical steroids are usually the first line of therapy. Another option is topical T-cell immunomodulators, such as tacrolimus or pimecrolimus. These drugs block T-cell activation and prevent release of inflammatory cytokines. However, these products carry warnings regarding the possible increased risk of cancer associated with their use.

Inflammatory acne may be treated with retinoic acid (vitamin A) derivatives, such as oral isotretinoin and topical tretinoin. These drugs reduce sebaceous gland size, reduce sebum production, and regulate cell proliferation and differentiation. Owing to teratogenicity, numerous stipulations have been placed upon isotretinoin prior to a prescription for this product being dispensed. In addition to its teratogenicity, additional concerns over depression and suicidal ideation, elevated triglycerides, hepatitis, back pain, and visual disturbances have raised concerns with isotretinoin. The retinoic acid derivatives may cause excessive skin dryness, cheilitis, pruritus, and photosensitivity. Additional drugs used to treat acne are described in Table 10-5.

TABLE 10-5. Pharmacotherapy in Acne

Drug	Mode of Application	Mechanism Comments	Comments
Benzoyl peroxide	Topical	Releases free radical oxygen to oxidize bacterial proteins in sebaceous follicles, decreasing the number of anaerobic bacteria and decreasing the irritating free fatty acids	Bleaches fabrics
Sulfur, resorcinol, and salicylic acid	Topical	Keratolytic and mildly antibacterial	
Antibacterials	Topical, oral	Examples: erythromycin, tetracyclines, clindamycin, metronidazole	
Azelaic acid	Topical	Antimicrobial activities	May cause erythema, burning, pruritus
Adapalene	Topical	Modulates cellular differentiation, keratinization, and inflammatory processes	Retinoid-like compound Less irritating than tretinoin
Tazarotene	Topical	Modulates differentiation and proliferation of epithelial tissue Anti-inflammatory activities	Retinoid
Tretinoin	Topical	Causes keratinocytes in follicle to be less adherent, for easier removal	A "flare" is seen after initial treatment Irritating to skin
Isotretinoin	Oral	Decreases sebum production; inhibits *Propionibacterium acnes* Inhibits inflammation Increased differentiation of keratinization	Cheilitis, skin desquamation, muscle stiffness, arthralgias, hypertriglyceridemia, aggressive/ violent behavior, teratogenicity

●●● ASTHMA

Drug Classes: B₂-selective Agonists, Mast Cell Stabilizers, Corticosteroids, Leukotriene Receptor Antagonists, and Methylxanthines

According to the National Institutes of Health, asthma is primarily a disease of inflammation, with secondary broncho-constriction. In addition to inhaled (or oral, if necessary) corticosteroids, mast cell stabilizers, such as cromolyn or nedocromil, are anti-inflammatory options for patients with mild disease. With these drugs, mast cells are no longer able to release inflammatory leukotrienes, cytokines, or hista-mine. Mast cell stabilizers are extremely safe agents; their anti-inflammatory effects are less than those of glucocorti-coids, but they may be used in conjunction with cortico-steroids in an effort to reduce corticosteroid dosages. Cough, dry throat, headache, and bitter taste (nedocromil) are asso-ciated with their use. Keep in mind that, although a thera-peutic response may be observed in 2 weeks, it will likely take 4 to 6 weeks until maximal benefits are seen (Box 10-2). Not all patients respond favorably to mast cell stabilizers, and children are more likely than adults to respond favorably.

Another strategy for asthmatics is to antagonize leuko-triene LTC₄ and LTD₄ receptors (see Fig. 10-3). Orally active leukotriene receptor inhibitors, such as montelukast and zafirlukast, may be used. In addition, inhibition of 5-lipoxy-

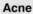

PATHOLOGY

Acne

The etiology of acne involves several pathophysiologic changes. (1) Androgen production increases sebaceous gland activity. (2) Sebum (glycerides, wax esters, and cholesterol) is produced in sebaceous glands. (3) The glycerides are metabolized by *Propionibacterium acnes* to fatty acids, which cause inflammation. (4) Plugging of the follicle and abnormal desquamation of follicular epithelial cells may further exacerbate inflammation.

Box 10-2. ADDITIONAL MAST CELL STABILIZERS USED IN TREATMENT OF SEASONAL ALLERGIES AND ASTHMA

Ocular	Pulmonary
Lodoxamide	Cromolyn
Pemirolast	Nedocomil

Nasal

Cromolyn

genase, the rate-limiting step in leukotriene synthesis, with the orally active drug zileuton, can also be used to treat asthma. However, not all patients respond favorably to this class of drugs, with elderly patients responding least well.

When used to treat asthma, inhaled corticosteroids alter gene transcription such that the number of β_2-receptors expressed in the lungs increases, mucus production decreases, inflammation is inhibited by decreased synthesis of pro-inflammatory cytokines, vascular permeability decreases, and cellular recruitment also decreases (fewer mast cells, macrophages, lymphocytes, and eosinophils). Corticosteroids are used in asthma to control and reverse inflammation, as well as for long-term suppression of inflammation. Although corticosteroids are the most effective anti-inflammatory agents used to treat asthma, it may take as long as 8 weeks until maximal effects are observed. Oral corticosteroids may be used for short-term control of acute exacerbations.

In addition to chronic airway inflammation, broncho-constriction occurs in asthma. Thus, bronchodilators are first-line treatments for asthmatics. Specifically, β_2-selective agonists, such as albuterol or pirbuterol, are used to treat acute bronchoconstriction. These drugs relax activated bronchial smooth muscle cells by inducing a G_s-mediated increase in cAMP. Side effects include tremors and tachycardia, but the consequences of severe bronchoconstriction can be life-threatening. In addition to the short-acting β_2-agonists mentioned above that are used for acute situations, longer acting agents such as levalbuterol, formoterol, and salmeterol are used prophylactically.

For some asthmatics, methylxanthines such as theophylline may be effective bronchodilators. Theophylline inhibits cAMP phosphodiesterase, indirectly elevating cAMP, analogously to the β_2-agonists. Theophylline has a narrow therapeutic index, and serum concentrations must be monitored periodically. Adverse effects include nausea and vomiting, headache, hyperglycemia, hyperkalemia, tachycardia, arrhythmias, tremors, severe neurologic toxicities (which can include seizures), and death. Theophylline is metabolized by hepatic microsomal P-450 isoenzymes, and concomitant use with P-450 inhibitors increases the risk of theophylline toxicity.

A final strategy reserved for patients whose symptoms are inadequately controlled with inhaled corticosteroids is that of omalizumab, a monoclonal antibody that blocks IgE receptors. Malignant neoplasms, injection site reactions, and the possibility of anaphylactic reactions are possible with this drug.

The NIH has established guidelines for treating asthma based on symptom severity. Step therapy guidelines are listed in Table 10-6.

●●● GOUT

Drug Classes: Colchicine, Uricosurics, and Xanthine Oxidase Inhibitors

Gout occurs when urate crystals are deposited within joints often because of underexcretion or overproduction of uric acid. Additionally, gout may occur as a secondary complica-

tion of myeloproliferative diseases or kidney disorders or as a result of enzymatic defects.

Anti-inflammatory NSAIDs, such as ibuprofen, ketorolac, and indomethacin, are effective to reduce gout joint pain. In addition to NSAIDs to manage joint pain, colchicine is often used. Even though colchicine relieves pain of acute gout attacks, it is not an analgesic. Instead, colchicine decreases motility of leukocytes and other inflammatory cells within joints by interfering with microtubule assembly. Ultimately, this reduces the deposition of urate crystals that perpetuate inflammatory responses. When properly administered, colchicine provides pain relief within 12 hours. However, colchicine treatment is limited by severe GI distress, bone marrow toxicity, and myopathy or peripheral neuritis.

Two strategies to diminish uric acid load are also effective treatments for gout. Uricosuric drugs (probenecid and sulfinpyrazone) are particularly effective for patients who are "underexcretors" of uric acid, since these drugs work by inhibiting uric acid transporters in renal proximal tubules that normally reabsorb uric acid. The net result of these drugs is that uric acid excretion is enhanced. These drugs are best used prophylactically and should not be used during acute attacks because kidney stones may form. Temporary urinary alkalization and good hydration for the first few days of therapy minimize the risk of kidney stones. Recall that salicylates inhibit the uricosuric effects of these drugs.

The second pharmacologic strategy to diminish uric acid load is to inhibit uric acid synthesis. Xanthine oxidase (Fig. 10-4) is the enzyme that converts soluble xanthine and hypoxanthine into insoluble uric acid. Allopurinol is a xanthine oxidase inhibitor that is particularly useful in patients who are "overproducers" of uric acid. The drug is also administered prophylactically to cancer patients who are receiving cytotoxic purine mimetics. Allopurinol is associated with an unusually high incidence of nonallergic skin rash when administered concomitantly with ampicillin.

●●● RHEUMATOID ARTHRITIS

Drug Classes: NSAIDs AND DMARDs

Rheumatoid arthritis (RA) is a chronic inflammation of the synovium of peripheral joints. It is primarily a disease

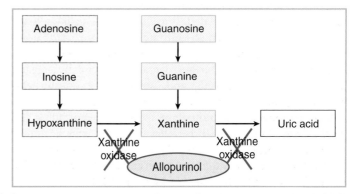

Figure 10-4. Mechanism of action for allopurinol, which leads to reduction in uric acid load.

TABLE 10-6. Stepwise Approach to Managing Asthma in Adults and Children Older Than 5 Years of Age

Classify Severity: Clinical Features Before Treatment or Adequate Control			Medications Required to Maintain Long-Term Control
Step	**Day Symptoms/ Night Symptoms**	**PEF or FEV₁/ PEF Variability**	**Daily Medication**
Severe persistent (step 4)	Continual/frequent	≤60%/>30%	*Preferred treatment:* High-dose inhaled corticosteroids + Long-acting inhaled β₂-agonists + if needed Corticosteroid tablets or syrup long term (Make repeated attempts to reduce systemic corticosteroids and maintain control with high-dose inhaled corticosteroids)
Moderate persistent (step 3)	Daily/>1 night/wk	>60% to <80%/ >30%	*Preferred treatment:* Low- to medium-dose inhaled corticosteroids and long-acting inhaled β₂-agonists *Alternative treatment:* Increase inhaled corticosteroids within medium-dose range *or* Low- to medium-dose inhaled corticosteroids and either leukotriene modifier or theophylline
Mild persistent (step 2)	>2/wk but <1/day/ >2 nights/mo	≥80%/ 20% to 30%	*Preferred treatment:* Low-dose inhaled corticosteroids *Alternative treatment:* Cromolyn, leukotriene modifier, nedocromil *or* Sustained-release theophylline to serum concentration of 5–15 μg/mL
Mild intermittent (step 1)	≤2 days/wk/ ≤2 nights/month	≥80%/<20%	No daily medication needed Severe exacerbations may occur, separated by long periods of normal lung function and symptoms A course of systemic corticosteroids is recommended

From Busse W, et al. National Asthma Education & Prevention Program: Expert Panel Report: Guidelines for the Diagnosis and Management of Asthma—Update Selected Topics 2002, p. 116. National Heart, Lung, & Blood Institute, U.S. Department of Health & Human Services, Bethesda, MD, NIH Pub. 02-5074, June 2003.

mediated by proinflammatory cytokines. Activated CD4+ T cells invade and infiltrate the joint. These cells release IL-2, IL-6, and interferon gamma, which chemoattract B cells and macrophages. Activated B cells (plasma cells) release rheumatoid factor, which initiates cartilage and bone damage. Activated macrophages within the synovium release IL-1 and TNFα, which further degrade the joint by causing synovial endothelial cells and fibroblasts to proliferate, neovascularize, and remodel the joint. These cytokines also activate osteoclasts to proteolyse the bone surrounding the joint. Thus, it is no surprise that NSAIDs, which inhibit cyclooxygenase-induced proinflammatory prostanoids and thromboxanes, are effective treatments for rheumatoid arthritis. Similarly, orally active glucocorticoids can be used to diminish chronic inflammation in patients with rheumatoid arthritis.

Disease-modifying antirheumatic drugs (DMARDs) are also used (Table 10-7). DMARDs are the only drugs capable of halting the underlying disease processes. Recent additions to DMARDs include monoclonal antibodies or receptor antagonists for circulating pro-inflammatory cytokines.

- Infliximab, a neutralizing antibody that targets tumor necrosis factor (TNF).
- Etanercept, a recombinant form of the TNF receptor that binds to circulating TNF, preventing interaction with endogenous receptors.
- Adalimumab, a monoclonal antibody that targets TNFα.
- Anakinra, an IL-1 receptor antagonist.

There is, however, a warning that all TNF inhibitors can cause serious infections and sepsis, especially when combined with IL-1 antagonists. These drugs may also increase the risk of cancer.

TABLE 10-7. Disease-Modifying Antirheumatoid Drugs (DMARDs)

Drug	Mechanism	Adverse Effects
Infliximab	Monoclonal antibody that neutralizes TNFα, thus suppressing TNF-induced proliferation of immune cells and macrophages	Hypersensitivity reaction Serious infection Heart failure Increased risk of cancer
Etanercept	Recombinant form of TNF receptor that binds up circulating TNF	Hypersensitivity reaction Serious infections Increased risk of cancer
Adalimumab	Monoclonal antibody for TNFα	Serious infections Increased risk of cancer Lupus-like syndrome
Anakinra	IL-1 receptor antagonist	Infection Headache Gastrointestinal distress
Gold salts (e.g., auranofin)	Gold salts reduce migration of macrophage phagocytosis and cause stabilization of lysosomes	Rash Leukocytopenia Proteinuria Pruritus Persistent diarrhea
D-penicillamine	Hypothesized to inhibit T helper cell function Decreases circulating IgM rheumatoid factor	Gastrointestinal distress, intolerance Autoantibodies Vasculitis Neurologic symptoms
Hydroxychloroquine	Inhibits locomotion of neutrophils and chemotaxis of eosinophils	Dermatitis Cardiomyopathy Hematologic abnormalities Visual disturbances
Sulfasalazine	Unknown	Allergic myocarditis Hemolytic anemia Exfoliative dermatitis
Methotrexate	Interferes with folic acid synthesis and inhibits proliferating inflammatory cells	Gastrointestinal distress Hepatotoxicity Bone marrow depression
Azathioprine	Inhibits purine synthesis	Bone marrow depression
Leflunomide	Inhibits pyrimidine synthesis	Diarrhea Hypertension Respiratory tract infection Alopecia Gastrointestinal upset
Cyclosporine	Inhibits IL-2 production and inhibits T-cell activation	Hypertension Hirsutism Renal dysfunction

●●● TOP FIVE LIST

1. Inflammation is a physiologic process that fights disease and promotes wound healing responses. Unchecked inflammation is a pathologic crisis that is often an underlying cause of atherosclerosis, inflammatory bowel disease, asthma, and rheumatoid arthritis.

2. Inflammatory mediators are often lipid second messengers. Oxygenated derivatives of arachidonic acid include prostaglandins, thromboxanes, and leukotrienes. Nonsteroidal anti-inflammatory drugs inhibit cyclooxygenase activity, the enzyme that forms prostaglandins and thromboxanes. Inhibitors of leukotriene synthesis (zileuton) and antagonists of leukotriene receptors (montelukast, zafirlukast) can be effective in asthmatics.

3. H$_1$ (histamine)-receptor blockers are effective for allergies and can be obtained over the counter or in prescription strengths.

4. Inflammatory acne is often treated with retinoic acid derivatives.

5. Monoclonal antibodies that target the cytokine TNFα are effective for patients with rheumatoid arthritis.

Gastrointestinal Pharmacology 11

CONTENTS

It's all about the pump. That is, the H$^+$/K$^+$ pump, which regulates stomach acidity (Fig. 11-1). Drugs that inhibit the pump are effective agents for both gastroesophageal reflux disease and peptic ulcer disease. These agents can either directly inhibit the pump or inhibit the second messengers (cAMP and calcium) that activate the pump.

●●● GASTROESOPHAGEAL REFLUX DISEASE

Gastroesophageal reflux disease (GERD), or "heartburn," affects nearly 60 million Americans on an intermittent basis, with 25 million people suffering daily symptoms. The typical cause of GERD is decreased lower esophageal sphincter tone, resulting in acid reflux. Substances including chocolate, caffeine, cholesterol, alcohol, and nicotine can all decrease esophageal sphincter pressure and exacerbate GERD. Drugs can also be culprits. Pharmacologic agents known to aggravate GERD are listed in Table 11-1.

Pharmacologic treatments for GERD include reducing stomach acidity by means of antacids, H$_2$ blockers, or proton pump inhibitors as well as prokinetic drugs that increase lower esophageal sphincter smooth muscle tone. Mild and transient GERD can be treated with over-the-counter

medications, whereas chronic, recalcitrant cases require prescription-strength medications.

Antacids

Antacids, including aluminum hydroxide, magnesium hydroxide, and calcium carbonate, can be quite effective against occasional GERD. Antacids increase gastrointestinal (GI) pH. However, as with any over-the-counter medication, adverse effects (Table 11-2) and drug interactions may occur (e.g., aluminum, magnesium, and calcium may form insoluble complexes with tetracyclines or fluoroquinolones, reducing bioavailability of the antibiotics). Since GI pH is elevated by antacids, absorption of numerous other drugs may be limited. It is recommended that antacid administration be separated from other drugs by at least 2 hours.

Alginic Acid

Alginic acid reduces the adverse effects of reflux by forming a viscous foam on the top of the gastric contents—a mechanical barrier—that protects the esophagus.

Unfortunately, the effects of antacids and alginic acid are short-lived so the drugs have to be administered four times daily (usually with meals and at bedtime).

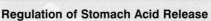

ANATOMY

Regulation of Stomach Acid Release

Neural release of acetylcholine and gastrin stimulates release of acid from the parietal cells of the gastric mucosa by activating the H$^+$/K$^+$-ATPase pump via a calcium-dependent protein kinase. In addition, acetylcholine and gastrin induce histamine release from enterochromaffin-like cells (ECLs), which then—through paracrine stimulation of H$_2$ receptors on parietal cells—also stimulates the H$^+$/K$^+$-ATPase pump. In contrast to acetylcholine and gastrin, H$_2$ receptors stimulate the H$^+$/K$^+$-ATPase pump via activation of adenylate cyclase to form cAMP and stimulate protein kinase A. Protein kinase A induces fusion of tubulovesicles within the canicular membrane of the parietal cell to release protons into the gastric lumen. Inhibition of muscarinic, gastrin, or histamine receptors will lead to inhibition of acid secretion by the pump. Additionally, activated PGE$_2$ receptors on parietal cells reduce pump activity via G$_i$ inhibition of adenylate cyclase.

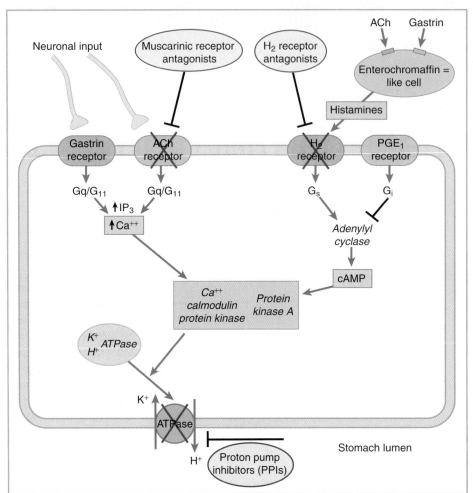

Figure 11-1. Sites of action of drugs that inhibit H^+/K^+ pump activity. This pump is responsible for transporting hydrogen ions (acid) into the stomach lumen.

TABLE 11-1. Drugs That Decrease Lower Esophageal Sphincter Tone and Contribute to GERD

Anticholinergics
Benzodiazepines
Ca^{++} channel blockers
Dopaminergic agents
Estrogens
Nitrates
Opioids
Progesterone
Theophylline

TABLE 11-2. Adverse Effects Associated with Antacids

Drug	Effect
Aluminum hydroxide	Constipation
	Binds to phosphate in gastrointestinal tract; may lead to bone damage
Magnesium hydroxide	Diarrhea
Calcium carbonate	Stimulates gastrin; acid rebound
	Hypercalcemia, milk alkali syndrome (hypercalcemia, alkalosis, kidney stones)

H_2 Blockers

Cimetidine, Famotidine, Nizatidine, and Ranitidine

Remember that the drug names all end in "-tidine."

Mechanism of action. Histamine H_2 receptor antagonists are now available both over the counter and with a prescription. These drugs antagonize parietal cell H_2 receptors, diminishing cAMP and resultant H^+/K^+ pump activity. H_2 receptor antagonists block basal levels of gastric acid secretion but not meal-stimulated secretion (which is gastrin-mediated). Over-the-counter doses are effective for intermittent heartburn if there is no evidence of esophagitis. Pharmacokinetic differences among common H_2 receptor antagonists are listed in Table 11-3.

Adverse effects. H_2 receptor antagonists are usually well tolerated. Adverse effects on the central nervous system are more common in elderly (anxiety, confusion, dizziness, headache). Cimetidine may cause some adverse endocrine effects, particularly in men (decreased libido, impotence,

TABLE 11-3. Typical H₂ Receptor Antagonists

Drug	Comment
Cimetidine	Significant P-450 inhibitor Can lead to toxic drug interactions as a result of inhibition of benzodiazepines, warfarin, and phenytoin
Famotidine	Does not interfere with P-450
Nizatidine	Does not interfere with P-450
Ranitidine	Weaker P-450 inhibition than cimetidine

TABLE 11-4. Typical Proton Pump Inhibitors

Drug	Comment
Omeprazole	Available over the counter as well as in prescription strengths for healing esophageal lesions
Lansoprazole	High bioavailability
Rabeprazole	Does not interfere with P-450
Pantoprazole	Also available as an intravenous formulation
Esomeprazole	S isomer (and active form) of omeprazole

gynecomastia). Owing to the superior acid inhibition and safety profile of proton pump inhibitors (see below), the use of prescription H_2 antagonists has markedly declined.

Proton Pump Inhibitors

Omeprazole, Lansoprazole, Rabeprazole, Pantoprazole, and Esomeprazole

Note that the drug names all end in "-prazole."

Mechanism of action. In cases of chronic GERD with evidence of esophagitis, proton pump inhibitors (PPIs), which directly inhibit the gastric mucosal cell H^+/K^+ pump, may be prescribed. These drugs bind irreversibly and covalently, via sulfhydryl groups, to the H^+/K^+ pump of esophageal and duodenal lesions to inhibit both basal- and meal-stimulated gastric acid production. As a result, the pH in the stomach is elevated and remains above pH 4, even postprandially (after meals).

Adverse effects. Overall, these drugs are well tolerated; GI disturbances are the most commonly reported adverse effects. Keep in mind, however, that hypochlorhydria (inadequate production of HCl by parietal cells) causes gastrin to be released and that resultant hypergastrinemia causes gastric tumors in rodents via a trophic effect on enterochromaffin-like cells. Long-term use of PPIs in humans has been associated with atrophic gastritis, which also may predispose patients to gastric tumors. Patients carrying *Helicobacter pylori* appear to be at greatest risk.

All currently used proton pump inhibitors are pro-drugs and are converted to the active drug in the parietal cell canaliculus (tubular "canals" in which HCl is secreted). Proton pump inhibitors are listed in Table 11-4.

Prokinetic Drugs

Metoclopramide and Bethanechol

Mechanism of action. In addition to proton pump inhibitors, severe GERD can be treated with prokinetic agents that increase lower esophageal sphincter tone, including dopamine antagonists (e.g., metoclopramide) or muscarinic cholinergic receptor agonists (e.g., bethanechol). Metoclopramide has antidopaminergic and cholinomimetic effects. The drug acts as dopamine receptor antagonist, with highest affinity for

CLINICAL MEDICINE

Patients May Self-medicate

Physicians should be aware that overuse of H_2 antagonists or proton pump inhibitors can mask underlying disease including Barrett's esophagus (a premalignancy leading to esophageal adenocarcinoma), peptic ulcer disease, or Zollinger-Ellison syndrome (an oversecretion of acid and pepsin). Furthermore, acid suppression by H_2 antagonists or proton pump inhibitors can lead to overgrowth of *Candida* or bacteria (including *C. difficile*) within the GI tract. H_2 antagonists are also recognized as independent risk factors for causing pneumonia.

D1, D4, and D5 receptors. As a result of its actions, metoclopramide inhibits smooth muscle relaxation normally produced by dopamine, which in turn enhances cholinergic responses in the myenteric plexus of the enteric nervous system. Additionally, metoclopramide increases lower esophageal sphincter tone and the force of peristaltic contractions. All together, gastric emptying is accelerated, which provides some symptomatic improvements.

Adverse effects. Unfortunately, metoclopramide is associated with a high incidence of adverse effects, many stemming from the drug's dopaminergic actions (extrapyramidal movements, gynecomastia, menstrual irregularities, galactorrhea). Its use is not recommended for more than 12 weeks because of the risk of tardive dyskinesia.

●●● PEPTIC ULCER DISEASE

Peptic ulcers of the duodenum and the stomach are the result of multiple inflammatory stresses that damage the GI mucosa; including *H. pylori*, NSAIDs (which diminish PGE_2 synthesis), and chronic glucocorticoids.

For patients with a history of peptic ulcer disease (PUD) who take NSAIDs, there are three options:

- COX-2 selective inhibitors should be utilized preferentially to NSAIDs
- synthetic PGE_1 analogs (misoprostol) with NSAIDs
- proton pump inhibitors with NSAIDs

Misoprostol enhances mucosal defenses by stimulating mucus and bicarbonate production. Additionally, misoprostol increases local blood flow by promoting vasodilation. Misoprostol is classified as pregnancy category "X" (absolutely contraindicated) because it induces uterine contractions and can cause miscarriage.

The primary therapeutic approaches to ulcer healing involve concomitant use of proton pump inhibitors and H_2 receptor blockers to alleviate symptoms plus two or more antimicrobials to eradicate *H. pylori*. The anti-infectives most often used in these multidrug regiments are

- Tetracycline
- Amoxicillin
- Clarithromycin
- Metronidazole

Frequently, bismuth subsalicylate (e.g., Pepto-Bismol) is also added. Bismuth subsalicylate protects the gastric tract by stimulating endogenous production of prostaglandins. Additionally, bismuth subsalicylate has antimicrobial actions against some strains of enteric bacteria. Adverse effects due to bismuth subsalicylate include dark-colored stools and tongue. Bismuth may interfere with absorption of tetracyclines. Owing to the salicylate component of bismuth subsalicylate, tinnitus (ear ringing) may occur. Patients with a history of asthma or sensitivity to salicylates should avoid using products containing this active ingredient. Bismuth subsalicylate may increase bleeding in patients taking anticoagulants. Use of bismuth subsalicylate is contraindicated in children because of the risk of Reye's syndrome.

Another option for managing PUD is sucralfate (ammonium salt of sulfated disaccharides), which forms a protective barrier at the ulcer lesion. Fortunately, the drug is not absorbed systemically, so adverse effects other than GI disturbances are uncommon. However, the drug must be administered 4 times a day—1 hour before meals and at bedtime. Numerous drug interactions are likely, since sucralfate binds nonspecifically to positively charged molecules, so it is recommended that its administration be separated from that of all other drugs by giving other agents at least 2 hours before sucralfate.

●●● INFLAMMATORY BOWEL DISEASE

Ulcerative colitis (limited to the colon and rectum) and Crohn's disease (may occur anywhere from mouth to rectum) are inflammatory bowel diseases (IBDs) that can be treated but not cured at present. One line of treatment focuses

MICROBIOLOGY

Peptic Ulcer Disease (PUD)

Even though individuals can be tested for *H. pylori* (release of $^{14}CO_2$ in breath from ^{14}C urea, IgG antibodies to *H. pylori*, or endoscopy followed by culture), a positive test may not correlate with PUD.

TABLE 11-5. Drugs Used to Manage Ulcerative Colitis

Drug	Comment
Sulfasalazine	Adverse effects are numerous and are related to those normally found with sulfonamides
Mesalamine	Has fewer side effects than sulfasalazine, since there is no sulfa moiety This drug is most efficacious in proximal regions of gastrointestinal tract
Olsalazine	Two molecules of mesalamine linked by a disulfide bond, which is cleaved by intestinal bacteria Associated with severe diarrhea
Balsalazide	Bacteria hydrolyze release of mesalamine in distal portions of the GI tract

on controlling inflammation, and another line of treatment involves immunosuppression. Some pharmacologic agents may induce remission, while others may also help maintain remission. Patients with severe gastric disease may have altered absorption of drugs, and doses may require adjustment. First-line treatment options for ulcerative colitis are described in Table 11-5. Note that most of these drugs are metabolized to mesalamine.

Initial therapeutic options for ulcerative colitis include sulfasalazine or mesalamine (5-aminosalicylic acid). Sulfasalazine is hydrolyzed by GI flora to both sulfapyridine (a sulfa antibiotic) and mesalamine. Therapeutic effects may be related to antibacterial properties of sulfapyridine and anti-inflammatory properties of mesalamine. Mesalamine inhibits cyclooxygenase and prostaglandin production and can be obtained in several formulations that deliver it to different regions of the small or large bowel.

Corticosteroids may be used when sulfasalazine or mesalamine derivatives are ineffective. Although sulfasalazine and corticosteroids are equally effective, anti-inflammatory effects occur more rapidly with corticosteroids. Corticosteroids may be administered intravenously, orally, or rectally to induce remission. Budesonide, approved for treating exacerbations of Crohn's disease, is extensively metabolized by "first-pass" metabolism in the liver, thereby limiting the adverse side effects generally associated with corticosteroid use. The pharmacology of corticosteroids is discussed in Chapter 10. Immunosuppressants, such as azathioprine, cyclosporine, and 6-mercaptopurine, are utilized when corticosteroids fail to induce remission of IBD. The pharmacology of these drugs is discussed in Chapters 5 and 10.

As a last resort, infliximab, a monoclonal antibody that targets TNFα may be used to manage severe Crohn's disease. This drug is administered intravenously to suppress inflammation mediated by TNF. Infliximab use is limited by the occurrence of serious infections and malignancies, including tuberculosis and lymphoma. Patients should avoid vaccinations with live virus vaccines while receiving this therapy. Owing to

TABLE 11-6. Drugs Used to Treat Nausea and Vomiting

Drug	Comment
Antimuscarinics/Antihistamines (mixed function)	
Scopolamine	Patch applied behind ear for motion sickness
	Predominantly blocks muscarinic cholinergic receptors in dorsal vagal complex
Dimenhydrinate	Drug of choice for children
	Metabolized to diphenhydramine (an antihistamine) moiety
Meclizine	Antihistaminic and anticholinergic actions
Diphenhydramine	Central blockade of H_1 receptors
Hydroxyzine	Antihistamine
Doxylamine	Antihistamine; often used to manage nausea and vomiting in pregnant women
Antidopaminergics	
Prochlorperazine	Phenothiazine that blocks dopamine receptors in chemoreceptor trigger zone
	Can cause sedation, liver dysfunction, and dystonias, especially in children with viral illnesses
Metoclopramide	Dopaminergic antagonist action raises the threshold of activity in the chemoreceptor trigger zone
Serotonin Receptor (5HT3) Antagonists	
Ondansetron	Block afferent vagal fibers in upper gastrointestinal tract as well as central vomiting center to prevent emesis
Granisetron	Generally well tolerated, do not induce sedation; minimal autonomic side effects
Dolasetron	
Alosetron	Often used postoperatively or for chemotherapy-induced nausea. Safe for children
	Note: All drug names end in "-setron"
Palonosetron	Only drug in this class that is approved for delayed nausea and vomiting associated with chemotherapy because of its long half-life
	Use with caution in those at risk for QT prolongation
Phosphated Carbohydrate Solutions	Used for mild symptoms
	May elevate blood sugar (like drinking a cola).
Cannabinoids	Used for chemotherapy-induced nausea when all other regimens have failed
	Act on receptors in the vomiting center of brain
	May cause numerous CNS adverse effects (mood changes, anxiety, memory loss, fear, confusion, motor incoordination, hallucinations, euphoria, sedation, paranoia)
	Can cause hypotension and tachycardia
	Tolerance may develop to side effects but not to antiemetic effects
Dronabinol	Δ_9THC, the active ingredient in marijuana
	Binds to cannabinoid receptors
	The endogenous cannabinoid receptor agonist in humans is arachidonylethanolamide
Nabilone	Fewer euphoric effects than dronabinol
Substance P/neurokinin-1 Receptor Antagonists	
Aprepitant	May be combined with 5 HT3 antagonists and dexamethasone for treatment of severe chemotherapy-induced nausea and vomiting
	While effective, inhibits CYP3A4 and induces CYP2C9, causing drug interactions
Corticosteroids	Inhibit production of prostaglandins, which can be highly emetogenic
	Effective, but adverse effects limit utility

receptor antagonists. It is easier to prevent nausea than to stop vomiting. Patients receiving chemotherapeutic agents require efficient treatment of nausea and vomiting. Often, severe emesis (vomiting) associated with chemotherapy requires use of drug combinations. Specific combination therapies include

- Metoclopramide + diphenhydramine + dexamethasone
- Prochlorperazine + lorazepam
- 5HT3 antagonists + dexamethasone + lorazepam

the biologic origin of this drug, hypersensitivities may occur. This medication may cause dizziness; caution is warranted while driving or performing activities that require alertness, coordination, or physical dexterity. Additional adverse effects include heart failure and lupus-like syndromes. Infliximab is usually given in combination with other immunosuppressants to reduce the likelihood that neutralizing antibodies will form to the anti-TNF monoclonal antibody.

●●● NAUSEA AND VOMITING

Nausea and vomiting, which can be triggered by gastrointestinal, infectious, neurologic, metabolic, or psychogenic diseases, can be treated with a multitude of drug classes (Table 11-6). They include mixed-function antimuscarinics/antihistamines, antidopaminergics, serotonin receptor (5HT3) antagonists, cannabinoids, and substance P/neurokinin

●●● DIARRHEA

The first line of defense in managing diarrhea is rehydration. Diarrhea is a complication of either increased intestinal secretions or decreased intestinal absorption of carbohydrates and resultant water. Increased chloride and water secretions frequently occur from bacterial or parasitic toxin-induced opening of cAMP-induced chloride channels. In fact, cholera toxin ADP-ribosylates the α-subunit of Gs, which inhibits the GTPase function of the stimulatory G protein, thus constitutively activating Gs to generate cAMP and open chloride channels.

Severe bacterial diarrhea, induced by *Shigella, Salmonella, Campylobacter, Cholera,* or *Staphylococcus,* can be treated with antibiotics, including tetracycline, ampicillin, and erythromycin. Noninvasive strains of *Escherichia coli* can be treated with rifaximin, a GI selective oral antibiotic. However, most diarrhea is self-limiting and often viral in nature (rotavirus is a frequent cause of acute gastroenteritis in

TABLE 11-7. Pharmacologics Therapies Used in Management of Diarrhea

Agent	Comment
Rehydrating solutions	Provide rehydration and electrolyte replacement to reduce mortality World Health Organization suggests rehydration is critical for preventing complications associated with diarrhea
Opiate derivatives Loperamide	Do not use opiates if bacterial enteritis is suspected Acts only on peripheral opioid receptors May also have antisecretory properties
Diphenoxylate Paregoric	Combined with atropine (to discourage opioid abuse) in a product called Lomotil Rarely used owing to abuse potential
Anticholinergics Atropine	Blocks vagal tone and prolongs gut transit time Used with diphenoxylate
Bismuth subsalicylate	Possesses antisecretory, antibacterial, and anti-inflammatory properties
Somatostatin analogs Octreotide	A somatostatin analog that blocks release of serotonin and other vasoactive peptides Used in symptomatic treatment of carcinoid tumors that secrete histamine, bradykinin, serotonin Can cause gallbladder and biliary tract complications Administered via injection
Adsorbents	Examples include kaolin, pectin, attapulgite, polycarbophil, and bile acid resins
Lactase enzymes	Used for osmotic diarrhea resulting from lactose intolerance
Proton pump inhibitors or H_2 blockers	May be used to manage chronic diarrhea that occurs *after* meals, which may be caused by increased acid secretion after eating Prescription doses should be tried and, if effective, relief will be noticed in 3 days

TABLE 11-8. Drugs That Speed Gastrointestinal Motility

Agent	Comment
Bulk-forming agents	Soften stool by retaining water
	Bowel obstruction can result if not consumed with adequate fluids
	Flatulence common
Psyllium hydrophilic colloids	
Methylcellulose	
Polycarbophil	
Malt soup extract	Often administered to children
Emollients	
Docusate	Facilitate mixing of aqueous and fatty materials within GI tract
	Used to prevent constipation or to reduce straining when stooling (e.g., after hemorrhoid surgery, childbirth)
Mineral oil	Oil coating on stools promotes easier passage
	Inhibits colonic reabsorption of water
	Oil may leak from anal sphincter
	Should not be used for more than 2 weeks or in debilitated patients (risk of aspiration)
Osmotic agents	Exert osmotic effects to pull water into intestines
	May cause flatulence, cramps, diarrhea, and electrolyte imbalances
Lactulose	Oral syrup formulation
Polyethylene glycol (PEG)	Often used for bowel evacuation before gastrointestinal procedures
	Also used for intermittent constipation
	Formulations that contain PEG plus electrolytes prevent salt imbalances and are preferred in patients with congestive heart disease, angina, and renal or liver disease
Glycerin	Suppositories often used for osmotic actions in children
Stimulants	Increase activity of gut by acting as irritants
	Should only be used intermittently
	May cause severe cramping and fluid and electrolyte disturbances
Bisacodyl	Oral and rectal formulations
Senna	Proposed laxative of choice for opioid-induced constipation
	May be associated with melanosis coli, a black pigment that infiltrates the colon wall
Casanthranol, castor oil	Stimulates secretions, decreases glucose absorption, promotes gastrointestinal motility
Saline cathartics	Magnesium and sodium salts
	Often used for bowel evacuation before gastrointestinal procedures
	May cause electrolyte disturbances
	Magnesium may accumulate in patients with renal dysfunction
	Sodium may worsen congestive heart failure

Some of these agents are not routinely recommended by health care professionals (castor oils). However, patients may use them as "old-time remedies", since many are available over the counter

children) and may well be a mechanism by which the body rids itself of harmful bacterial or viral toxins. Additional therapies used to manage diarrhea are listed in Table 11-7 and include opiate derivatives and anticholinergic agents.

CONSTIPATION

Constipation is not a disease; rather, it represents another underlying pathologic condition. It may be associated with metabolic or endocrine disorders (diabetic neuropathies, hypothyroidism); pregnancy (decreased gut motility); and neurogenic, psychogenic, or drug-induced events. Drugs used to speed GI motility are listed in Table 11-8. Remember that obstructions (impaction) should be removed before laxatives are used and that chronic use of laxatives can result in electrolyte imbalances and reduced peristaltic motility.

IRRITABLE BOWEL SYNDROME

Another potentially debilitating GI condition, irritable bowel syndrome (IBS), may be associated with either constipation or diarrhea. In fact, often symptoms will fluctuate between the two extremes. Note that IBS and IBD (Crohn's and ulcerative colitis) are very different conditions. It is of note that the etiology of irritable bowel syndrome is still undefined and that patients often experience symptoms of depression and anxiety (treated with selective serotonin receptor inhibitors [SSRIs] or tricyclic agents [TCAs]). Antispasmodic muscarinic receptor antagonists (dicyclomine or hyoscyamine) are often used to manage abdominal cramping.

For constipation, patients can be treated with multiple regimens, including increased dietary fiber, exercise, increased fluid intake, and stool softeners. For constipation-predominant IBS in women, an aggressive treatment involves tegaserod, a 5HT4 receptor partial agonist, which speeds GI mobility. Tegaserod should be discontinued if stomach pain worsens, if blood is present in stools, or if severe diarrhea occurs. This drug is also being used off-label for managing gastroparesis and GERD.

Loperamide and diphenoxylate/atropine are often recommended for diarrhea-predominant IBS. Alosetron, a 5HT3 antagonist is approved for use in women with IBS. For unknown reasons, bioavailability in men is 50% lower than in women. This drug is a last resort and is appropriate for only a small percentage of patients with the most severe disease because of the serious constipation and ischemic colitis that sometimes result. In fact, because of these serious adverse effects, alosetron was temporarily removed from the marketplace but was later reintroduced in a lower dose with stricter guidelines.

●●● COMPLEMENTARY AND ALTERNATIVE MEDICINE

Increasingly greater evidence illustrates the utility of probiotics—healthy bacterial microorganisms—for managing diarrhea, IBD, and IBS. *Lactobacillus* and *Bifidobacterium* are the two most commonly studied genera.

Level 1 evidence supports the use of probiotics for preventing and treating diarrhea, including antibiotic-associated diarrhea, *Clostridium difficile* pseudomembranous colitis, and rotaviral gastroenteritis. The mechanisms of action for probiotics may include

- Competing with harmful bacterial species for space and nutrients in the colon.
- Secreting bacteriocins that act as "antimicrobial" agents to eliminate harmful pathogens.
- Producing short-chain fatty acids that lower colonic pH.
- Stimulating the immune system to secrete IgA antibodies and protective cytokines.

New lines of evidence suggest that inflammatory bowel diseases are caused by abnormalities within normal gut flora. Such alterations may be caused by

- Persistent infection (at the moment *Mycobacterium paratuberculosis* is a leading candidate).
- Slight imbalances among "normal" GI flora.
- Defective mucosa that is continuously stimulated by gut bacteria.
- A lack of oral tolerance to one's own normal GI flora (essentially, an allergy develops to one's own normal flora).

Numerous clinical trials have found probiotics effective at maintaining remission in patients with ulcerative colitis, Crohn's disease, and pouchitis (inflamed surgical pouch following IBD bowel resection). Anecdotal evidence suggests that probiotics may be effective to induce remission in these inflammatory bowel diseases too.

Clinical evidence also finds probiotics effective for restoring appropriate gut function in patients with both constipation-predominant and diarrhea-predominant IBS. Some investigators have found increased GI colonization by clostridia in patients with IBS, a situation that probiotics may help resolve.

●●● TOP FIVE LIST

1. Histamine H_2 blockers and proton pump inhibitors limit GERD.
2. Antibiotics that eradicate *H. pylori* are given concomitantly with H_2 blockers and PPIs to treat peptic ulcer disease.
3. Ulcerative colitis and Crohn's disease are two severe forms of IBD treated with anti-inflammatory and immunosuppressive drugs.
4. Combinatorial drug therapy (antidopaminergic, antihistaminic, antimuscarinic, serotonin receptor antagonistic, corticosteroid) often is used to treat severe nausea and vomiting.
5. The first line of defense for diarrhea is rehydration.

Endocrine Pharmacology 12

CONTENTS

It's all about the axis, that is, the hypothalamus/pituitary axis. The keys to understanding endocrine pharmacology are the feed-forward and feed-back mechanisms that govern how "releasing" factors in the hypothalamus control the release of hormones in the pituitary that then target multiple organs within the body. This interplay of hormonally regulated signals is summarized in Table 12-1. Pharmacologically, pathologic alterations in these hormones can be corrected by recombinant or synthetic analogs of these hormones.

●●● ANTERIOR PITUITARY HORMONES

Adrenal Disorders

Stress triggers the hypothalamus to release corticotropin-releasing hormone (CRH), which is a positive stimulus for the secretion of adrenocorticotropin hormone (ACTH) from the anterior pituitary (Fig. 12-1). Circulating ACTH stimulates the adrenal gland to release glucocorticoids that control basic body functions and metabolic activities (Table 12-2). The released glucocorticoids feed back to negatively regulate the hypothalamus and the anterior pituitary to diminish release of CRH and ACTH and complete the feedback loop.

PHYSIOLOGY

The Hypothalamus Is Connected to the Pituitary . . .

Neurosecretory neurons originating within the hypothalamus release oxytocin and vasopressin from the posterior pituitary. In contrast, nerve fibers converge on the median eminence within the hypothalamus releasing hypothalamic hormones that travel via portal vessels to the anterior pituitary. Once there, these hypothalamic hormones trigger the release of pituitary hormones. These anterior pituitary hormones include growth hormone, adrenocorticotropic hormone (ACTH), thyroid-stimulating hormone (TSH), prolactin, dopamine, follicle-stimulating hormone (FSH), and luteinizing hormone (LH). These anatomic connections are depicted in Figure 12-1.

ANATOMY

The Adrenal "Zone"

The adrenal *cortex* is composed of three histologic zones with separate functions. The outer zone is the zona glomerulosa, which produces mineralocorticoids such as aldosterone. The middle zone, zona fasciculata, produces glucocorticoids such as cortisol. The inner zone, zona reticularis, primarily produces precursors of estrogens and androgens. Remember that the adrenal *medulla* releases epinephrine and norepinephrine.

TABLE 12-1. Signals on the Hypothalamic-pituitary Axis

Hypothalamus	Pituitary	Target Organ	Hormones/Cell Signal
Corticotropin-releasing hormone (CRH)	Adrenocorticotropic hormone (ACTH)	Adrenal cortex	Glucocorticoids, mineralocorticoids androgens
Thyrotropin-releasing factor	Thyroid-stimulating hormone (TSH)	Thyroid	Thyroxins (T_3, T_4)
Growth hormone–releasing factor and growth hormone inhibitory hormone (somatostatin)*	Growth hormone	Liver Adipose	Insulin-like growth factor (IGF-1) (mediates most growth effects of growth hormone)
Dopamine*	Prolactin	Mammary glands	Breast milk production
Gonadotropin-releasing hormone	Follicle-stimulating hormone and luteinizing hormone	Ovary Testes	Estrogen, progesterone, testosterone
Oxytocin†	Oxytocin	Uterus Mammary tissue	Induction of labor, lactation
Vasopressin†	Vasopressin	Renal tubules	Water reabsorption via aquaporin channels
		Smooth muscle	↑ cAMP

*While nearly all the hypothalamic hormones listed stimulate release of pituitary hormones, dopamine and somatostatin are exceptions. In this context, dopamine acts as an *inhibitory factor*, preventing release of prolactin and somatostatin prevents release of growth hormone.
†Vasopressin and oxytocin are synthesized within cell bodies located in the hypothalamus, but long axons transport the hormones for release by the posterior pituitary.

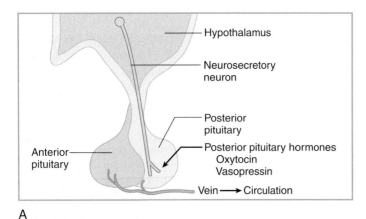

Figure 12-1. A, The posterior pituitary releases hormones directly from the hypothalamus. **B,** Hormones secreted by the anterior pituitary gland are released from resident cells in response to signals from the hypothalamus.

TABLE 12-2. Actions of Glucocorticoids

Glucocorticoid Effect	Target Tissue
Stimulates gluconeogenesis	Liver
Increases hepatic glycogen	Liver
Increases blood glucose	Liver
Stimulates lipolysis	Adipose
Protein catabolism	Muscle
Reduces inflammation and suppresses immune responses	Macrophages and lymphocytes
Stimulates gastric acid secretions	Stomach

Cushing's Syndrome (Hypercortisolism)

Aminoglutethimide, Metyrapone, High-dose Ketoconazole, and Mitotane

Cortisol serves as the primary glucocorticoid in humans. Increased levels of cortisol from the adrenal gland can lead to hypertension, hyperglycemia, impotence, hirsutism, osteoporosis, and mood changes. Patients may also exhibit moon faces. Increased cortisol concentrations can be a result of overproduction of ACTH due to an overactive hypothalamus (Cushing's disease) or from an adrenal or ectopic tumor that secretes ACTH. First-line treatment, where warranted, is surgical resection of the tumor. For patients who are not surgical candidates or during the interim until surgery can be

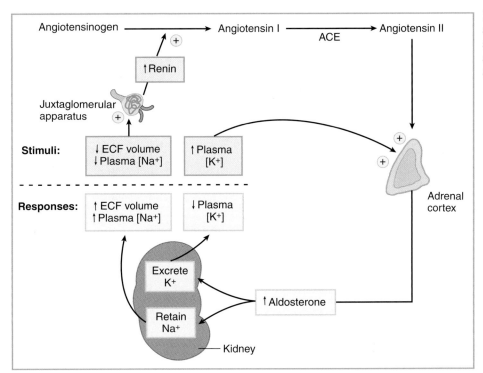

Figure 12-2. Role of renin and angiotensin in regulating aldosterone secretion by the adrenal cortex. Renin is an enzyme that converts angiotensinogen to angiotensin.

PHYSIOLOGY

Aldosterone and the Adrenal Gland

In contrast to glucocorticoids, which are stimulated via ACTH from the anterior pituitary, the mineralocorticoids are regulated by means of ion sensors within the adrenal gland itself. A decrease in plasma Na^+ concentration or a decrease in extracellular fluid (ECF) volume induces the adrenal gland to secrete aldosterone, which causes the kidney to retain sodium and excrete potassium and protons. The retention of Na^+ leads to an antidiuretic effect, which restores ECF volume.

The adrenal gland can also be stimulated to secrete aldosterone via circulating angiotensin II (Fig. 12-2). Production of angiotensin II is itself a consequence of ion sensors within the juxtaglomerular apparatus of the afferent arteriole, which releases renin, the rate-limiting enzyme that degrades angiotensinogen to angiotensin I. Angiotensin I is hydrolyzed by angiotensin-converting enzyme (ACE) to angiotensin II. Angiotensin II is both a potent vasoconstrictor and a stimulus for release of aldosterone.

When necessary, mineralocorticoid replacement therapy can be accomplished with aldosterone mimetics such as fludrocortisone. In contrast, spironolactone and eplerenone are pharmacologic agents that act as aldosterone receptor antagonists.

performed, pharmacologic intervention with drugs that inhibit cholesterol metabolism is the course of therapy.

Steroid-modifying drugs including aminoglutethimide and metyrapone and high doses of ketoconazole can be used to treat Cushing's syndrome. Each of these drugs inhibits one or more enzymes involved in cortisol synthesis (Fig. 12-3).

Aminoglutethimide inhibits cholesterol desmolase, the first and rate-limiting step responsible for converting cholesterol to pregnenolone. Metyrapone inhibits 11-hydroxylase activity, the last step in cortisol synthesis. Ketoconazole, at much higher doses than normally used for antifungal activity, inhibits both 11- and 17-hydroxylases.

Adverse effects of aminoglutethimide include extreme sedation, gastrointestinal (GI) disturbances (nausea), and severe skin rashes. Adverse effects occuring with metyrapone include nausea, vomiting, hirsuitism, acne (enhanced production of androgens due to cortisol blockage), and hypertension (because of accumulation of 11-deoxy-cortisol). Therefore, the two drugs are often used together for maximal efficacy and to allow dose reductions of each. Ketoconazole can also be used at high doses. Notice that antagonism of 17-hydroxylase with ketoconazole can lower testosterone levels, causing gynecomastia and reduced libido in men. Ketoconazole also elevates hepatic enzymes.

Other drug strategies for managing Cushing's disease include adrenolytics (drugs that cause atrophy of the adrenal gland) like mitotane. Mitotane therapy typically requires hospitalization so that plasma and urinary cortisol levels can be closely monitored. Steroid replacement therapy may be required in these patients. Lethargy, somnolence, and other adverse central nervous system effects are experienced by most patients. Also used to manage hypercortisolism are neuromodulators (e.g., cyproheptadine, bromocriptine, valproate, and octreotide—although none of these agents has been consistently effective) and glucocorticoid blockers (spironolactone, mifepristone). Remember that neither glucocorticoid blocker is specific for antagonizing only the glucocorticoid receptors. Spironolactone also blocks aldos-

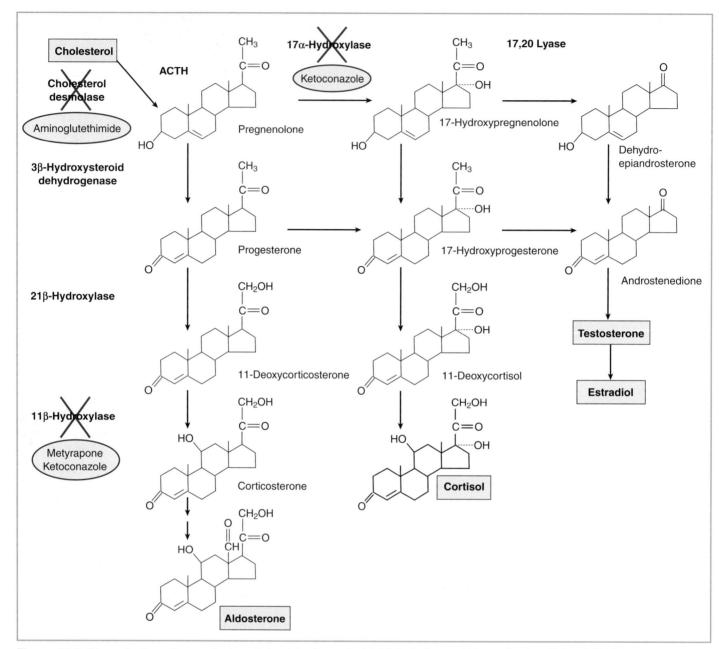

Figure 12-3. Biosynthetic pathway of adrenal steroids. Drugs that inhibit cholesterol biosynthesis will, by definition, lower production of cortisol and thus are first-line treatments for Cushing's disease. However, note that these drugs affect testosterone and alderosterone production.

terone receptors, and mifepristone (better known as RU-486 or the "abortion pill") is an antagonist of progesterone receptors.

Addison's Disease (Adrenal Insufficiency)

Hydrocortisone and Fludrocortisone

Symptoms of adrenal insufficiency are observed only after greater than 90% of the adrenal gland is nonfunctional. The most common cause of adrenal insufficiency is chronic glucocorticoid use (hypothalamic-pituitary axis suppression due to feedback inhibition). Specifically, pharmacologic levels of glucocorticoids can negatively regulate the hypothalamus and diminish ACTH levels. This is particularly important in

patients who abruptly stop taking high-dose glucocorticoid (immunosuppressive) treatment, since their adrenal glands are no longer capable of producing adrenal steroids. Another condition of adrenal insufficiency is Addison's disease, in which diminished ACTH leads to diminished adrenal gland function.

The major uses of corticosteroids with glucocorticoid activity are as immunosuppressives and as adjuvants to combinatorial cancer chemotherapeutic regimens (see Chapter 5). In cases of adrenal insufficiency, hydrocortisone is usually given for its combined glucocorticoid and mineralocorticoid effects. Major side effects of chronic corticosteroid therapies are listed in Box 12-1. If mineralo-

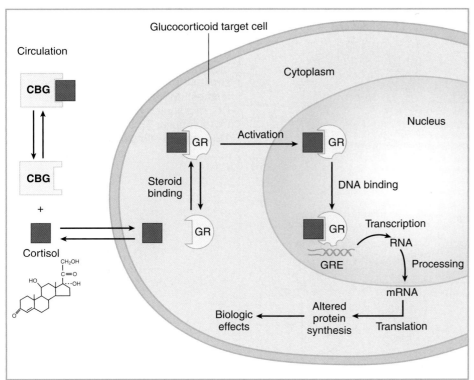

Figure 12-4. Cell and molecular biologic features of cytosolic glucocorticoid receptors. Upon binding to the cortisol (purple box), the receptor assumes a shape that permits DNA binding. CBG, cortisol-binding globulin; GR, glucocorticoid receptor; GRE, glucocorticoid response element.

Box 12-1. SIDE EFFECTS OF CHRONIC CORTICOSTEROID TREATMENT

Sodium retention
Edema
Muscle wasting
Growth suppression
Cataracts
Peptic ulcer disease
Osteoporosis
Hypokalemia
Increased risk of infections
Iatrogenic (treatment-induced) Cushing's syndrome

BIOCHEMISTRY

Cholesterol as the Master Steroid

To appreciate the drugs that regulate adrenal dysfunction, an understanding of cholesterol metabolism is required. As depicted in Figure 12-3, cholesterol is the precursor of all adrenal steroids. Cholesterol and its metabolites are the substrates for multiple enzymes. Thus, inhibition of specific enzymes in these interrelated metabolic pathways can decrease specific metabolic and reproductive steroids at the expense of others. Cholesterol desmolase and the 17α- and 11β-hydroxylases are critical pharmacologic targets. Cholesterol is also the precursor of vitamin D and bile acids (not depicted in Fig. 12-3).

---

corticoid replacement is also needed for adrenal insufficiency, fludrocortisone is administered. Side effects associated with fludrocortisone are typically those associated with Na⁺ retention and fluid overload.

Hirsutism

Finasteride and Flutamide

The zona reticularis of the adrenal gland is a site of steroid dysregulation that leads to hirsutism. Overproduction of adrenal androgens in females can lead to husky voice, menstrual irregularities, and male pattern baldness. Treatments include finasteride, which inhibits 5α-reductase to prevent conversion of testosterone to dihydrotestosterone. Flutamide, which inhibits tissue uptake of androgens, decreases binding of androgen to cytosolic receptors. (These drugs are discussed further under Men's Reproductive Disorders.)

PHYSIOLOGY

Steroid-mediated Signal Transduction

The mechanism of action of cell-permeable (lipophilic) glucocorticoids is mediated by cytosolic steroid-binding receptors, as depicted in Figure 12-4. When bound to glucocorticoids, the steroid-binding receptor translocates to the nucleus. Binding the glucocorticoid also changes the confirmation of the steroid receptor, exposing a selective DNA binding domain. This transactivating complex binds to specific glucocorticoid regulatory elements on the 5′ untranslated region of DNA to repress or enhance transcription of immunosuppressive or anti-inflammatory cytokines, respectively. Hence, steroid receptors act as transcription factors.

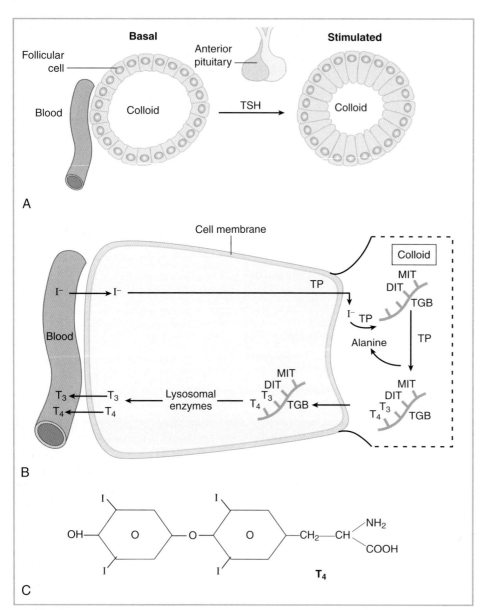

Figure 12-5. A, Thyroid hormone biosynthesis. Thyrotropin from the anterior pituitary stimulates thyroid follicular cells to produce thyroxine. **B**, Detailed biosynthesis of thyroxin (T_3/T_4). Chemical structure of T_4 (T_3 simply loses one of the iodines). MIT, monoiodinated tyrosine; DIT, diiodinated tyrosine; TGB, thyroglobulin; TP, thyroperoxidase; TSH, thyroid-stimulating hormone.

Thyroid Disorders

Thyroid-stimulating hormone (thyrotropin; TSH) from the anterior pituitary stimulates follicular cells of the thyroid to produce thyroxine (Fig. 12-5). The activated thyrotropin receptor is coupled via G_s to produce cAMP, which regulates expression of precursors to thyroxine. Specifically, iodide (I^-) is removed from the circulation by the thyroid gland and oxidized to iodine (I) via actions of the enzyme thyroperoxidase. Iodine then crosses into the colloid, a secretory matrix comprised of a large glycoprotein, thyroglobulin. Iodine molecules bind to the numerous tyrosine residues found on thyroglobulin. Through the activity of thyroperoxidase, monoiodinated tyrosines (MITs) combine to form diiodinated tyrosines (DITs). MITs can combine with DITs within the colloid to form a molecule that when released is known because the T_3 hormone. Likewise, when two DITs combine within the colloid, the molecule when released from the thyroid is known as T_4. Before T_3 or T_4 is released, thyro-

globulin must be removed from the hormones. This occurs in the follicular cells, because the T_3 or T_4 precursors are endocytosed back into the follicular cells, where functional T_3 and T_4 are subsequently released from the glycoprotein through actions of lysosomal enzymes. Finally, newly synthesized thyroid hormones are released into the circulation.

T_3 and T_4 can be thought of as master regulators of metabolism, oxygen consumption, energy, and growth and development. Both hyper- and hypodysregulation of thyroid function leads to major, but opposite, changes in metabolism and heart function. Signs and symptoms of hyper- and hypothyroidism are reviewed in Table 12-3.

Graves' Disease (Hyperthyroidism)
Radioactive Iodide and Thionamides (Propylthiouracil and Methimazole)

Causes of hyperthyroidism include TSH-secreting pituitary tumors, pituitary resistance to thyroxine, and thyroid goiters. Graves' disease, an autoimmune syndrome in which anti-

TABLE 12-3. Symptoms of Hyper- and Hypothyroidism

Hyperthyroid Symptoms	Hypothyroid Symptoms
Nervousness	Lethargy, slow cerebration
Weight loss	Weight gain
Diarrhea	Constipation
Tachycardia	Bradycardia
Insomnia	Sleepiness
Increased appetite	Anorexia
Heat intolerance	Cold intolerance
Oligomenorrhea (sparse and infrequent menstrual cycles)	Menorrhagia (heavy menstrual cycles)
Muscle wasting	Weakness
Goiter	Dry, coarse skin
Exophthalmos (bulging eyes)	Facial edema

Box 12-2. THYROXINE-DRUG INTERACTIONS

- Drugs that induce cytochrome P-450 enzymes, such as phenytoin, carbamazepine, and rifampin, may increase metabolism and biliary excretion of thyroxine.
- Calcium and iron products chelate oral thyroxine preparations in the GI tract, diminishing their effectiveness. Raloxifene may also decrease absorption of thyroid hormones.
- Soy flour, soy isoflavones, high-fiber diets, and some legumes inhibit absorption of thyroxine.
- Warfarin doses should be decreased because thyroxine may increase degradation of vitamin K clotting factors.
- Effects of β-agonists, stimulants, and decongestants should be monitored, since thyroxine potentiates sympathetic effects on the heart.
- Thyroid hormones may increase the dose requirement for insulin and oral hypoglycemic drugs.

bodies to the thyrotropin receptor stimulate thyroxine production and release, is another cause of hyperthyroidism. Note that patients with hyperthyroidism often have weight loss despite an increased appetite. When patients come to the emergency room with severe hyperthyroidism—thyrotoxicosis (thyroid storm)—the first steps are to stabilize the patient. Symptoms are controlled with β-blockers, aspirin, and corticosteroids. Then, the underlying clinical problem is addressed as discussed below.

Treatments for hyperthyroidism include surgery and radioactive iodide isotopes (^{131}I), which destroy overactive thyroid tissue. However, a consequence of thyroid removal or destruction is hypothyroidism.

Pharmacologic treatments that may be used until surgical removal of thyroid tissue or as management during a thyrotoxic crisis include drugs that are substrates for thyroid peroxidase, which block oxidation of iodide in the thyroid gland and prevent subsequent synthesis of T_3 and T_4. These drugs are known as thionamides (propylthiouracil and methimazole). Patients using these drugs are at risk for maculopapular and pruritic rashes, arthralgia, and fever. Hypersensitivity reactions can be severe and may include thrombocytopenia, pancytopenia, aplastic anemia, and agranulocytosis. Hypersensitivity reactions occur suddenly, often within the first 3 months of therapy; therefore, white blood cell counts should be monitored closely. Patients should be counseled to see their physician if they experience any flu-like symptoms.

Another pharmacologic treatment of hyperthyroidism involves use of potassium iodide. Sudden exposure to excess serum iodide inhibits oxidation or organification of iodide, thus diminishing thyroid hormone biosynthesis. The exact mechanism of this action is unknown. For a short period of time, T_3 and T_4 release is inhibited. However, within 2 weeks of continued exposure to large amounts of iodide, the thyroid gland escapes this blockade and hormone biosynthesis continues.

Hypothyroidism

Synthetic Thyroxine (Levothyroxine, T_4; Liothyronine, T_3)

Hypothyroidism during pregnancy can result in miscarriage or mental retardation (cretinism). The cause of the hypothyroidism usually is inadequate iodine levels during the first trimester of pregnancy, and it can be prevented. Pregnant women should ingest approximately 220 µg of iodine, a little higher than the typical average daily intake of 160 µg. As many as 6 of 100 miscarriages may be due to thyroid insufficiency. Also of importance, 10% of all women over 65 years of age develop hypothyroidism. Women are five times more likely to develop thyroid insufficiency than men are.

Treatments for hypothyroidism include natural thyroid extracts or synthetic thyroxine. Natural thyroid extracts contain a mixture of T_3 and T_4 from animal sources (hog, sheep, cow). Absorption and bioavailability are unpredictable, and hypersensitivity reactions can occur. On the other hand, synthetic thyroxine (levothyroxine) contains T_4 only and this drug is chemically stable, relatively nonantigenic and easily converted to the more active T_3 form with defined kinetics. Levothyroxine is highly protein bound and has a relatively long half-life ($t_{1/2}$) of 9 days in hypothyroid patients. It may take up to 30 days to reach a steady-state level of replacement. Drugs such as rifampin, carbamazepine, and phenytoin can increase metabolism and removal of synthetic T_4 via P-450 induction.

There are also T_3 synthetic thyroxins. Liothyronine contains T_3. This drug has a shorter half-life, leading to faster dose titration. This drug is also quickly eliminated in cases of overdose. However, liothyronine also has a slightly higher incidence of cardiac adverse effects compared with T_4 synthetic drugs. Liothyronine may be preferred in those patients who lack the ability to convert T_4 to T_3. The many drug interactions for thyroxines are listed in Box 12-2.

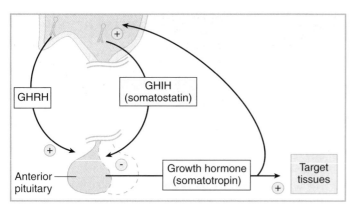

Figure 12-6. Growth hormone feedback inhibition. GHIH, growth hormone inhibitory hormone (somatostatin); GHRH, growth hormone–releasing hormone.

Growth-related Disorders

Sermorelin and Mecasermin (Dwarfism) Octreotide and Pegvisomant (Acromegaly, Gigantism)

Sermorelin is given for growth hormone deficiency, and octreotide and pegvisomant are used to treat growth hormone excess.

Growth hormone–releasing hormone (GHRH) induces the anterior pituitary to secrete growth hormone (somatotropin). Growth hormone induces its own feedback inhibition by stimulating growth hormone *inhibitory* hormone (GHIH or somatostatin) release from the hypothalamus (Fig. 12-6). Recombinant DNA versions of growth hormone can be used to treat growth hormone deficiency (dwarfism). A variety of different recombinant products are available and differ from each other in terms of route of administration (IM or SC) and frequency of injection (3 to 7 times per week). A growth hormone–releasing hormone drug, sermorelin (consisting of the first 19 amino acids of GHRH) is available for patients who have a hypothalamic deficiency. An insulin-like growth factor (IGF) therapy, mecasermin, has been approved for children with severe IGF-1 deficiency. These children may not necessarily have a growth factor deficiency but may be resistant to the effects of growth hormone. Mecasermin is administered subcutaneously before meals to avoid a hypoglycemic response. This is yet another example of how targeting a signal transduction cascade (IGF-1 tyrosine kinase receptors) yields a novel therapeutic strategy.

In contrast, a synthetic pharmacologic growth hormone inhibitory hormone, octreotide, is effective for managing growth hormone excess (acromegaly or gigantism). The drug is 40 times more potent at inhibiting growth hormone secretion than is endogenous somatostatin. However, octreotide is associated with abdominal cramps, reduced gallbladder contractility and gallstones, reduced serum levels of vitamin B_{12}, and altered absorption of dietary fats. A newer, more specific therapy utilizes a growth factor receptor antagonist such as pegvisomant to treat acromegaly. Injection site reactions, flu-like symptoms, diarrhea, and elevated liver enzymes can occur. Hepatoxicity must therefore be closely monitored.

Prolaction Disorders

Dopamine Receptor Agonists

Dopamine receptor agonists include bromocriptine, pergolide, and the newer agents cabergoline, pramipexole, and ropinirole. A more detailed discussion of dopamine agonists can be found in Chapter 13.

Hyperprolactinemia (increased prolactin secretion) in women presents as menstrual dysfunction, lack of ovulation, and inappropriate lactation. Hyperprolactinemia can also induce lactation in men. The most common cause of hyperprolactinemia is drug-induced. Drugs that have been implicated most often are those with dopamine receptor antagonist properties (e.g., haloperidol metoclopramide). In addition, even selective serotonin reuptake inhibitors (SSRIs) and oral contraceptives can induce hyperprolactinemia. Pharmacologic treatment of hyperprolactinemia utilizes dopamine receptor agonists, of which there are many examples: bromocriptine, pergolide, and the newer agents cabergoline, pramipexole, and ropinirole. Dopamine receptor agonists reduce prolactin secretion by the anterior pituitary. Adverse effects include GI distress (abdominal pain, diarrhea) and dizziness, headache, and fatigue. Patients should be warned that all dopamine receptor agonists can cause sudden sleep attacks. Newer drugs seem to target the D_2-like receptor subtypes preferentially over the D_1-like receptors and seem to have a lower incidence of side effects.

Sometimes it is desirable to facilitate breast milk production in lactating women. Metoclopramide, a dopamine receptor antagonist that leads to prolactin release from the anterior pituitary, has been used on a short-term basis for this purpose.

●●● POSTERIOR PITUITARY HORMONES

Desmopressin

As depicted in Figure 12-7, vasopressin (also known as antidiuretic hormone or ADH) controls fluid balance in response to osmoreceptor stimulation. Desmopressin is a long-acting,

---

PHYSIOLOGY

Vasopressin

Increased blood osmolarity, sensed by osmoreceptors within the hypothalamus, activates release of vasopressin (also called antidiuretic hormone, ADH) from the posterior pituitary. As depicted in Figure 12-7, circulating vasopressin activates G_s-coupled V_2 vasopressin receptors within the tubules of the nephron to produce cAMP. Activation of cAMP-regulated protein kinase A (PKA) leads to insertion of additional aquaporin water channels in the luminal membrane of renal tubules that reabsorb water and limit diuresis, thereby reducing blood osmolarity. Desmopressin is a long-acting, synthetic, nasally administered ADH analog that is used to treat diabetes insipidus, a medical condition characterized by decreased ADH levels, resulting in large volumes of dilute urine.

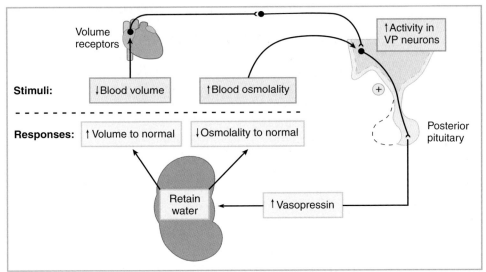

A

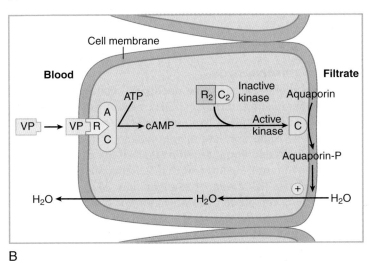

B

Figure 12-7. Feedback control mechanisms (**A**) and signaling cascades (**B**) regulated by vasopressin. VP, vasopressin; AC, adenylyl cyclase; R_2C_2, inactive protein kinase A holoenzyme (R, regulatory subunit, and C, catalytic).

synthetic analog of vasopressin. Oral and nasal spray formulations are available and are used to treat both diabetes insipidus and enuresis. In both situations, it is desirable to form less urine. Desmopressin accomplishes this by enhancing water reabsorption from renal tubules. The adverse effect is "water intoxication" or hyponatremia. Patients should be cautioned to ingest only enough fluid to satisfy their thirst.

Oxytocin

Oxytocin is the other hormone released from the posterior pituitary. Its primary role is to induce labor and stimulate contraction of smooth muscles in the breast during lactation to facilitate milk ejection. Clinically, oxytocin is used to facilitate labor. Unborn infants must be monitored closely for signs of fetal distress during oxytocin infusions because of severe contractions. Because of structural similarities with vasopressin, oxytocin causes fluid retention in the mother.

●●● WOMEN'S REPRODUCTIVE HEALTH AND DISORDERS

Pregnancy

Oxytocin, Dinoprostone, Misoprostol, β₂-Agonists

As mentioned above, oxytocin, synthesized in the hypothalamus and released from the posterior pituitary, induces or augments labor. Prostaglandin E analogs, such as dinoprostone and misoprostol, can also be given vaginally to "ripen" the cervix and augment labor.

In contrast, β₂-agonists, such as ritodrine and terbutaline, can be used to mitigate uterine contractions and manage preterm labor. However, tachycardia, palpitations, and hyperglycemia can result. Magnesium sulfate, which antagonizes Ca^{++} to prevent actin-myosin interactions, and Ca^{++} channel blockers (e.g., nifedipine) can also be used to suppress uterine contractions. In cases of premature birth, glucocorticoids

Box 12-3. DRUG SAFETY DURING PREGNANCY

Category A	Controlled studies in women fail to demonstrate a risk to the fetus in the first trimester; possibility of fetal harm appears remote
Category B	Either animal studies do not indicate a risk to the fetus and there are no controlled studies in pregnant women *or* animal studies indicate a fetal risk but controlled studies in pregnant women fail to demonstrate a risk
Category C	Either animal studies indicate fetal risk and there are no controlled studies in women *or* there are no available studies in animals or women
Category D	There is positive evidence of fetal risk but there may be situations where benefits might outweigh the risks
Category X	Definite fetal risk based on animal or human studies or human experience; the risk clearly outweighs any benefit in pregnant women

TABLE 12-4. Some Drugs to Avoid During Pregnancy

Drug	Consequence
Salicylates	Delay onset of labor, increase bleeding during delivery, premature closure of patent ductus arteriosus
Benzodiazepines	Cleft palate (first trimester); CNS depression, withdrawal symptoms (especially diazepam) (third trimester)
Lithium	Cardiac defects (first trimester)
Isotretinoin	Craniofacial, CNS, cardiac abnormalities
Tetracyclines	Stained teeth, skeletal system abnormalities
Antineoplastics	Teratogenic
Androgens	Ambiguous genitalia
Fluoroquinolones	Cartilage damage
Thalidomide	Teratogenic

such as betamethasone are given to mothers during labor to hasten fetal lung development and decrease the incidence of respiratory distress syndrome.

As discussed above, to facilitate lactation, metoclopramide, a drug with dopamine receptor antagonist actions, can be administered to stimulate prolactin release. In contrast, methylergonovine or methysergide, an ergot alkaloid, can be used to suppress lactation. As expected, ergot alkaloids should never be given to nursing mothers. Ergot alkaloids can cause chest pain and vasoconstriction.

Pregnancy and the FDA

For more than 20 years, the FDA has required that all new drugs be assigned a pregnancy category that illustrates the

TABLE 12-5. Differing Pharmacologic Effects of Progestins Used in Oral Contraceptives

	Relative Effects		
Progestins	Progestinic	Estrogenic	Androgenic
Desogestrel and levonorgestrel	++++	—	+++
Norgestrel and norgestimate	++	—	++
Ethynodiol diacetate and norethindrone acetate	++	+++	++

++++, Pronounced effect; +++, moderate effect; ++, low effect; +, slight effect; —, no effect.

safety for use during pregnancy. This rating scale is shown in Box 12-3, and specific drugs to avoid are listed in Table 12-4.

Contraception

Oral Contraceptives

It's all about the negative feedback. Estrogens suppress follicle-stimulating hormone (FSH), preventing development of a dominant follicle that ultimately leads to ovulation. Progestins suppress luteinizing hormone (LH), blocking ovulation. In addition, progestins thicken the cervical mucus, reduce ovum movement, and thin the endometrium, thereby reducing the likelihood of implantation. Most oral contraceptives are composed of combinations of synthetic estrogens and progestins. For the most part, the estrogen is ethinyl estradiol (EE, the major estrogen produced by the ovaries) or mestranol, which is metabolized by the liver into EE. On the other hand there are substantial differences in pharmacologic effect among various progestins used in oral contraceptive standard. Progestins may differ in their relative estrogenic and androgenic effects (Table 12-5).

Various formulations achieve mono-, bi-, or triphasic dosing levels throughout the female cycle. The "phasic" formulations were designed to reduce progestin exposure in the earlier stages of the menstrual cycle to lower the incidence of adverse effects.

Oral contraceptives can also be administered to achieve hormonal balance, regulate menstrual cycling, and control endometriosis. The major effects of both too much and too little estrogenic and progestin activities are listed in Table 12-6; these are the types of common side effects observed when patients begin taking oral contraceptives.

It is not uncommon for users of users of oral contraceptives to experience the following adverse effects: migraine, breast tenderness, elevated blood pressure, adverse effects on lipids, nausea and vomiting, intolerance of contact lenses, weight gain, hirsutism, and chloasma (brown patches of irregular size and shape on the face). Estrogen-containing oral contraceptives decrease breast milk production and are to be avoided in breast-feeding women.

TABLE 12-6. Symptoms of Estrogen and Progestin Excess and Deficiency

Estrogen		Progestin	
Excess	**Deficiency**	**Excess**	**Deficiency**
Nausea, bloating	Early or mid-cycle breakthrough bleeding	Increased appetite	Late breakthrough bleeding
Cervical mucorrhea	Spotting	Weight gain	Amenorrhea
Polyposis	Hypomenorrhea	Tiredness, fatigue	
Chloasma (age spots)		Hypomenorrhea or Hypermenorrhea	
Hypertension		Acne, oily scalp	
Migraine		Hair loss, hirsutism	
Breast fullness or tenderness		Breast regression	
Edema		Depression	
		Vaginal yeast infection	

TABLE 12-7. Symptoms Experienced by Oral Contraceptive Users That Could Indicate Serious Adverse Effects (Mnemonic: ACHES)

Symptom	Condition
Abdominal pain	Gallstones, blood clot, pancreatitis
Chest pain, shortness of breath, coughing blood	Blood clot in lung, myocardial infarction
Headaches	Stroke, hypertension, migraine
Eye problems	Stroke, hypertension, vascular occlusion
Severe leg pain	Blood clot

Oral contraceptives are contraindicated in patients with thrombotic disorders, cardiovascular disease, impaired liver function, breast cancer, pregnancy, and in heavy tobacco smokers. Adverse drug reactions include thrombotic disease, pulmonary emboli, myocardial infarction, cerebral hemorrhage, gallbladder disease, and hepatic tumors. The risk of deep vein thrombosis and pulmonary emboli dramatically increases with smokers who use high-dose estrogen formulations. Symptoms of severe adverse events are listed in Table 12-7.

Drugs that induce cytochrome P-450 metabolism, such as rifampin and griseofulvin, speed estrogen metabolism and thus significantly diminish the efficacy of oral contraceptives. Patients should be counseled to use additional, alternative contraceptives or switch to high-dose estrogen contraceptives.

For patients in whom estrogen is contraindicated (those who smoke or are breast-feeding), progestin-only (mini-pills) contraceptives are available (norethindrone, norgestrel). However, for maximal effects, progestin-only pills must be started on the first day of menses and taken at the same time each day. This type of contraception has a higher incidence of irregular bleeding and ectopic pregnancy compared with combination oral contraceptives. Keep in mind that with progestin-only pills, ovulation may not be suppressed.

In addition to oral contraceptives, progestins can be deposited intramuscularly for long-lasting contraception. Drugs such as medroxyprogesterone can be administered every 3 months via intramuscular injection. Depot medroxyprogesterone has been associated with significant, sometimes irreversible, loss of bone density. Similarly, levonorgestrel-containing intrauterine devices (IUDs) can be inserted for long-lasting contraception (5 years).

Other combinatorial estrogen plus progestin formulations have been developed including the vaginal ring, which releases ethinyl estradiol (EE) and etonogestrel; the transdermal patch (EE and norelgestromin); and the combination oral contraceptive Yasmin, which contains EE plus drospirenone. Drospirenone is a progestin whose mechanism resembles that of spironolactone. As a result, there is less water retention and associated weight gain. Patients should not take drospirenone with other medications that retain potassium, since the drug has mineralocorticoid activity that influences water and electrolyte balance. Oral contraceptives have now been formulated for 3-month hormonal therapy (EE plus levonorgestrel).

Menstrual Disorders

Premenstrual syndrome (PMS) is a group of symptoms related to the menstrual cycle. Women who experience severe dysmenorrhea (painful menstrual cramps) are often treated with ethinyl estradiol (EE)–containing hormonal contraceptives. Table 12-8 lists treatment options for managing symptoms of severe premenstrual syndrome.

TABLE 12-8. Premenstrual Syndrome

Symptom	Treatment
Dysmenorrhea and cramps	Oral contraceptives, NSAIDs
Migraines	Low-dose estrogen, NSAIDs
Breast tenderness (mastodynia)	Vitamin E, bromocriptine (dopamine agonist), leuprolide (gonadotropin-releasing hormone agonist)
Insomnia	Antihistamines, tricyclic antidepressants
Anxiety	Benzodiazepines
Depression/irritability	Selective serotonin reuptake inhibitors
Weight gain, bloating	Spironolactone, drospirenone
Mood swings	Lithium, carbamazepine, valproate

Menopause

Hormonal Replacement Therapy (HRT)

Permanent amenorrhea occurs when ovarian follicles no longer respond to FSH. This loss in ovarian function leads to a decline in ovarian estrogen secretion. Menopausal women still make some adrenal-derived estrogens (estrone, E1) from androstenedione; however, these forms of estrogen are only one third the potency of EE and there are no cyclic variations throughout the monthly cycle as there formerly were with EE.

Women entering menopause often experience vasomotor instability (hot flashes) as the lack of estrogen leads to surges in LH and FSH, which affect thermoregulation of the hypothalamus. Additionally, menopausal women are frequently bothered by urinary and vaginal irritation (dryness, atrophy, dyspareunia).

Hormone replacement therapies composed of estrogens (conjugated, synthetic, natural) and progestins are used to manage symptoms. Topical vaginal formulations are treatments of choice for women with symptoms of urogenital irritation. For those with hot flashes, systemic hormone replacement therapies are necessary. Formulations most often include either oral tablets or transdermal patches, although depot oil injections, lotions, and gels are also available. Women with an intact uterus also receive progestins with their estrogen replacement therapy—either in a continuous fashion or in a cyclic manner during the second half of the month. The continuous progestin formulations prevent bleeding, while the cyclic formulations cause bleeding reminiscent of menstrual cycles. The reason progestins are added to estrogen replacement therapies is that, without progestins, estrogen therapy is associated with a higher risk of endometrial cancer.

CLINICAL MEDICINE

Risks Associated with Hormone Replacement Therapy

Outcomes from the Women's Health Initiative (WHI) trial found that hormone replacement therapy increased the risk of heart disease, breast cancer, and stroke (although the risk of colon cancer was reduced).

Specifically, during the WHI, an oral combination product containing conjugated estrogens with medroxyprogesterone was utilized. Additional studies have suggested that not only does hormone replacement therapy increase the *risk* of breast cancer, it also makes the cancer more difficult to detect by increasing breast tissue density.

Currently, it is recommended that hormone replacement therapy (1) be used at the lowest possible dose, for the shortest possible time, in women with vasomotor symptoms and (2) be avoided in women with a significant risk of breast cancer or heart disease. Moreover, continuous use of progesterone may increase the risk of breast cancer compared with intermittent use. When discontinuing hormone replacement therapy, it is recommended that the drugs be gradually tapered for 6 to 8 weeks to reduce the likelihood of vasomotor adverse effects.

Adverse effects of hormone replacement therapy include nausea, vomiting, breakthrough vaginal bleeding, edema, breast tenderness or enlargement, gallbladder disease, elevated blood pressure, thromboembolic disease, hyperkalemia, and glucose intolerance. Patients should notify their health care professional if they experience pain in the groin or calves, sharp chest pain, shortness of breath, abnormal vaginal bleeding, sudden or severe headache, dizziness or fainting, visual or speech disturbance, yellowing of skin or eyes, breast lumps, or severe depression, since these symptoms can be signs of serious adverse effects.

PHYSIOLOGY

Clasts versus Blasts

Bone tissue is continually in a state of dynamic flux. This is due, in part, to the fact that osteoclasts signal osteoblasts and osteoblasts signal osteoclasts.

Osteoclasts release proteases that dissolve bone mineral and collagen matrix, a process known as bone resorption. The process serves to clear away damaged bone. Simultaneously, osteoclasts secrete growth factors that act as chemoattractants for osteoblasts.

Osteoblasts fill in bone cavities with new bone matrix. Osteoblasts release cytokines to attract osteoclasts and continue the dynamic remodeling of bone. The entire process can be hormonally regulated to modulate release or absorption of calcium into bone matrix and thus indirectly regulate serum calcium levels.

Medroxyprogesterone is the most commonly used progestin during menopause, but norethindrone acetate and progesterone also are used. Progesterone causes some women to be sedated because it is metabolized to allopregnanolone, a

TABLE 12-9. Hormonal Regulators of Bone

Hormone	Mechanism	Predominant Effect
Parathyroid hormone	Secreted from parathyroid gland in response to low serum calcium concentrations; increases osteoclast activity	Stimulates bone resorption
Calcitonin	Secreted from thyroid to inhibit osteoclast bone resorption	Prevents bone loss
Vitamin D	Increases calcium absorption (GI tract) and increases calcium reabsorption (kidney)	Prevents bone loss
Estrogen	Blocks the IL-6 receptor, a potent cytokine associated with bone resorption; inhibits PTH activity; increases apoptosis of osteoclasts	Prevents bone loss

BIOCHEMISTRY

Organ-Specific Modification of Vitamin D(s)

Ergosterol (provitamin D_2) $\xrightarrow{\text{UV light}}$ Ergocalciferol (vitamin D_2) $\xrightarrow{\text{Liver}}$ 25-Hydroxyergocalciferol (25-[OH]-D_2) $\xrightarrow{\text{Kidney}}$ 1,25-Dihydroxyergocalciferol (1,25-[OH]$_2$-D_2)

7-Dehydrocholesterol (provitamin D_3) $\xrightarrow[\text{UV light}]{\text{Skin via}}$ Cholecalciferol (vitamin D_3) $\xrightarrow{\text{Liver}}$ Calcifediol (25-[OH]-D_3) $\xrightarrow{\text{Kidney}}$ Calcitriol (1,25-[OH$_2$]-D_3)

TABLE 12-10. Variations among Calcium Salts

Calcium Salt	Elemental Calcium (%)
Calcium carbonate	40
Calcium citrate	24
Calcium lactate	18

compound that acts at GABA-A receptors (see chapter 13). Capsule formulations contain peanut oil and therefore are contraindicated in women who are allergic to peanuts.

Osteoporosis

Calcium Supplements, Hormone Replacement Therapy, Selective Estrogen Receptor Modulators (Raloxifene), Bisphosphonates, and Calcitonin

Osteoporosis affects nearly 45 million Americans, of whom nearly 70% are women. Osteoporosis is a gradual loss of bone mass, leading to "trauma-less" fractures, the most common of which occur in vertebrae and the most serious in the hip. The main physiologic regulators of bone density are listed in Table 12-9.

Treatment of osteoporosis usually begins with prevention. Calcium and vitamin D supplements should be encouraged as well as weight-bearing exercise. Caffeine and nicotine should be discouraged. Each calcium salt contains differing amounts of elemental calcium (Table 12-10). This is important because most adult women require between 1000 and 1200 mg elemental calcium daily. Therefore, intake of supplements must be adjusted to ensure the optimal dose of calcium.

Calcium carbonate is relatively insoluble and requires an acidic environment to be absorbed. On the other hand, calcium citrate is readily soluble and does not require a low pH for absorption, so calcium citrate is a preferred calcium supplement in patients with low gastric acid production (e.g., patients with achlorhydria or who take antacids, H$_2$-blockers, proton pump inhibitors or are post-bariatric surgery). High doses of calcium may cause constipation and kidney stones (the latter usually occur only in the presence of large amounts of oxalate). Calcium can interfere with absorption of a variety of drugs:

- Iron
- Tetracyclines
- Fluoroquinolones
- Bisphosphonates
- Phenytoin
- Fluoride

Inadequate levels of vitamin D or inadequate sun exposure cause abnormal bone mineralization (rickets in children, osteomalacia in adults). Vitamin D$_2$ and vitamin D$_3$ are metabolized via actions of the liver and kidneys to their active forms, 1,25-dihydroxyergocalciferol and calcitriol, respectively.

Calcitriol is the most potent form of vitamin D. Vitamin D_3 is the form found in many multivitamins, but it must be metabolized by the liver and kidneys to its more active form, calcitriol. Calcitriol is used especially by patients with renal or hepatic dysfunction. Adverse effects associated with vitamin D excess begin with weakness, headache, and bone pain and progress to polyuria, polydipsia, weight loss, and symptoms associated with hypercalcemia (cardiac arrhythmias).

Raloxifene is a selective estrogen receptor modulator (SERM) that can be used to promote bone mineralization. This drug acts as an agonist at some tissues and as an antagonist at other tissues. Specifically, raloxifene functions as an estrogen agonist in bone and liver but acts as an estrogen receptor antagonist in breast and uterine tissues. Thus, raloxifene diminishes endometrial and breast cancer development while stimulating bone mineralization. As a bonus, raloxifene improves HDL/LDL ratios. This is not the first SERM drug discussed. Tamoxifen, described in Chapter 5, is a SERM and is antagonistic for breast tissue but agonistic for uterine tissue as well as bone. Compared with hormone replacement therapy (HRT), raloxifene does not stimulate uterine or endometrial tissues, does not require coadministration of progestins, and does not cause breast swelling or tenderness.

Despite its low risk of causing reproductive cancers, raloxifene still can increase the risk of deep vein thrombosis and thromboemboli. Raloxifene also can decrease the absorption of thyroxine; therefore, for the large subset of women who experience hypothyroidism and osteoporosis, raloxifene and thyroid hormone administration should be separated by 12 hours. Raloxifene may cause hot flashes and leg cramps.

Another therapeutic approach for osteoporosis is the bisphosphonates. These drugs actively adsorb to the hydroxyapatite of bone to become part of the bone matrix. These "reenforced" bones are more resistant to the proteolytic actions of osteoclasts. Alendronate or risedronate are available in once a week formulations. Ibandronate is the first once monthly bisphosphonate therapy to be approved. Notice that most of the bisphosphonates end in "-dronate." The bioavailability of bisphosphonates is poor; food and antacids further diminish absorption through the GI tract. Therefore, the drugs should be taken with water, first thing in the morning, on an empty stomach, at least 30 minutes before breakfast. Patients must also be instructed to maintain an upright position for at least 30 minutes after taking the drug to minimize esophageal irritation. The major adverse side effects are esophageal erosion and peptic ulcer disease. Rare but serious eye problems have also been reported. Other bisphosphonates are used to treat Paget's disease or hypercalcemia of malignancy, including etidronate, pamidronate, tiludronate, and zoledronic acid. Recently, serious jaw necrosis has been reported by cancer patients using some intravenous bisphosphonate therapies. Overall, bisphosphonates reduce the risk of vertebral fractures significantly.

Synthetic salmon calcitonin also can be administered to limit bone loss. Calcitonin inhibits osteoclast-induced bone resorption via activation of G_s-mediated cAMP. Calcitonin helps to maintain homeostasis by opposing the actions of parathyroid hormone (PTH). Calcitonin also has antinociceptive properties, with analgesia occurring in as little as 5 days. Hypersensitivity reactions (anaphylactic shock, laryngeal edema, angioedema, bronchospasm) may occur due to an immune response to the foreign antigen.

Another new therapy for osteoporosis is a recombinant truncated form of parathyroid hormone (teriparatide), administered subcutaneously. Although somewhat of a paradox, continuous administration of PTH causes bone resorption, whereas intermittent dosing preferentially stimulates new bone formation. Teriparatide is administered SC daily and thus stimulates bone formation. However, this parathyroid analog has been associated with osteosarcoma, and long-term safety is a concern. Patients should discontinue use after 2 years. Patients often experience dizziness or tachycardia following injections, although these effects typically subside after the first few doses. Teriparatide is the only drug that stimulates new bone formation; other drugs simply slow bone loss.

●●● MEN'S REPRODUCTIVE DISORDERS

Erectile Dysfunction

Phosphodiesterase-5 Inhibitors

Phosphodiesterase-5 inhibitors include sildenafil, tadalafil, and vardenafil. Note that the names all end in "-afil."

Erectile dysfunction can be caused by numerous abnormalities: endocrine, neurologic, vascular, psychological, and structural. Medications can also contribute. The most common drugs used to treat erectile dysfunction are the phosphodiesterase-5 (PDE5) inhibitors, which facilitate vasodilation. These phosphodiesterase inhibitors prevent catabolism of cGMP. Remember that nitric oxide–induced smooth muscle relaxation and resultant vasodilation is cGMP-dependent. For the most part, differences between agents are pharmacokinetic in nature (Table 12-11). Keep in mind that since tadalafil has a long duration of activity, any side effects that occur may last for extended periods of time.

TABLE 12-11. Pharmacologic Treatments for Erectile Dysfunction

Parameter	Drug		
	Sildenafil	**Tadalafil**	**Vardenafil**
Duration of activity	Up to 5 hr	Up to 36 hr	Up to 5 hr
Time to onset	60 min	30 min	16 min
Common side effects	Headache Flushing Bluish vision	Headache Dyspepsia Back pain	Headache Flushing

Dosage must be lowered for all three PDE5 inhibitors in patients who take potent P-450 CYP3A4 inhibitors, and these drugs are contraindicated in patients who use nitrates. Additionally, the PDE5 inhibitors must be used cautiously, if at all, in patients who take α-blockers for hypertension or benign prostatic hyperplasia because of the risk of hypotension and dizziness. Men should seek medical attention if priapism (continuous erection of the penis) develops, since permanent damage could ensue. There are increasing concerns about visual disturbances, including optic neuritis. PDE5 inhibitors may inhibit PDE6, which is the phosphodiesterase found in photoreceptors.

Alprostadil, a PGE_1 analog, enhances cavernous arterial blood flow and is another option for treating erectile dysfunction. This drug comes in various injectable formulations as well as urethrally inserted pellets. Penile fibrosis and pain can occur with regular use. Priapism also may occur.

Hypogonadism/Andropause

Testosterone replacement therapy has long been used as a treatment for male hypogonadism. Testosterone replacement therapy in aging, but otherwise healthy, men is receiving new attention in the management of andropause (weakness, fatigue, reduced muscle mass, osteoporosis, sexual dysfunction, depression, insomnia, and memory impairment associated with aging in men).

Testosterone replacement therapies come in numerous forms: transdermal patches, gels, subcutaneous pellets, injectables, and transbuccal delivery systems. The oral dose form is noticeably absent from this list. Oral testosterone formulations are avoided because of hepatic injury. Adverse effects associated with testosterone replacement therapy include acne, cardiovascular disease, gynecomastia, testicular atrophy, and advancement of benign prostatic hypertrophy or prostate cancer.

Benign Prostatic Hypertrophy

α-Adrenergic Receptor Blockers and 5α-Reductase Inhibitors

α-Adrenergic receptor blockers include doxazosin, prazosin, terazosin, tamsulosin, and alfuzosin. Examples of 5α-reductase inhibitors are dutasteride and finasteride.

α-Adrenergic receptor blockers and 5α-reductase inhibitors are the drugs of choice for managing symptomatic benign prostatic hypertrophy. First-generation α-receptor blockers (doxazosin, prazosin, and terazosin) relax not only prostatic smooth muscle but also vascular smooth muscle, thereby accounting for some of their side effects (hypotension, dizziness). On the other hand, newer α-receptor blockers (tamsulosin and alfuzosin) are more selective for prostatic smooth muscle but may be associated with decreased ejaculation. Alfuzosin prolongs the cardiac QT interval, and CYP3A4 P-450 inhibitors increase alfuzosin concentrations.

5α-Reductase inhibitors, drugs that inhibit conversion of testosterone to more active dihydrotestosterone, such as dutasteride and finasteride, are also used to manage benign prostatic hypertrophy. In fact, since it takes 6 to 9 months for 5α-reductase inhibitors to reach their maximal effects, they are often combined with α-receptor blockers, at least for a few months, since the α-receptor blockers alleviate troublesome voiding symptoms almost immediately. Adverse effects associated with decreased production of dihydrotestosterone are sexual in nature (impotence, decreased libido, gynecomastia). These drugs are contraindicated in pregnant women—meaning that men should not give blood for 6 months after taking these medications and pregnant health care workers should avoid handling the tablets owing to the risk of fetal anomalies in male fetuses.

Numerous drugs and natural products may be responsible for worsening urinary symptoms in men; examples include

- Opiates
- Anticholinergics (tricyclic antidepressants, sedating antihistamines, muscle relaxants)
- Sympathomimetics (pseudoephedrine, ma huang, ephedrine)

PHYSIOLOGY

Dysfunctional Signaling Leads to Type 2 Diabetes

Insulin resistance is due to unknown genetic or environmental changes and is often associated with obesity, aging, and sedentary lifestyle. The molecular mechanisms underlying type 2 insulin resistance are unknown but are speculated to include inappropriate phosphorylation of insulin receptor substrates (IRSs) that uncouple insulin receptors from downstream targets. Impaired insulin receptor signaling results in diminished transcription of critical gene products (GLUT4 protein) essential for proper plasma membrane internalization and processing of glucose. Dysfunctional lipid or glucose metabolism (free fatty acids, glycosphingolipids) may ultimately be responsible for impaired insulin receptor signaling. Notably, there has been a rise in type 2 diabetic symptoms in adolescents worldwide, correlating with a change in diet as "Western-style" fast food restaurants became more prevalent.

BIOCHEMISTRY

Sites of Insulin Action

Insulin facilitates glucose utilization by
- Increasing glucose uptake by *peripheral tissues*
- Increasing glycogen synthesis, decreasing gluconeogenesis in the *liver*
- Increasing lipogenesis, decreasing lipolysis in *adipose tissue*
- Increasing protein synthesis in *muscle*

●●● PANCREATIC DISORDERS

Diabetes Mellitus

Insulin, Sulfonylureas and Meglitinides, Biguanides and Thiazolidinediones, and α-Glucosidase Inhibitors

Diabetes mellitus is the inability to properly manage glucose metabolism (glucose intolerance) owing to either the inability to produce and secrete insulin as a result of autoimmune destruction of pancreatic β-cells (type 1) or the inability of peripheral tissues to respond to circulating insulin as a result of diminished or impaired insulin receptor signaling (type 2).

For the most part, patients with type 1 diabetes are managed by insulin replacement therapy and diet, whereas patients with type 2 diabetes are initially managed by diet and oral agents that improve insulin secretion or insulin sensitivity. As elevated glucose levels progressively damage pancreatic β-cells, patients with type 2 diabetes often are subsequently managed with insulin therapy.

A multiplicity of interconnected metabolic disorders is ultimately responsible for the high morbidity and mortality of uncontrolled diabetes. Insulin deficiency and insulin resistance both lead to hyperglycemia. Often, hyperlipidemia and hypertension are accompanying problems that you must address. Tight glucose control is known to reduce both microvascular and macrovascular diabetic complications (neuropathies, gastroparesis, parasthesias, etc.). However, tight glucose control also increases the risk of hypoglycemic events.

Patients with type 1 diabetes have polyuria, nocturia, polydipsia, unexplained weight loss, weakness, and dry skin. In contrast, patients with type 2 diabetes are often obese and have increased appetite, blurred vision, frequent urinary tract infections, and numbness or tingling in extremities (peripheral neuropathy).

Insulin

Insulin is administered subcutaneously via multiple formulations in patients with type 1 diabetes and in approximately 30% of patients with type 2 diabetes who are insulin-dependent because of progressive dysfunction of pancreatic β-cells.

Differences between insulin formulations are largely pharmacokinetic. There are insulin formulations that cover ranges of action from 3 to 24 hours. Rapid or short-acting formulations are taken with meals, in contrast to intermediate- and long-acting preparations that are used to manage glucose throughout the day. Synthetic insulin homologs include lispro, insulin-aspart, glargine, and glulisine. These synthetic insulins have one or two amino acid changes that keep insulin in a monomeric state (lispro), increase absorption (aspart), diminish degradation (glargine), or lead to faster onset of action (lispro, aspart, and glulisine) compared with regular (natural or unadulterated) insulin. Some formulations of insulin contain protamine and zinc or acetate to prolong efficacy. Allergic reactions may develop to protamine. In contrast to the subcutaneous formulations mentioned above, regular insulin can be administered intravenously too. The major adverse reaction to all insulin formulations is hypoglycemia, associated with sweating, tachycardia, palpitations, tremors, confusion, and seizures. Immediate ingestion of sugar (glucose tablets) can resolve symptoms within 15 minutes. Weight gain is a long-term adverse effect associated with increased insulin levels because insulin is lipogenic (promotes fat storage).

Oral Agents for Type 2 Diabetes

Patients with type 2 diabetes are managed pharmacologically by

- Increasing pancreatic insulin secretion with sulfonylureas or meglitinides and/or
- Decreasing hepatic gluconeogenesis with biguanides and/or
- Improving insulin sensitivity in peripheral tissues with thiazolidinediones and/or
- Preventing breakdown of complex carbohydrates into simple sugars with α-glucosidase inhibitors.

Each of these oral therapeutic approaches is discussed below.

Sulfonylureas and Meglitinides

Examples of sulfonylureas are glyburide, glipizide, and glimepiride. Meglitinides include repaglinide and nateglinide.

The mechanism of action of both sulfonylureas and meglitinides is to inhibit ATP-dependent K^+ channels in pancreatic β-cells, which results in membrane depolarization and subsequent calcium influx. This calcium influx leads to augmented insulin release in functional β-cells. These drugs are known as insulin secretogogues.

CLINICAL MEDICINE

Monitoring of Patients with Diabetes

Fasting glucose plasma concentration >126 mg/dL is diagnostic of diabetes. Postprandial glucose level >200 mg/dL after a glucose tolerance test (ingestion of 75 g glucose) is also consistent with diabetes. Glucose levels >180 mg/dL can result in urinary glucose excretion.

In addition to plasma or urinary glucose determination, glycosylated hemoglobin (HbA_{1C}) can be used for long-term monitoring of diabetic patients. Intermittent diabetic screenings should be initiated in patients over 30 years of age who are at risk for diabetes (are obese; have a family history; belong to a high-risk population, e.g., African American, Hispanic, Native American; are hypertensive or hyperlipidemic).

Many devices are being developed for noninvasive blood glucose testing or to minimize the pain and inconvenience of routinely checking plasma glucose concentrations. In addition to insulin and proper control of blood sugar, tight blood pressure management and cholesterol control are important. Aggressive blood pressure control reduces adverse cardiovascular events and decreases the risk of macrovascular diabetic complications. Many patients with type 2 diabetes are also given ACE inhibitors for renal protection, and β-blockers and statins for cardiovascular protection.

Glyburide, glipizide, and glimepiride are second-generation sulfonylureas. Initially, 60% to 70% of patients respond to sulfonylureas, but many patients go on to develop secondary pancreatic β-cell failure. Like insulin therapy, the major adverse side effect of sulfonylureas is hypoglycemia. Other common adverse effects include nausea, vomiting, dyspepsia, pruritus, erythema, urticaria, and skin rash.

Meglitinides prescribed for patients with type 2 diabetes include repaglinide and nateglinide. The main difference between sulfonylureas and meglitinides is that meglitinides have a rapid onset of action as well as a short duration of activity. This makes meglitinides ideal for patients with postprandial hyperglycemia. Thus, these drugs are taken just before meals, to reduce postprandial hyperglycemia. Note that if a meal is skipped, the drugs should be skipped too. Hypoglycemia is the most common adverse effect but occurs less often than with sulfonylureas. Since meglitinides do not contain a sulfa chemical moiety, they can be taken by patients with sulfa allergies.

Because repaglinide is extensively metabolized by the cytochrome P-450 3A4 isotype, drugs that induce or inhibit this P-450 should be avoided or closely monitored. Specifically, drugs that inhibit P-450 3A4 (azoles, erythromycin, fluoxetine, paroxetine, cimetidine, protease inhibitors, gemfibrozil) can increase the risk of repaglinide-induced hypoglycemia. In contrast, drugs that induce P-450 3A4 transcription (rifampin, barbiturates, carbamazepine, phenytoin, St John's wort) can reduce the therapeutic efficacy of repaglinide.

Biguanides

Metformin

The major mechanism of action for biguanides is inhibition of hepatic glucose production. These drugs may also decrease intestinal glucose absorption and increase peripheral insulin sensitivity. They are first-line agents in obese patients with type 2 diabetes. Unlike sulfonylureas, which promote weight gain (by increasing insulin levels), biguanides may promote weight loss. Metformin is a biguanide and is often used in combination with sulfonylureas for maximal effectiveness. The major adverse effect associated with metformin is diarrhea and other GI distress. Lactic acidosis also is a concern, and the drug should be avoided by those at risk (those with acutely decompensated congestive heart failure, renal or liver disease, or alcoholism; those who are more than 80 years of age; those who have been given radiologic contrast media).

Thiazolidinediones

Pioglitazone and Rosiglitazone

Thiazolidinediones are a great example of how target identification has led to a group of useful drugs. Peroxisome proliferator-activated receptor gamma (PPARγ) is a nuclear receptor and transcriptional regulator for insulin-responsive genes that control glucose and lipid metabolism (Fig. 12-8). Thus, therapeutics that selectively activate PPARγ can be used to bypass dysfunctional insulin receptors. Specifically,

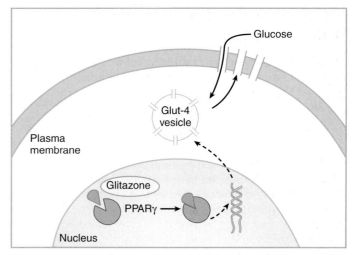

Figure 12-8. Mechanism of action for thiazolidinediones. These drugs activate the peroxisome proliferator-activated receptor gamma (PPARγ), a nuclear receptor found in adipose, skeletal muscle, and liver. PPARγ activates transcription of insulin-response genes that control glucose and lipid metabolism as well as synthesis of the glucose transporter, GLUT4. Newly transcribed and translated GLUT4 is packaged within vesicles for insertion into the plasma membrane. Functional GLUT4 reduces insulin resistance in muscle by increasing glucose uptake, thereby removing glucose from the circulation.

pioglitazone and rosiglitazone reduce blood glucose levels by decreasing insulin resistance in skeletal muscle and adipose tissues. Drugs that activate PPARγ increase expression of GLUT4, the transporter that moves glucose into cells. Thiazolidinediones can be used as a monotherapy along with diet and exercise for patients with type 2 diabetes. In addition, thiazolidinediones are often combined with sulfonylureas and biguanides but must be used cautiously with insulin, since this combination may cause fluid retention and congestive heart failure. As a bonus, pioglitazone reduces triglyceride levels while elevating HDL.

α-Glucosidase Inhibitors

Acarbose and Miglitol

The α-glucosidase inhibitors, such as acarbose and miglitol, delay the breakdown of ingested complex carbohydrates into glucose by inhibiting α-glucosidase, an enzyme found within the brush border epithelium of the small intestine. These drugs are particularly useful to diminish postprandial hyperglycemia.

The major side effects of these drugs are gastrointestinal owing to their mechanism of action. Specifically, diarrhea occurs from unabsorbed carbohydrates, as well as abdominal pain, flatulence, and intestinal obstruction. Patients with concomitant inflammatory bowel disease should not use these drugs.

New Drugs for Diabetes
Pramlintide and Exenatide

As new targets (hormones and receptors) are discovered, new opportunities for drug therapies are created. Two new

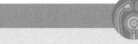

Diabetic Ketoacidosis

Patients with diabetes do not respond well to cortisol- or catecholamine-induced stress. When an insulin deficit is coupled with increased levels of a stress hormone and a precipitating factor (acute illness, surgery), the vicious cycle of diabetic ketoacidosis may begin.

Exacerbated hyperglycemia induces osmotic diuresis and dehydration. Insulin deficiency induces fat mobilization and release of fatty acids, which are oxidized to acidic ketones. Diminished glomerular filtration rate (GFR) because of dehydration further worsens glucose and ketone elimination, worsening hyperosmolality. Osmotic diuresis also causes loss of potassium, sodium, phosphate, and bicarbonate. This hypovolemia decreases tissue perfusion, leading to lactic acid accumulation, which further worsens the ketoacidosis. Vomiting may result, which further exacerbates dehydration. This metabolic ketoacidosis leads to hyperventilation, known as Kussmaul's respiration (shallow but fast) as well as "acetone breath." Over time, Kussmaul's breathing may reduce P_{CO_2} levels, leading to a compensatory respiratory alkalosis.

Diabetic ketoacidosis presents with lethargy, hyperventilation, tachycardia, fruity breath, altered mental status, nausea, thirst, decreased urine output (secondary to a decrease in GFR), and dry mucous membranes. Patients have elevated ketone levels as well as a significant anion gap. Patients require immediate treatment including rehydration, rapid-onset forms of insulin, and careful management of electrolyte and acid-base balance. Typically, patients with type 1 diabetes mellitus are at risk of diabetic ketoacidosis.

injectable drugs have been approved for treating diabetes. Pramlintide can be used adjunctively for type 1 and type 2 diabetic patients. Pramlintide is a synthetic analog of amylin, a neuroendocrine hormone that boosts insulin secretion. Physiologically, amylin slows gastric emptying, suppresses glucagon secretion and postprandial hyperglycemia, and enhances satiety. Pramlintide allows insulin doses to be reduced. However, the risk of severe hypoglycemia is increased.

Exenatide is now approved for patients with type 2 diabetes. The drug was developed after studying glucagon-like peptide-1 from the Gila monster. Exanatide is similar in function to the gastrointestinal hormone glucagon-like peptide-1 (GLP-1) and is referred to as an incretin-mimetic. Exenatide stimulates release of insulin, slows gastric emptying, suppresses glucagon secretion to reduce postprandial hyperglycemic, and may help produce satiety responses that are impaired in type 2 diabetics. Adverse effects include nausea and bloating as a result of slowed gastroparesis. Hypoglycemia may also be problematic so doses of oral hypoglycemic drugs should be reduced. Importantly, no other diabetic medications stimulate insulin secretion *and* cause weight loss.

●●● COMPLEMENTARY AND ALTERNATIVE MEDICINE

Fenugreek is a cooking spice that is sometimes used therapeutically to enhance breast milk production. Hypoglycemic actions are possible, and the herbal product should be used cautiously by diabetics. Additionally, the herb may have anticoagulation properties, which could be problematic in patients taking anticoagulants or those with bleeding disorders. Since fenugreek is a member of the legume family, there also is a theoretical risk of cross-hypersensitivity in patients who are allergic to peanuts.

St. John's wort is used by some women who experience mild depression at various times throughout their monthly cycles. However, drug interactions occur between this natural supplement and selective serotonin reuptake inhibitors, tricyclic antidepressants, monoamine oxidase inhibitors, L-tryptophan, and dopaminergic agonists, potentially leading to serotonin syndrome (confusion, agitation, fever, tremor, spasm).

Other alternative therapies used by some women include dong quai for controlling hot flashes and black cohosh for alleviating cramps, hot flashes, and vaginal dryness. These alternative therapies have adverse side effects. Dong quai has a laxative effect, may cause photosensitivity, and increases bleeding tendencies, while black cohosh may upset the stomach and its long-term effects are unknown. Black cohosh should not be confused with blue cohosh, which is relatively toxic and induces uterine contractions or menstruation. Phytoestrogens from soy products (isoflavones) may also help hot flashes. Accepted therapies for treating premenstrual syndrome include aerobic exercise and calcium, magnesium, and vitamin E supplementation.

Many men treat benign prostatic hypertrophy with saw palmetto. The natural product seems to aid in management of nocturia, weak urinary stream, and difficulty postponing the urge to urinate. However, despite its efficacy, prescription medications usually work better. Saw palmetto may increase the risk of bleeding in patients taking anticoagulants or antiplatelet agents.

●●● TOP FIVE LIST

1. The anterior pituitary releases multiple factors that control growth (growth hormone), adrenal function (adrenocorticotropic hormone), thyroid function (thyroid-stimulating hormone), and reproductive organs (luteinizing hormone, follicle-stimulating hormone, prolactin). The posterior pituitary produces vasopressin (antidiuretic hormone) and oxytocin, which control fluid balance and labor, respectively.

2. Thyroid storm (thyrotoxicosis) can be managed with a combination of thionamides, β-blockers, aspirin, and corticosteroids.

3. For osteoporosis in women, selective estrogen receptor modulators (SERMs), bisphosphonates, and Ca⁺⁺ supplements may be safer treatments than traditional hormone

replacement therapy (HRT), which can have significant cardiovascular side effects.

4. Preventing breakdown of cGMP by means of phospho-diesterase inhibitors is an effective therapy for erectile dysfunction.

5. Type 1 diabetes may be controlled by diet and insulin, while type 2 diabetes may be managed by a combination approach with sulfonylureas, meglitinides, biguanides, thiazolidinediones, and α-glucosidase inhibitors.

Central Nervous System 13

CONTENTS

It's all about managing chemical imbalances in the brain. In most cases, neurologic and psychiatric disorders are the manifestation of perturbed neurochemical homeostasis. Unlike the autonomic nervous system (ANS), the central nervous system (CNS) is not a simple—essentially binary—organization. That is, the ANS is a simple opposition system in which the parasympathetic objective is "rest and digest," while the sympathetic is "fight or flight" (see Chapter 6). The CNS in contrast is complex and characterized by neurochemical nuances. The CNS, beyond its complex organization of billions of cells with a seemingly infinite number of connections, is noteworthy for its diverse number of neurotransmitter systems. There are more than 20 different neurotransmitter systems and multiple receptors for each neurotransmitter. Therefore, there is tremendous diversity in organization, structure, and function of the brain. When any one of the systems goes awry, it can be manifested as a distinct clinical entity—whether neurologic (epilepsy, Parkinson's disease) or psychiatric (depression, Alzheimer's disease). In many cases, we do not know or understand the underlying pathology (e.g., schizophrenia) or etiology (e.g., loss of nigrostriatal dopamine neurons in Parkinson's disease). However, years of clinical trial and error, as well as rational drug design, have brought us to the point where we have effective drug therapies. Although simplified, Table 13-1 provides an overview of key neurotransmitters in the CNS and clinical manifestations thought to occur as a result of chemical imbalances.

●●● CNS PHARMACOLOGIC MOLECULAR TARGETS

As discussed in Chapters 2 and 6, there are a variety of molecular drug targets composed of selective protein subtypes: ion channels, 7TM-GPCRs (7-transmembrane, G protein–coupled receptors), neurotransmitter channels, and signal transduction and biosynthetic enzymes (Fig. 13-1). Because there are so many different types of molecular targets and diseases of unknown etiology, CNS therapies generally treat the symptoms rather than the cause. In addition, selective receptor agonists have been developed to treat patients with one disorder, while selective receptor antagonists are used to treat patients with another disorder. For example, dopamine agonists are used for Parkinson's disease, whereas dopamine antagonists are a central component of

TABLE 13-1. Simplified View of Chemical Imbalances in the Brain

Neurotransmitter	Too Much	Too Little
Norepinephrine	Anxiety, panic, anorexia, excitability, insomnia	Depression, ADD/ADHD
Dopamine	Psychoses, Tourette's syndrome/tics, chorea	Parkinson's disease, ADD/ADHD, depression
Acetylcholine	Delirium/confusion, psychoses	Alzheimer's disease
Serotonin	Sleep, hallucinations, decreased appetite, anxiety	Depression, OCD, pain sensitivity, anxiety
Glutamate	Seizures, neuronal degeneration	Schizophrenia, depression, cognitive impairment
γ-Aminobutyric acid (GABA)	CNS depression, respiratory depression, sedation	Seizures, movement disorders

ADD, attention deficit disorder; ADHD, attention deficit hyperactivity disorder; OCD, obsessive compulsive disorder.

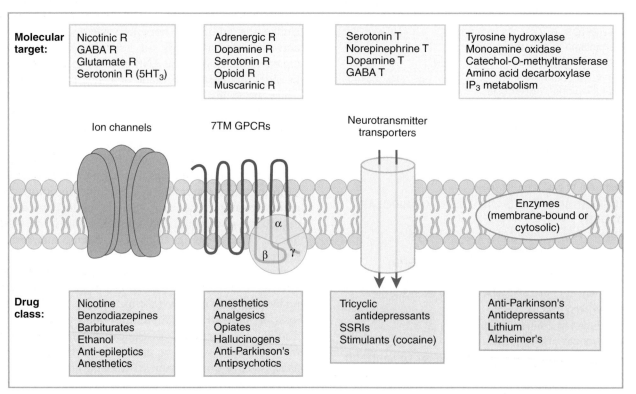

Figure 13-1. Drugs and molecular targets in the CNS. This figure summarizes the receptors, channels, transporters, and enzymes that are subject to regulation in CNS disorders. Specific pharmacologic classes are listed at the bottom. Note that in the case of ion channels, the channel itself is the receptor and binding of the ligand opens the channel. R, receptor; T, transporter.

antipsychotic neuroleptic therapies. Alternatively, it also is common to tackle a given CNS disorder with drugs having widely disparate mechanisms of action. As an example, both barbiturates and inhalant anesthetics are used as general anesthetics despite the fact that these are two distinct, and seemingly independent, classes of compounds. Finally, it will come as no surprise that many of these compounds produce untoward side effects. Adverse effects occur because receptors are widely distributed and serve not only different functions but also are differentially localized. Therefore, patient compliance becomes an important factor in delivering pharmacologic therapies for CNS disorders.

Another important aspect of CNS pharmacotherapy is the balance between stimulation versus inhibition. This occurs at two levels. Of course, we must consider agonists versus antagonists at any given receptor system. Indeed, this is a common theme throughout this text. However, we must also carefully balance opposing neuronal systems. We first visited this concept when considering the autonomic nervous system and opposing sympathetic and parasympathetic pathways (see Chapter 6). The same concept applies in the CNS. For example, GABA (γ-aminobutyric acid) is the major inhibitory neurotransmitter in the brain. This is opposed, in large measure, by excitatory glutamatergic systems (where glutamate is the neurotransmitter). Therefore, pharmacotherapeutic approaches must balance the therapeutic and toxicologic aspects of disrupting this delicate relationship.

●●● ANESTHETICS

Mechanisms of Anesthetic Action

In this case, it's all about excitable membranes. Given that nerve activity, pain, the autonomic nervous system, voluntary muscle control, involuntary muscle reaction (twitching, spinal reflex), and conscious thought are all dependent on membrane depolarization, they can all be regulated by common drugs. Therefore, it is obvious that if you interfere with membrane biophysics, you will create an altered state—figuratively and literally. As a result, the field of anesthesia is designed around decreasing membrane reactivity in such a way as to decrease pain or reduce consciousness, all without decreasing bodily processes to the point where the patient no longer breathes.

The central intent of general anesthesia is to create a reversible surgical state characterized by loss of consciousness and pain sensation (or involuntary response). In practice, this is accomplished in two general ways—through inhalation agents (anesthetic gases) and intravenous agents (predominantly GABA modulators). The mechanisms of action of the general anesthetics have been a point of contention since the first public demonstration of ether anesthesia in 1846. Until recently, it was assumed that these agents nonspecifically modulated membrane fluidity characteristics and so stabilized membrane activity—inhibiting action potentials. Of course, molecular biology and signal transduction pathways provide us with more satisfying and physiologic mechanisms. There is growing evidence that whatever their mechanism of action, anesthetics work by modulating ligand-gated ion channels (see Fig. 13-1) either by activating GABA channels (hyperpolarizing cells) or by blocking excitatory receptors (like NMDA-glutamate receptors).

Inhalation Anesthetics

Halothane, Desflurane, Sevoflurane, and Isoflurane

Note that these drug names all end in "-ane."

Inhalation anesthetics are represented by the prototypical halogenated hydrocarbons halothane, desflurane, sevoflurane, and isoflurane (Table 13-2). (Early general anesthetics such as ether [which is highly flammable] and chloroform [which has toxic properties] are no longer used as general anesthetics.)

The use of general anesthetics is driven by two important concepts—minimal alveolar concentration (MAC) and the blood:gas partition coefficient. MAC is the concentration of anesthetic agent that renders 50% of patients immobile during surgery. As noted in Table 13-2, this is measured as the percentage of the agent in inspired air. MAC is a direct measure of the potency of a drug. This is therefore the value that is considered in choosing the dose for administration. MAC is influenced by the age and physiologic state of the patient and by the presence of other pharmacologic agents. In fact, although nitrous oxide produces only weak anesthetic effects, it is widely used adjunctively for its "second gas" effect to enhance coadministered anesthetic agents.

The blood:gas partition coefficient is a function of solubility of the agent in blood and is a measure of how quickly the inhalation anesthetic will equilibrate between lungs and blood and ultimately the target site in the brain. Therefore, an agent with a low blood:gas coefficient (e.g., desflurane) will equilibrate quickly because it prefers to be in the gas phase. The blood:gas coefficient is *inversely* related to the rate of induction of anesthesia and recovery from anesthesia. In other words, the lower the blood:gas coefficient, the faster the induction and the faster the recovery. Keep in mind that there are other important partitioning coefficients (such as the blood:fat ratio) that determine the long-term fate of an agent (volume of distribution). Similarly, the rate of metabolism is an important factor. All inhalational general anesthetics decrease blood pressure, depress ventilatory responses to CO_2, increase intracranial pressure, and relax skeletal muscles.

Nitrous oxide is a weak anesthetic agent. To induce general anesthesia as a single agent would require high concentrations (essentially >100%) of nitrous oxide, which are possible only under hyperbaric conditions. It is used frequently in outpatient dentistry because it provides analgesia and sedation at concentrations that can be reached under normal atmospheric pressure.

Intravenous Anesthetics

Thiopental, Methohexital, Propofol, and Ketamine

Parenteral anesthetics (Table 13-3) are noteworthy in that they are administered intravenously and act quickly. In

TABLE 13-2. Inhalation Anesthetic Agents

Drug	MOA	MAC	Blood:Gas Coefficient	Side Effect	Comment
Halothane	Ion channels	0.75	2.3	↓ BP	Malignant hyperthermia; tolerated by children; bronchodilator; metabolized by cytochrome P-450; hepatitis
Isoflurane	Ion channels	1.2	1.4	↓ BP	Widely used
Enflurane	Ion channels	1.6	1.8	↓ BP	Reduced use in recent years
Sevoflurane	Ion channels	2.0	0.65	↓ BP	Rapid onset and recovery; tolerated by children; bronchodilator
Desflurane	Ion channels	6.0	0.45	↓ BP	Rapid onset and recovery

BP, blood pressure; MAC, minimum alveolar concentration; MOA, mechanism of action.

TABLE 13-3. Parenteral Anesthetics

Drug	Mechanism of Action	Side Effect and Comments
Thiopental	Barbiturate (↑ GABA receptor activity)	In common use ↓ Cerebral metabolic rate ↓ BP and respiration
Methohexital	Barbiturate (↑ GABA receptor activity)	↓ Cerebral metabolic rate ↓ BP and respiration
Propofol	Nonbarbiturate ↑ GABA activity ↓ Glutamate activity	In common use Rapid onset and recovery Antiemetic
Etomidate	↑ GABA receptor activity	*Increases* BP (choice for patients at risk for hypotension) Ultra-short-acting
Ketamine	Blocks glutamate (NMDA receptor)	Selected pediatric uses Delirium during postoperative recovery (dissociative anesthetic)

BP, blood pressure.

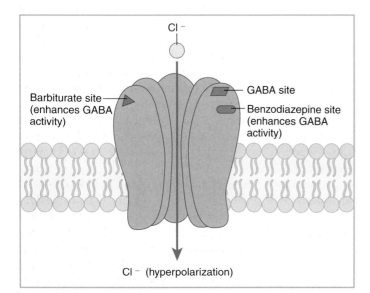

Figure 13-2. GABA-stimulated chloride channel.
The GABA (γ-aminobutyric acid) receptor is a ligand-gated chloride channel. Stimulation of this receptor leads to opening of the channel and the subsequent rush of chloride into the cell. This flow of chloride down its concentration gradient (into the cell) causes hyperpolarization of the cell and inhibits cell firing. In addition to a GABA binding site, the GABA receptor contains a benzodiazepine binding site as well as an independent binding site for barbiturate. Indeed, current thinking suggests a direct interaction between ethanol and the GABA receptor. Given the central importance of GABA as a CNS inhibitory neurotransmitter, it is not surprising that regulation of the GABA receptor is a key therapeutic strategy (anxiolytics, sedative-hypnotics, anesthetics, antiepileptics).

addition, in nearly all cases, their mechanisms of action are more precisely characterized because they have known binding sites on ligand-gated ion channels (Fig. 13-2). The predominant class is the barbiturates (thiopental, methohexital). These agents work by enhancing GABA-stimulated chloride

channel activity. These chloride channels (GABA ligand-gated chloride channel; see Fig. 13-2) open and lead to an influx of chloride that inhibits neuronal firing.

Although the precise mechanism of action of propofol is currently unknown, this agent is also thought to work through GABA receptors. Propofol has a fast onset of action and a fast recovery time with less of a "hangover" effect than that of barbiturates. This property is useful for outpatient surgeries because it allows patients to be discharged rapidly. Another advantage of propofol is its antiemetic properties, which make it a good choice for patients at risk of postoperative nausea and vomiting. The propofol emulsion contains egg phospholipids and is contraindicated in patients with known hypersensitivity. This white emulsion is facetiously termed "milk of amnesia." Thiopental and propofol are the two commonly used intravenous anesthetics. Etomidate, like propofol, has a rapid onset and short duration; however, it *increases* blood pressure, making it useful for patients at risk for hypotension.

Unlike the parenteral agents that stimulate GABA receptors, ketamine is a dissociative anesthetic that binds to the "PCP" binding site on the N-methyl-D-aspartate (NMDA-type) glutamate receptor. Ketamine blocks (antagonizes) this stimulatory ion channel receptor. Indeed, ketamine is a version of phencyclidine (PCP; "angel dust") and can elicit delirium (hallucinations) and vivid dreams during recovery. It also has a strong amnesic effect. Ketamine causes less respiratory depression than do other general anesthetics and stimulates heart rate, blood pressure, and cardiac output by sympathomimetic actions. These properties are useful in patients at risk for hypotension but not for the patient at risk of myocardial infarction. Ketamine also is advantageous because of its inherent analgesic properties. Ketamine has significant abuse liability and is sometimes abused at "rave" clubs. Ketamine is frequently used for its anesthetic and analgesic effects on dogs, cats, rabbits, and other small animals.

Effects of Anesthesia on Nerve Fibers

Recall that nerve fibers come in a variety of types based on size and function (A, B, and C fibers). Local anesthetics are particularly safe and efficacious because they target the smaller fibers (Aδ, B, and C fibers) that are responsible for sensory (pain, temperature) and autonomic functions without affecting motor functions and proprioception (Aα, Aβ, and Aγ). That's why you can chew following dental procedures but cannot feel anything.

Local (Regional) Anesthesia

Lidocaine, Bupivacaine, Cocaine, Benzocaine

Local anesthesia is accomplished through the use of such agents as lidocaine, bupivacaine, and cocaine by administration directly to the site where their action is needed. They act via direct interactions with voltage-gated Na$^+$ channels that are responsible for action potentials. In fact, one of their key characteristics is that they are readily ionizable compounds (weak bases) that cross cell membranes in the uncharged state, become protonated (and stuck) inside the cells, and interact with an intracellular component of sodium channels. Thus, local anesthetics reversibly block action potentials responsible for nerve conduction. While lidocaine and bupivacaine are the two most widely used clinical agents, there are a variety of other local anesthetics with unique characteristics. Indeed, cocaine remains a commonly used drug for nasal surgery because of its anesthetic and vasoconstrictive effects. Benzocaine is a protypical over-the-counter local anesthetic that is used for such varied applications as hemorrhoidal itching and oral pain (toothache or teething).

●●● MUSCLE RELAXANTS

A key problem in general anesthesia is achieving a *depth* of anesthesia that not only removes consciousness but also prevents reflex muscle responses (reflex twitching) during surgery. Unfortunately, this muscle paralysis is one of the last effects achieved by general anesthesia and can require doses approaching toxic levels. To address these concerns, muscle relaxants (neuromuscular blockers) are used as adjuvants to anesthesia. This permits the use of lower (and safer) concentrations of general anesthetic during surgery. Similarly, these agents may be employed to achieve flaccid paralysis in cases of assisted ventilation.

Neuromuscular Blockers

Tubocurarine, Atracurium, Vecuronium, Succinylcholine, Pancuronium, and Mivacurium

Recall from Chapter 6 that the neuromuscular junction (NMJ) is controlled by the somatic nervous system and acetylcholine-releasing nerves. In fact, as discussed previously, the nicotinic acetylcholine receptor at the NMJ is amenable to selective pharmacologic manipulation.

Surgical paralysis can be achieved through two approaches: competitive inhibition with NMJ nicotinic receptor antagonists (tubocurarine, atracurium, and vecuronium) or depolarization blockade with succinylcholine (Table 13-4). The first approach uses curare derivatives. Curare is a mixture of plant alkaloids containing the prototypical compound D-tubocurarine. These paralytic drugs work by competitive antagonism of the NMJ nicotinic receptor. Because of the side effects associated with first-generation drugs, they have largely been replaced by short-acting versions (atracurium and vecuronium).

The second approach to adjuvant paralysis makes use of succinylcholine. This agent is actually an agonist that leads to depolarization blockade and paralysis. This counterintuitive concept is worthy of brief discussion. Like acetylcholine, succinylcholine binds to the NMJ nicotinic receptor and stimulates muscle contraction. However, unlike acetylcholine, it is not degraded as rapidly and so remains in the synapse and *over*stimulates the receptor. The NMJ nicotinic receptor is unique in that it is exquisitely sensitive to overstimulation and responds by desensitizing—essentially shutting down as the receptors desensitize. Therefore, the succinylcholine agonist provides a short-term phase I activation of the NMJ that can lead to muscle fasciculations. This is rapidly followed by a phase II desensitization that is characterized by flaccid paralysis. The advantage of this approach is that it is short-acting and readily reversed. This is another example of the

TABLE 13-4. Neuromuscular Blockade

Drug	Mechanism of Action	Comment
Succinylcholine	Depolarization blockade; phases I and II	Fundamentally different mechanism of action (compared to curare-like drugs)—overstimulates receptor first and then desensitizes the receptor Very short duration
Atracurium	Competitive nicotinic blockade	Short duration of action
Pancuronium	Competitive nicotinic blockade	Long duration
Vecuronium	Competitive nicotinic blockade	Long duration
Mivacurium	Competitive nicotinic blockade	Very short duration

importance of receptor theory (receptor desensitization; see Chapter 2) having direct clinical relevance.

Spasmolytics

Dantrolene, Diazepam, and Baclofen

An important aspect of anesthesia involves the need for spasmolytics—agents to block muscle contraction directly—in the case of malignant hyperthermia. Malignant hyperthermia is a genetic defect that is uncovered during inhalant anesthesia (particularly with halothane). It appears to lead to a situation in which Ca^{++} is released from the sarcoplasmic reticulum and not sequestered. Therefore, the muscle cannot stop contracting. This leads to very high O_2 consumption and a lethal elevation in body temperature. Since it is not mediated by nerve signals, it cannot be prevented by classical NMJ blockade. Therefore, it requires the use of an agent that acts directly on muscle—dantrolene. Dantrolene blocks the release of calcium from the sarcoplasmic reticulum and thereby prevents the malignant hyperthermia. Other agents that can be used as spasmolytics include diazepam (a $GABA_A$ agonist) and baclofen (a $GABA_B$ agonist). As a word of caution, dantrolene is extremely hepatotoxic. Another common clinical indication for antispasmotics is the use of botulinum toxin for cosmetic purposes (anti-wrinkle) and spasticity associated with multiple sclerosis, cerebral palsy, and dystonias. In this case, botulinum toxin works by poisoning the nerves and disrupting acetylcholine release (by blocking vesicle trafficking to the plasma membrane).

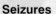 ANTICONVULSANTS

Underlying Pathophysiology of Epilepsy

Epilepsy is a disorder of the cerebral cortex that is characterized by intermittent, unpredictable, and repeated seizures. The seizure is an uncontrollable coordinated firing of neurons. In fact, the seizure is the physical manifestation of abnormal electrical activity in the brain. This activity can be manifested in a variety of ways but is most commonly thought of, by the general patient population, as the tonic-clonic twitching of a

grand mal episode. Interestingly, certain types of medications may contribute to seizures by lowering the seizure threshold, including antipsychotics, antidepressants, analgesics, some antibiotics, and bowel preparations that alter electrolyte balance.

Treatment of Seizure Disorders

Carbamazepine, Lamotrigine, Oxcarbazepine, Phenytoin, Topiramate, Valproic Acid, Zonisamide, Ethosuximide, Phenobarbital, Diazepam, Clonazepam, Tiagabine, Gabapentin, Pregabalin, Levetiracetam, and Vigabatrin

Epilepsy is treated with four general approaches that all work by inhibiting neuronal firing. The difficulty is controlling unregulated impulses without generating the types of inhibition that produce anesthesia. Current therapeutic approaches focus on (1) blocking Na^+ channels, (2) blocking Ca^{++} channels, (3) antagonizing excitatory glutamate receptors, and (4) enhancing GABA activity. However, the precise mechanisms of action vary among the drugs and are depicted in Figure 13-3. In fact, some compounds undoubtedly act in multiple ways.

Most of the first-line antiepileptic drugs act by slowing channel function. Notably, carbamazepine, lamotrigine, oxcarbazepine, phenytoin, topiramate, valproic acid, and zonisamide work by slowing the reversal of sodium channel inactivation (following depolarization). This effectively hyperpolarizes cells and slows their activity.

Carbamazepine has some unique pharmacokinetic properties that are noteworthy given its widespread use. Food enhances its bioavailability, and absorption is variable. In addition, it is not only rapidly metabolized by hepatic P-450 enzymes to an active metabolite, oxcarbazepine, but it is also a hepatic P-450 *auto*-induce—that is, it induces its own metabolism. Drug interactions are frequent, and side effects are numerous. Phenytoin, in spite of a similar mechanism of action, has unique characteristics. Dissolution is the primary rate-limiting step, and absorption varies by manufacturer and formulation. It has a variable metabolism because it is metabolized by zero-order kinetics—like alcohol, a constant amount of drug is metabolized per unit time—the concept of $t_{1/2}$ cannot be applied. When the dose of phenytoin increases, the time for drug elimination increases proportionally. Predictable dose-dependent side effects include nystagmus, ataxia, and altered mental status. Idiosyncratic side effects include drowsiness, lethargy, acne, and peripheral neuropathies. A signature side effect is gingival hyperplasia—overgrowth of tissues of the gums. Drug interactions are also common. Lamotrigine antagonize glutamate excitatory neurotransmitter activity (by blocking sodium channels). This decreases the excitatory "tone" in the CNS. The largest drawback to lamotrigine is a potentially fatal rash (Stevens-Johnson syndrome).

Topiramate and valproate not only block sodium channels but also facilitate GABA activity. Topiramate can cause CNS side effects at high doses (ataxia, confusion) and can produce kidney stones (careful hydration is required) as well as

---

CLINICAL MEDICINE

Seizures

Seizures are more than the prototypical grand mal episode. For instance, seizures are categorized as *partial* (originating from a single part of the cortex) and *generalized* (involving widespread parts of the brain in both hemispheres). The hallmark of the partial seizure is that it does not include loss of consciousness. Within this categorization scheme are a number of types of seizure. These include the tonic-clonic grand mal and petit mal or absence seizures (generalized). Additionally, more discrete disorders include simple and complex partial seizures (focal disturbances—motor, sensory, speech, or affective disorders).

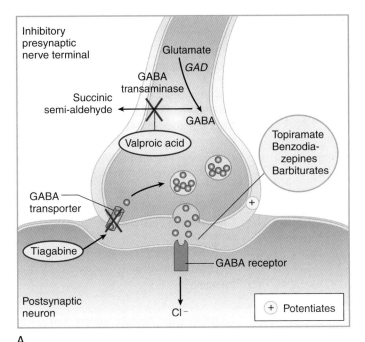
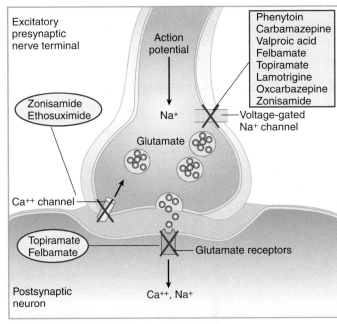

A   B

Figure 13-3. Mechanisms for antiepileptic drugs. Note that many of these drugs are thought to have multiple mechanisms of action. GAD, glutamic acid decarboxylase; GABA, gamma amino butyric acid.

myopia and glaucoma. Valproate is confusing because it has multiple sites of action: it is reported to be an inhibitor of the GABA transaminase (increasing GABAergic "tone"), a blocker of sodium channels, as well as a potential inhibitor of calcium channels. Pharmacologically, valproate is important because it is an inhibitor of hepatic P-450 enzymes. This may lead to potential severe drug interactions. It also has gastrointestinal and CNS effects in its own right.

Ethosuximide, zonisamide, and, to a lesser extent, valproic acid block Ca^{++} channels (T-currents) in the thalamus. Thalamic activity is thought to contribute in a substantive way to absence seizures. Note that the dual-channel activity of valproic acid (Na^+ and Ca^{++} channels) may explain its broad spectrum of activity (Table 13-5). Ethosuximide is a drug of choice for absence seizures. Zonisamide may cause serious rashes, kidney stones, and hyperthermia. It is also contraindicated in patients with known sensitivity to sulfa drugs.

Finally, as will be discussed in the section on Sedative-hypnotic and Anxiolytic Agents, the primary inhibitory system in the brain is mediated by GABA. Therefore, drugs that enhance GABA activity tend to suppress seizure activity. Prototypical agents are the barbiturates (e.g., phenobarbital) and benzodiazepines (e.g., diazepam, clonazepam) that enhance GABA receptor activity (they are allosteric activators of the GABA receptor). These actions increase chloride conductance and hyperpolarize neurons. In addition, newer agents such as gabapentin and tiagabine work by enhancing GABA activity. Gabapentin is well tolerated with few drug interactions and is also used for many other approved and unlabeled indications: to treat nerve pain, as a mood stabilizer, for migraine prevention, and for preventing menopausal

hot flashes. A structural analog of gabapentin, pregabalin, has recently been approved for treatment of partial seizures and neuropathic pain. Tiagabine inhibits reuptake of GABA, thereby enhancing synaptic inhibitory activity. Like gabapentin, tiagabine is well tolerated; unlike gabapentin, it is sensitive to drugs that induce P-450 enzymes as well as to displacement by drugs that are highly protein bound. An additional therapeutic target is GABA transaminase—the enzyme responsible for destroying GABA. This enzyme is inhibited by both valproic acid and vigabatrin. As a result, levels of the inhibitory GABA neurotransmitter are increased. A new drug, levetiracetam, has a fundamentally different mechanism of action from any of the other antiepilepsy medications. This drug does not modulate any known inhibi-

CLINICAL MEDICINE

Treatment for Epilepsy

Many health issues should be addressed in patients taking antiepileptic drugs. Bone density may be reduced in drugs that induce hepatic P-450 microsomal enzymes (carbamazepine, phenytoin, phenobarbital, oxcarbazepine, and topiramate). Patients, especially women, taking these drugs should take calcium and vitamin D supplements because some antiepileptic drugs interfere with vitamin D metabolism. Additionally, antiepileptic drugs that induce cytochrome P-450s reduce the efficacy of many other drugs, including oral contraceptives. Often combinations of antiepilepsy medications are required to suppress seizures.

TABLE 13-5. Antiepileptic Drugs

Drug	Mechanism of Action	Indication	Side Effects/Notes
Carbamazepine	Blocks Na$^+$ channel	Partial and generalized seizures	CNS depression; teratogenic; hepatotoxic; P-450 inducer
Oxcarbazepine	Blocks Na$^+$ channel; metabolite of carbamazepine	Partial seizures	Less induction of P-450s compared with carbamazepine; hyponatremia
Valproic acid	Blocks Na$^+$ channel Blocks GABA transaminase May block Ca^{++} channel	Widely used; broad range of clinical indications	GI distress; hepatotoxicity; teratogenic; *inhibits* drug metabolism
Ethosuximide	Blocks Ca^{++} channel	Absence seizures	GI distress
Phenobarbital	Potentiates GABA activity	Generalized and partial seizures	CNS depression; induces P-450s; abuse potential
Phenytoin	Blocks Na$^+$ channel	Psychomotor and generalized seizures	CNS depression; hepatotoxicity; gingival hyperplasia; teratogenic; induces P-450s
Gabapentin	Potentiates GABA activity	Partial seizures	Sedation
Pregabalin	Analog of gabapentin	Partial seizures and neuropathic pain	
Lamotrigine	Blocks Na$^+$ channel Blocks glutamate release	Generalized and partial seizures	Sedation; hepatotoxicity; severe rash
Topiramate	Blocks glutamate receptor Blocks Na$^+$ channel Enhances GABA activity	Partial and generalized seizures	Sedation; nervousness; ocular effects; hyperthermia (children); metabolic acidosis
Tiagabine	Potentiates GABA activity by blocking GABA reuptake	Partial seizures	Dizziness; tremor
Zonisamide	Blocks Na$^+$ and Ca^{++} channels	Partial seizures	Well tolerated; somnolence; ataxia; hyperthermia (children); contraindicated in sulfonamide allergies
Levetiracetam	Unknown MOA but binds to a presynaptic vesicle protein	Partial seizures	Well tolerated; lack of energy; behavioral problems

CLINICAL MEDICINE

Mood Disorders

Affective (mood) disorders include mania and depression (anxiety is covered in a separate section). *Depression*, by itself, is characterized by an altered state with decreased mood (melancholy, despondency) or inability to derive pleasure in everyday activities (anhedonia). This might also include, among other things, decreased appetite, feelings of worthlessness, and suicidal ideation. On the other hand, *mania* is characterized by a combination of euphoric mood, uncontrolled speech, and psychomotor agitation. This can also include inflated self-esteem, lack of intellectual and cognitive focus, and wild flights of fancy. In keeping with the notion that mania and depression seem to be at opposite ends of a behavioral spectrum, there is a clinical disease, known as *bipolar disorder*, in which a single patient cycles between the two states.

BIOCHEMISTRY

Biogenic Amines

Recall from Chapter 6 that the catecholamines (dopamine, norepinephrine, and epinephrine) are all derived from the same precursor—the amino acid tyrosine. Therefore, different cells in the CNS express different aspects of the biosynthetic pathway and can be characterized as either dopaminergic, noradrenergic (norepinephrine-containing), or adrenergic. In a related biosynthetic pathway, another aromatic amino acid, tryptophan, can be used to synthesize the neurotransmitter serotonin. Collectively, these neurotransmitters (along with histamine) are known as the biogenic amines.

●●● ANTIDEPRESSANTS AND TREATMENT OF BIPOLAR DISORDER

Biogenic Amine Theory of Affective Disorder

On the basis of current effective treatments (tricyclic antidepressants and selective serotonin reuptake inhibitors), the biogenic amine theory of affective disorders has been

tory (GABAergic) or excitatory (sodium channel, glutamate) systems. Although its mechanism of action is currently unknown, it does bind to a novel presynaptic protein that may be involved in vesicle trafficking.

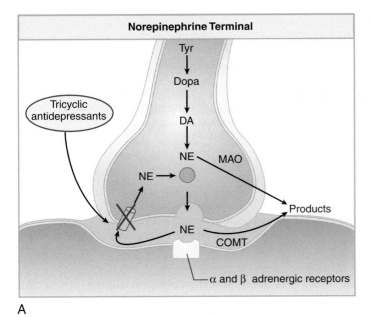
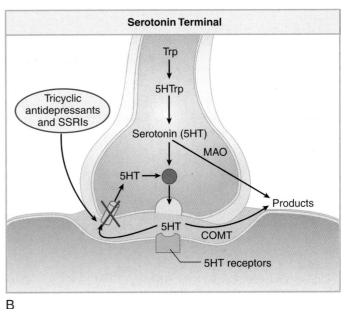

A   B

Figure 13-4. Biogenic amine reuptake inhibitors. Antidepressants (and selected psychomotor stimulants) act by blocking reuptake of biogenic amines (serotonin, norepinephrine, and dopamine) into the nerve terminal. This increases the levels of synaptic neurotransmitter and enhances neuronal activity. The tricyclic antidepressants block both norepinephrine and serotonin transporters, while the SSRIs show a preference for serotonin transporter. Stimulants like cocaine and amphetamine work on all transporters but exert their reinforcing effects by, respectively, blocking the dopamine transporter or reversing this transporter to allow the passive flow of dopamine from the cell. Other centrally acting drugs (anti-Parkinson's drugs) work by inhibiting the metabolism of the biogenic amines by MAO and COMT. COMT, catechol-O-methyltransferase; DA, dopamine; dopa, dihydroxyphenylalanine; 5HT, 5-hydroxytryptamine (serotonin); 5HTrp, 5-hydroxytryptophan; MAO, monoamine oxidase; NE, norepinephrine; Trp, tryptophan; Tyr, tyrosine.

developed. The basic concept is that decreases in norepinephrine and serotonin activities within the CNS are responsible for the psychiatric disorder. The theory is noteworthy because most effective therapies for depression *do not* modulate dopamine activity. This is in contrast to the antipsychotic agents that focus on dopamine, as will be discussed.

Tricyclic Antidepressants

Imipramine, Amitriptyline, Amoxapine, Desipramine, Doxepin, Maprotiline, Nortriptyline, and Trazodone

Given the prevailing biogenic amine hypothesis for depression, all effective therapeutics modulate the metabolism of dopamine, norepinephrine, and serotonin (Fig. 13-4). Historically, first-generation antidepressants were the tricyclics—so-named for their common three-ringed chemical structures (Table 13-6). (Be aware that there are also tricyclic antipsychotic drugs such as the phenothiazines, e.g., chlorpromazine and thioridazine. This unfortunate dual nomenclature can lead to confusion, although the term tricyclic is most commonly reserved for antidepressants.)

The prototype tricyclic antidepressant is imipramine. This compound acts by blocking the reuptake of norepinephrine and serotonin into their respective nerve terminals. As a result, the actions of the neurotransmitters are prolonged within the synapse. Related therapeutic agents are amitriptyline, amoxapine, desipramine, doxepin, maprotiline, and

nortriptyline. The tricyclic antidepressants are important pharmacotherapeutics for several reasons. First, they are beneficial treatments for major depression. Second, tricyclic antidepressants are useful for many other conditions, including nerve pain, headache, panic disorders, eating disorders, and enuresis. Third, they have marked side effects because of their mechanisms of action. Since they have a broad binding spectrum (most have antimuscarinic activities in addition to their reuptake blockade profile), as well as the potential to block norepinephrine reuptake in the peripheral (sympathetic) nervous system (see Chapter 6), they can elicit unwanted autonomic effects. In fact, the side effects represent a major obstacle to patient compliance. Potential adverse effects include (among the most severe) orthostatic hypotension, sodium channel blockade (cardiac conduction delays), tachycardia, palpitations, seizures, and sedation. There is also a wealth of minor side effects ("anticholinergic" side effects) associated with blockade of muscarinic receptors. Moreover, the tricyclic antidepressants have strong—and predictable—interactions with a variety of other pharmacotherapeutic agents. Because they block the reuptake of neurotransmitters, they work synergistically with noradrenergic and serotonergic agents (direct agonists) and with modulators of biogenic amine metabolism (see Monoamine Oxidase Inhibitors, below). In addition, there are additive adverse effects with other drugs that exhibit pharmacologically similar properties (e.g., sedation, cardiac conduction blockade). In spite of these concerns, the drugs remain efficacious. Although the tricyclic

TABLE 13-6. Antidepressant Drugs

Drug	Mechanism of Action	Indication	Side Effects/Comment
Tertiary Amine Imipramine (desipramine is a metabolic product) Amitriptyline (nortriptyline is a metabolic product) Doxepin	Tricyclic antidepressant; Blocks amine reuptake	Depression	Hypotension, antimuscarinic activities (dry mouth/eyes, constipation, urinary retention, nausea)
Triazolopyridine Trazodone	Blocks amine reuptake	Depression	No muscarinic activity; can cause priapism; antagonist at histamine receptor so causes sedation
SSRIs Citalopram (escitalopram is a metabolic product)	SSRI	Depression	Generally safer than tricyclics; nausea, vomiting, sexual dysfunction
Fluoxetine	SSRI	Depression	See citalopram; agitation
Sertraline	SSRI	Depression	See citalopram
Fluvoxamine		OCD	
Paroxetine			
NE/Serotonin-selective Duloxetine Venlafaxine	NE, serotonin	Depression, neuropathic pain	Increases blood pressure; hepatitis, cholestatic jaundice Increases blood pressure
Aminoketone Bupropion	NE, DA (*no serotonin*)	Depression	Lowest incidence of sexual side effects; agitation, anorexia, insomnia; lowers seizure threshold
MAO Inhibitor Phenelzine	MAO inhibitor	Depression	Risk of hypertensive crisis with tyramine-containing foods, dizziness, drowsiness, agitation, nausea

DA, dopamine; MAO, monoamine oxidase; NE, norepinephrine; SSRI, selective serotonin reuptake inhibitor; OCD, obsessive-compulsive disorder.

antidepressants have similar therapeutic efficacy, they have differing pharmacokinetic characteristics that make each uniquely valuable for individual patients.

Another commonly used antidepressant whose mechanism is similar to the tricyclics but whose chemical structure is markedly distinct is trazodone. In addition to inhibiting norepinephrine and serotonin reuptake, trazodone also acts as an antagonist at histamine receptors. This property causes sedation and is useful for treating depression with an anxiety component. As an adverse effect, trazodone may cause priapism (painful and persistent erection of the penis).

Selective Serotonin Reuptake Inhibitors (SSRIs)

Fluoxetine, Citalopram, Escitalopram, Venlafaxine, Sertraline, Fluvoxamine, Paroxetine, and Duloxetine

Unlike the tricyclic antidepressants (which block norepinephrine and serotonin uptake), SSRIs block serotonin reuptake (see Fig. 13-4) with essentially no activity toward norepinephrine and dopamine. As a result, they have few side effects and a favorable therapeutic index. Related compounds in this family of serotonin-selective reuptake inhibitors (SSRIs) are fluoxetine, citalopram, escitalopram, venlafaxine, sertraline, fluvoxamine, and paroxetine (see Table 13-6). They all share the favorable features of fluoxetine with varying pharmacokinetic profiles. An unexplained feature of antidepressants is the observation that it can take 2 to 3 weeks to obtain effective treatment of the depression. While the reasons for this remain obscure, they surely involve an adaptation or remodeling of neuronal activity. SSRIs are no more efficacious than tricyclic antidepressants; however, SSRIs are generally safer and have fewer side effects. It is important, though, to slowly taper SSRIs to avoid withdrawal symptoms that can worsen underlying depression or cause mania to emerge. Withdrawal symptoms are most likely to occur following rapid discontinuation of short-acting SSRIs (i.e., paroxetine), and withdrawal symptoms often resemble influenza (Box 13-1).

It is important to realize that serotonin is not the complete story, because later generation molecules (e.g., venlafaxine, duloxetine) are aimed at inhibiting both serotonin and

Box 13-1. SYMPTOMS ASSOCIATED WITH RAPID WITHDRAWAL OF SSRIS (MNEMONIC: FLUSH)

*F*lu-like—fatigue, diarrhea, nausea, diaphoresis
*L*ightheadedness
*U*neasiness, restlessness
*S*leep, sensory disturbances
*H*eadache

norepinephrine. While venlafaxine displays some selectivity for serotonin, duloxetine is almost equally balanced between the two neurotransmitters. Adverse effects include nausea, insomnia, sexual dysfunction, fatigue, and elevated blood pressure. Indeed, in terms of the serotonin role, it is now clear that the antidepressant bupropion has virtually no activity at the serotonin transporter and weak activity at the norepinephrine and dopamine transporters. Bupropion has few significant drug interactions, may be efficacious in patients who have not responded to SSRIs, and is not associated with sexual dysfunction. However, bupropion lowers the seizure threshold and should not be used when there is a history of recent head injury or epilepsy. As an aside, bupropion is an example of a drug that was "repackaged" by the pharmaceutical industry for a different clinical indication. In this case, bupropion is also used to reduce craving in patients attempting to stop smoking.

Monoamine Oxidase Inhibitors (MAOIs)

Phenelzine and Tranylcypromine

As noted in Chapter 6 and Figure 13-4, the primary mechanism for intracellular degradation of catecholamines (dopamine, norepinephrine, and epinephrine) and serotonin is accomplished through the activity of monoamine oxidase (primarily the MAO-A isoform in the case of norepinephrine and serotonin in the CNS). (Note that the MAO-B isoform, a dopamine-selective enzyme, is a pharmacotherapeutic target in Parkinson's disease—through the use of selegiline.) Irreversible inhibition of the MAO-A enzyme by phenelzine leads to an increase in intracellular concentrations of primarily norepinephrine and serotonin. This can then "leak" out of the nerve terminal and increase synaptic concentrations of neurotransmitter. These drugs are not first-line therapies because MAO-A is also needed to break down other compounds, most notably tyramine. Tyramine is found in cheeses, red wines, avocados, chocolate, and many other foods (Box 13-2). Ingestion of these foods leads to a dramatic rise in the tyramine, (which is metabolized into a norepinephrine-like molecule), and indirectly produces sympathomimetic symptoms (e.g., hypertension, tachycardia, stroke). Numerous foods are contraindicated in patients taking MAO inhibitors owing to the risk of tyramine-induced hypertensive crisis. Additionally, there are numerous medication restrictions for patients taking MAO inhibitors, since any drug that enhances central activity of norepinephrine, dopamine,

or serotonin may cause hypertensive crisis or serotonin syndrome (Box 13-3).

Treatment of Mania and Bipolar Disorder

Lithium

Lithium is given for mood *stabilization*. Bipolar disorder is characterized by mood swings—mania to depression. Treatment with traditional antidepressants is not effective (and is contraindicated) because it can trigger hypermania. Fortuitously, it was discovered that treatment with lithium salts (mainly lithium carbonate) is efficacious in managing mood swings. Until recently, lithium's mechanism of action was obscure, but we now know that it blocks the key bioactive lipid second messenger IP_3 (inositol trisphosphate).

Box 13-2. FOODS CONTAINING TYRAMINE

Fermented foods (cheese, yogurt, sour cream, sauerkraut)
Wine and beer
Chocolate and coffee
Preserved fish (sardines, anchovies, herring)
Dried fruits
Avocado

Box 13-3. DRUGS CONTRAINDICATED WHILE TAKING MONOAMINE OXIDASE INHIBITORS (MAOIs)

Amphetamines	Levodopa
Appetite suppressants	Local anesthetics containing
Asthma inhalants	sympathomimetic
Buspirone	vasoconstrictors
Cocaine	Meperidine
Cyclobenzaprine	Methyldopa
Decongestants	Methylphenidate
Dextromethorphan	Other antidepressants
Dopamine	Reserpine
Ephedrine	Stimulants
Epinephrine	Sympathomimetics
Guanethidine	Tryptophan

CLINICAL MEDICINE

Serotonin Syndrome

Serotonin syndrome is a hyperserotonergic state that is potentially fatal and is caused by serotonin-enhancing drugs (generally a combination of two or more drugs). The syndrome manifests with a variety of psychiatric and nonpsychiatric symptoms including euphoria, drowsiness, rapid eye movements, hyperreflexia, clumsiness, restlessness, feeling drunk and dizzy, contraction and relaxation of the jaw, sweating, intoxication, muscle twitching, rigidity, high body temperature, mental status changes, shivering, diarrhea, loss of consciousness, and death.

Specifically, it blocks the dephosphorylation of inositol monophosphate that is an obligatory step in regenerating the precursor to IP_3 (Fig. 13-5).

Cleavage of PIP_2 is triggered by G protein–coupled receptors (GPCRs) coupled to phospholipase C like those found throughout the brain. Therefore, inhibition of IP_3 metabolism would be expected to have widespread effects on

---

BIOCHEMISTRY

Phosphatidylinositol Bisphosphate

The cleavage of phosphatidylinositol bisphosphate (PIP_2) by phospholipase C yields diacylglycerol (DAG) and inositol trisphosphate (IP_3). IP_3 goes on to trigger release of calcium, which activates calcium-dependent protein kinases—calcium/calmodulin-dependent protein kinase II (CaMPKII). DAG is a regulator of lipid-dependent protein kinases (known as PKCs).

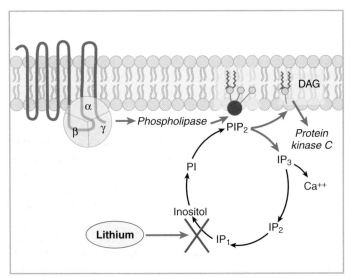

Figure 13-5. Site of action of lithium.

---

numerous systems (including neuronal activity). How this stabilizes mood is unknown, but it is clear that lithium has a narrow therapeutic window with a wide range of side effects. Early and usually transient adverse effects include vomiting, diarrhea, tremor, muscle weakness, and lethargy. Long-term adverse effects include diabetes insipidus, hypothyroidism, and cardiac abnormalities. Lithium is also the subject of many drug-drug interactions and is teratogenic. Because the therapeutic index of lithium is so narrow, its concentrations in the blood must be monitored to achieve optimal steady-state concentration. Likewise, thyroid, CBC, creatinine, and cardiac function should be checked at baseline and monitored periodically.

●●● ANTIPSYCHOTICS

Psychoses are mental disturbances of perceived reality, cognition, and diminished mood. *Schizophrenia* is the prototypical disorder that has positive and negative attributes—these represent gain or loss of function, respectively, rather than desirable or undesirable traits. Positive symptoms include hallucinations, bizarre behaviors, and delusions. Negative symptoms include diminished speech, blunted affect, and anhedonia (lack of interest in pleasurable activities). It is important to realize, however, that all psychoses are not schizophrenia and aspects of this disorder can be observed in drug abuse as well as in Alzheimer's disease.

Dopamine Hypothesis of Schizophrenia

Based on the pharmacologic profiles of first-generation treatments for psychoses (the neuroleptic tricyclic antipsychotics such as chlorpromazine and thioridazine), the hypothesis was developed that schizophrenia is the outward manifestation of an overactive dopamine system, possibly overactivity within the mesolimbic or mesocortical regions of the brain (Table 13-7 and Fig. 13-6). Dopamine receptors are

---

TABLE 13-7. Actions of Central Dopamine Pathways

Dopamine Tract	Origin	Innervation	Function	Dopamine Antagonist Effects
Nigrostriatal	Substantia nigra	Basal ganglia	Extrapyramidal system movement	Movement disorders (parkinsonism, tardive dyskinesia, extrapyramidal reactions)
Mesolimbic	Ventral tegmental area	Limbic areas Amygdala, olfactory tubercle	Arousal, memory Stimulus processing	Antipsychotic
		Septal nuclei, cingulate gyrus	Motivational behavior	
Mesocortical	Ventral tegmental area	Frontal and prefrontal cortex	Cognition, communication, social function, response to stress	Antipsychotic
Tuberoinfundibular	Arcuate nucleus of the hypothalamus	Dopamine acts on cells in the anterior pituitary	Regulates prolactin release	Increased prolactin release (galactorrhea, menstrual disorders)

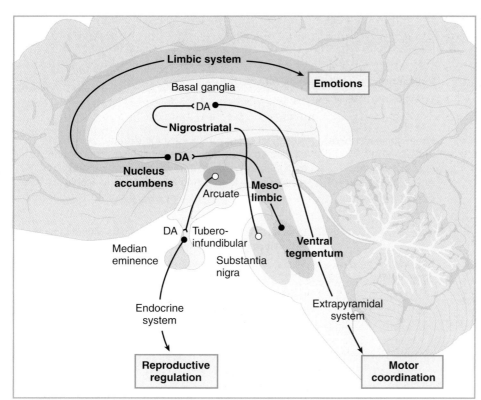

Figure 13-6. Dopaminergic pathways in the brain. The mesolimbic pathway is thought to be disrupted in schizophrenia. However, pharmacologic manipulations of the mesolimbic pathway can result in adverse effects within the nigrostriatal pathway (extrapyramidal movements) and the tuberoinfundibular pathway (galactorrhea, menstrual irregularities).

represented by five gene products: D_1 through D_5. However, they are classified into two functional groups: the D_1 class (D_1 and D_5) and the D_2 class (D_2, D_3, and D_4). In particular, agents that antagonize or block dopamine receptors (particularly the D_2 receptor class—D_2, D_3, and D_4) are effective treatments for this disorder (Table 13-8). In addition, agents that stimulate dopamine receptors or otherwise enhance its actions (e.g., cocaine), can lead to psychotic symptoms or exacerbate schizophrenic symptoms. While this notion certainly has merit, it is clearly simplistic in its scope. There are newer generation drugs that target serotonergic receptors (particularly the $5HT_2$ receptor) that are clinically efficacious. The older term *neuroleptic* refers to the ability of these drugs to reduce spontaneous activity and excessive behaviors. In addition, the ability of these agents to reduce initiative, diminish emotion, and blunt affect also resulted in their early classification as *tranquilizers*. It is now clear, however, given the range of activities, that these drugs are more appropriately referred to as antipsychotics.

Antipsychotic Therapeutics

Haloperidol, Chlorpromazine, Fluphenazine, Prochlorperazine, Thioridazine, Clozapine, Olanzapine, Risperidone, Ziprasidone, Quetiapine, and Aripiprazole

First-generation antipsychotic compounds are essentially drugs that block dopamine D_2-type receptors. Prototypes include haloperidol and the phenothiazines (chlorpromazine, fluphenazine, prochlorperazine, and thioridazine; also known

as tricyclic antipsychotic drugs). As mentioned at the outset, however, newer, "atypical" antipsychotics (clozapine, olanzapine, risperidone, ziprasidone, and quetiapine) display less antidopaminergic activity and exhibit preference for serotonin 2A ($5HT_2A$; 5-hydroxytryptamine 2A) receptor antagonism.

Typical antipsychotic drugs tend to be effective in reducing the positive symptoms of schizophrenia. That is, they blunt some of the "gained" symptoms such as hallucinations and delusions. Although this helps the patient return to societal relationships, it may not alleviate the anhedonia and depression-like characteristics of the negative symptoms. The *atypical* antipsychotics, on the other hand, are more effective for alleviating both the positive and the negative symptoms of schizophrenia. Antipsychotics, like antidepressants, can require weeks before clinical efficacy is achieved. Antagonists like the traditional first-generation phenothiazines and haloperidol antagonists can have profound side effects (see Table 13-8). On the dopamine side, antagonism blocks essential nigrostriatal communications and can lead to extrapyramidal side effects similar to symptoms of Parkinson's disease (see Neurodegeneration and Movement Disorders, below). Extrapyramidal reactions—dystonias (trismus, glossospasm, oculogyric crisis, torticollis), paresthesias, pseudoparkinsonism, and even irreversible tardive dyskinesia—may occur owing to supersensitivity of blocked dopamine receptors. With the exception of tardive dyskinesia, most extrapyramidal side effects can usually be managed with antimuscarinics and antihistamines. Table 13-8 also details problems encountered with typical antipsychotics because of

TABLE 13-8. Antipsychotic Drugs

Drug	Mechanism of Action*	Indication	Side Effects/Notes
Typical Antipsychotics			
Butyrophenone			
Haloperidol	D_2	For all antipsychotics: Schizophrenia Acute psychotic illness (delirium) Severe agitation	All typical antipsychotics exhibit extrapyramidal side effects: acute dystonias, parkinsonism, neuroleptic malignant syndrome, tardive dyskinesia, motor restlessness, long-acting IM injections available
Phenothiazines			
Chlorpromazine	$5HT_2$		Less severe extrapyramidal side effects, antimuscarinic side effects, sedation, hypotension
Prochlorperazine	D_2	Effective for nausea and vomiting	Mild side effects, drowsiness
Fluphenazine	D_2		See haloperidol
Thioridazine	D_2		Less severe extrapyramidal side effects, antimuscarinic side effects, sedation, hypotension
Thioxanthene			
Thiothixene	D_2		Also used to treat intractable hiccups
Atypical Antipsychotics			
Clozapine	$5HT_2/D_4$		Less severe extrapyramidal side effects, antimuscarinic side effects, sedation, hypotension, agranulocytosis, metabolic syndrome (weight gain, diabetes, lipid imbalances)
Olanzapine	$5HT_2/D_2$		Less severe extrapyramidal side effects, antimuscarinic side effects, elevates blood glucose, causes weight gain
Risperidone	$5HT_2/D_2$		Less severe extrapyramidal side effects
Ziprasidone	$5HT_2/D_2$		Less severe extrapyramidal side effects, sedation, rare increase in the cardiac QT, interval less weight gain than other atypical drugs
Quetiapine	$D_2 = 5HT_2$		Less severe extrapyramidal side effects, sedation, hypotension, cataracts
Aripiprazole	$D_2 = 5HT_2$ agonist/ antagonist		Hypotension, somnolence

*The order of the receptors reflects the drug's relative preference (the first receptor has the stronger affinity). All are receptor antagonists (except aripiprazole).

the "dirty" and nonselective nature of these compounds: antihistamine-like symptoms (sedation), atropine-like antimuscarinic actions (dry eyes/mouth, blurred vision, constipation, urinary retention), α-adrenergic blockade–induced orthostatic hypotension, and sedation.

Fortunately, newer *atypical* antipsychotics do not routinely cause movement disorders. However, these drugs come with their own unique adverse effects: clozapine may cause agranulocytosis and therefore requires biweekly blood counts. Risperidone is associated with stroke when used in the elderly. Although at high doses, risperidone has caused extrapyramidal effects, tardive dyskinesia has not proved to be a problem. Ziprasidone prolongs the QT interval on ECGs, but causes less weight gain than other atypical antipsychotics. In fact, new warnings have been added to the atypical

antipsychotics concerning weight gain, development of diabetes, and unfavorable lipid profiles. The newest addition to the antipsychotic armamentarium is aripiprazole, a drug said to be a "dopamine stabilizer." Aripiprazole is a partial agonist at some dopamine receptors and an antagonist at serotonin receptors. This drug appears to have the best side effect profile observed to date.

●●● NEURODEGENERATION AND MOVEMENT DISORDERS

These disorders represent tremendous unmet medical needs. In the case of Parkinson's, Huntington's, and Alzheimer's diseases, we have partially effective therapies for treating symptoms, but the therapies cannot cure the diseases.

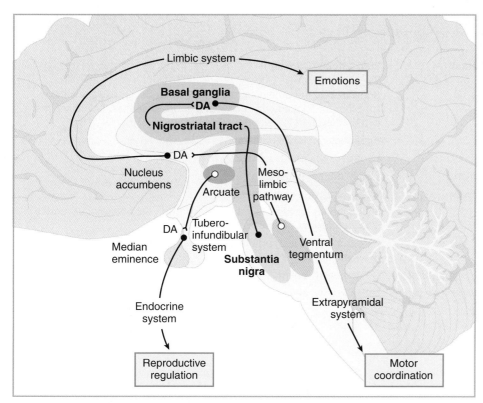

Figure 13-7. Dopaminergic pathways disrupted in Parkinson's disease. Drugs that treat Parkinson's disease facilitate actions of dopamine in the nigrostriatal tract. Adverse effects of these drugs are due to their nonspecific actions in the mesolimbic/mesocortical pathways (psychosis, hallucinations).

Parkinson's Disease

Levodopa, Bromocriptine, Pergolide, Ropinirole, Pramipexole, Selegiline, Tolcapone, Entacapone, Trihexyphenidyl, Benztropine, and Apomorphine

Note: Levodopa is used in combination with carbidopa as a metabolism modifier.

Parkinson's disease is characterized by loss of dopaminergic neurons (Fig. 13-7) in the basal ganglia. The mainline treatments (Table 13-9) are based on

- Replacing the lost dopamine with an excess of precursor (levodopa).
- Directly stimulating dopamine receptors with an agonist (bromocriptine, pergolide, ropinirole, and pramipexole).
- Inhibiting dopamine breakdown (selegiline, tolcapone, and entacapone).
- Blocking muscarinic activity (trihexyphenidyl, benztropine).

The logical treatment for Parkinson's disease would be to administer dopamine. Unfortunately, dopamine does not cross the blood-brain barrier. Levodopa, however, does enter into the brain and is the immediate precursor of dopamine synthesis (see Chapter 6). When administered, levodopa therefore increases dopamine content in surviving nigrostriatal neurons and alleviates the symptoms of lost neurons. However, there are several significant problems with levodopa. First, it is rapidly metabolized in the periphery by an amino acid decarboxylase. Therefore, it is administered as a combination therapy with carbidopa—a potent decarboxylase inhibitor that does not cross the blood-brain barrier and does not affect CNS metabolism. Carbidopa prevents

peripheral breakdown (or degradation) of levodopa, permitting more of it to enter the CNS. Second, levodopa exhibits a short half-life. This causes patients to cycle between normal and parkinsonian states (the so-called on-off phenomenon). Third, levodopa therapy has a limited lifetime of effectiveness (generally less than 5 years). This fact is probably due to continuing loss of nigrostriatal neurons to the point where there is no remaining neuronal infrastructure for converting levodopa to dopamine and subsequently releasing the neurotransmitter. In fact, it has been hypothesized that the very degradation of dopamine generates free radicals that may contribute to oxidative damage and neuronal loss in the nigrostriatal regions. Dose-limiting toxicities include dyskinesias (aberrant and uncontrollable movements), nausea, and psychoses (hallucinations and confusion).

ANATOMY & PATHOLOGY

Parkinson's Disease

Parkinson's disease is characterized by a specific loss of dopaminergic neurons originating in the substantia nigra. The etiology of the disease is unknown but is thought to involve oxidative stress (perhaps caused by reactive O_2 species originating from the breakdown of dopamine) as well as environmental factors. These neurons, projecting to the corpus striatum, are responsible for modulating movement (in a tonic fashion). Sadly, disease symptoms do not occur until greater than 80% of neurons have died, limiting treatment options and long-term prognosis.

TABLE 13-9. Drugs for Treatment of Parkinson's Disease

Drug	Mechanism of Action	Side Effects/Comment
Levodopa	DA precursor	Administered in combination with peripheral decarboxylase inhibitor (carbidopa); fluctuations in clinical response, nausea, hallucinations and confusion in the elderly
Bromocriptine	Partial DA agonist	Hypertension, nausea, fatigue
Pergolide	DA agonist (D_1/D_2)	Hypertension, nausea, fatigue
Ropinirole	DA agonist (D_2-selective)	Well tolerated, nausea, fatigue
Pramipexole	DA agonist (D_2-selective)	Well tolerated, nausea, fatigue
Selegiline	MAO-B inhibitor	May enhance adverse levodopa reactions in patients with advanced disease; anxiety, insomnia
Entacapone/tolcapone	COMT inhibitors	Rare but severe liver problems with tolcapone; nausea, dizziness, drowsiness
Trihexyphenidyl	Muscarinic receptor antagonist	Limited utility; antimuscarinic side effects, sedation, mental confusion
Benztropine	Muscarinic receptor antagonist	Limited utility, antimuscarinic side effects, sedation, mental confusion

COMT, catechol-*O*-methyltransferase; DA, dopamine; MAO, monoamine oxidase.

The direct dopamine agonists offer an alternative to levodopa therapy for maintaining dopaminergic "tone." Bromocriptine and pergolide are prototypical agents. Bromocriptine is a D_2-receptor agonist and a partial D_1 agonist. Because partial agonists do not elicit a full biological response (they have reduced efficacy), they antagonize the full agonist potential of the endogenous dopamine. Pergolide is an agonist at both the D_1 and D_2 receptor subtypes. The later generation ropinirole and pramipexole are more selective for D_2 receptor subtypes. Because their duration of action is longer than that of levodopa, dopamine agonists may be beneficial for patients experiencing the "on-off" symptoms of levodopa. All these dopamine receptor agonists have troubling psychotic side effects, nausea, and fatigue, as well as orthostatic hypertension. Recall that the antipsychotic agents work by blocking excess dopaminergic activity. Therefore, it is not surprising that dopamine agonists can lead to psychotic side effects. The newer drugs (pramipexole and ropinirole) exhibit more rapid onset kinetics and less gastrointestinal disturbance. They are limited, however, by the risk of producing sleep disorders (sudden sleep attacks). Pergolide may also cause damage to cardiac valves related to its cumulative dosage and duration of use.

The latest addition to clinical therapy for Parkinson's disease is apomorphine. This drug, a dopamine receptor agonist, is said to be a "rescue" drug. It is used to treat "off" periods in patients who have been using standard dopamine agonist therapy for 3 to 5 years. Apomorphine is administered as a subcutaneous injection and works quickly—within 5 to 10 minutes. The drug is hampered by substantial nausea and vomiting as well as severe hypotension.

Inhibitors of dopamine metabolism are another potential treatment for Parkinson's disease. Just as carbidopa inhibits levodopa metabolism, tolcapone and entacapone (inhibitors of catechol-*O*-methyltransferase; COMT) and selegiline (an MAO-B inhibitor) block the degradative metabolism of dopamine (see Fig. 13-4). These drugs, then, increase the half-life of the neurotransmitter in synapses. The side effects for tolcapone are similar to the levodopa/carbidopa combination: nausea, orthostatic hypertension, and psychotic episodes. Tolcapone is noteworthy for causing hepatotoxicity, an adverse event that is much less problematic with entacapone. Selegiline targets the dopamine-selective MAO-B and may have neuroprotective antioxidant effects. Importantly, selegiline lacks the peripheral side effects of the MAO-A inhibitors. Taken together, all the drugs that prevent dopamine breakdown are used to extend the actions of levodopa to prevent the end-of-dose "wearing-off" effect and to lower the levodopa dose.

Finally, Parkinson's disease can be treated with anticholinergic agents. The rationale is that symptoms of the disease are manifested when the loss of dopaminergic neurons creates unopposed cholinergic activity within the striatum. Therefore, some therapies target this cholinergic activity with anticholinergics such as trihexyphenidyl or benztropine. These compounds have modest clinical utility and are limited by considerable antimuscarinic side effects (sedation, urinary retention, blurred vision, and confusion). These therapies are effective for treating parkinsonian tremor, especially early in therapy when symptoms are mild. Although numerous drugs possess anticholinergic properties, only those that cross the blood-brain barrier will be effective treatments for Parkinson's disease.

As a clinical correlate, there are a number of drug therapies that elicit Parkinson-like symptoms when administered in excessive concentrations. Noteworthy are the typical antipsychotics like haloperidol and fluphenazine. As explained under Antipsychotics, the typical antipsychotics work by blocking dopamine receptors (predominantly D_2). At sufficient concentrations, dopaminergic blockade begins to

TABLE 13-10. Acetylcholinesterase Inhibitors for Treatment of Alzheimer's Disease

Drug	Comment
Donepezil	Nausea, vomiting, diarrhea, insomnia; however, best tolerated drug
Rivastigmine	Nausea, vomiting, diarrhea, insomnia
Galantamine	Nausea, vomiting, diarrhea, insomnia
Tacrine	Not widely used because of dose-limiting side effects—GI disturbances, anorexia, nausea, vomiting, diarrhea, potential hepatotoxicity

resemble the loss of neurons typical of Parkinson's disease. Care, then, must be taken to monitor doses and side effects for patients receiving antipsychotic therapy.

Alzheimer's Disease

Tacrine, Donepezil, Rivastigmine, Galantamine (Acetylcholinestrase Inhibitors), and Memantine (NMDA Receptor Antagonist)

Alzheimer's disease is characterized by a progressive loss of cognitive function. Neuropathologically, this disorder is defined by the deposition of insoluble extracellular protein deposits (plaques composed of aggregates of β-amyloid) and formation of intracellular neurofibrillary tangles composed of the filamentous tau (τ) protein. There are currently no effective treatments for Alzheimer's disease. However, based on the observation that the earliest neurotransmitter lost appears to be acetylcholine, some therapies are aimed at increasing acetylcholine. Specifically, four inhibitors of acetylcholinesterase are approved for use in patients with Alzheimer's disease: tacrine, donepezil, rivastigmine, and galantamine (Table 13-10). These drugs are relatively selective for the CNS form of acetylcholinesterase and are also used to improve cognitive function in patients with vascular dementia (e.g., for strokes or transient ischemic attacks). However, when these drugs do improve cognition in Alzheimer's patients, they only modestly extend the period of independent living, and they treat symptoms and not the underlying cause of the disease. Moreover, based on their mechanism (cholinesterase inhibition) they can elicit effects similar to the SLUD syndrome discussed in Chapter 6: nausea, vomiting, and diarrhea. Of the group, tacrine is associated with hepatotoxicity and is rarely used.

Memantine is unique among the drugs used to manage Alzheimer's disease in that it is an NMDA receptor antagonist. Since it has been postulated that overexcitation of glutamate may play a role in Alzheimer's disease, memantine may prevent adverse effects associated with abnormal glutamate transmission. It has been beneficial for even advanced forms of Alzheimer's disease and is better tolerated than cholinesterase inhibitors.

Multiple Sclerosis

Interferon-β and Glatiramer

Multiple sclerosis is characterized by loss of the myelin sheath that surrounds axons. Demyelination disrupts transmission of nerve impulses, leading to a host of symptoms, including weakness in the limbs, abnormal gait, and incoordination. Therapies are limited. During acute attacks corticosteroids may be utilized.

To prevent relapses and progression of the disease, three different immunomodulatory drugs may be used: interferon-β_1a/interferon-β_1b or glatiramer. These drug types are administered subcutaneously or intramuscularly. Although the precise mechanism of the interferons is unknown, numerous immunomodulatory actions have been suggested. Adverse effects of interferons resemble flu-like symptoms (fever, chills, myalgias), which can be minimized by pretreatment with acetaminophen. Shortness of breath and tachycardia may also occur. Unfortunately, neutralizing antibodies to the interferons develop quickly and may negate their benefit. Glatiramer is an intriguing compound in that it is a synthetic polypeptide composed of the precise amino acid sequence of myelin basic protein that is targeted by the immune system of patients with multiple sclerosis. This creates a situation in which the pharmacologic therapy mimics the antigenic properties of myelin basic protein; therefore, in the presence of the drug, the immune system attacks the pharmacologic agent rather than the body. Adverse effects usually consist of irritation at the injection site, but systemic reactions (chest tightness, flushing, palpitations, dyspnea) may occur transiently within a few minutes postinjection. None of these therapies offers a cure, and benefits are relatively modest.

Because multiple sclerosis takes its toll on numerous organ systems, pharmacologic therapies used to manage the many secondary symptoms of multiple sclerosis are shown in Table 13-11.

GENETICS

Huntington's Chorea

Huntington's disease is a genetic disorder that is characterized by choreiform movements—abnormal voluntary movements (jerky motor incoordination). It is caused by the inheritance, in non-Mendelian fashion, of trinucleotide repeats in the protein *Huntingtin*. For reasons that remain obscure, this trinucleotide expansion (long tracts of glutamine residues) leads to selective loss of medium spiny neurons that project from the striatum to the globus pallidus. This leads to a loss of inhibitory activity and increased excitatory drive that promotes uncontrolled movements. Unfortunately, there are no drugs to slow progression of the disease (death occurs within 15 to 20 years). In addition, there are no effective drugs to treat the movement symptoms, because the loss of neurons is so selective that global treatments produce too many side effects. Huntington's disease is invariably accompanied by depression with occasional paranoia and psychosis. These symptoms are treated with standard antidepressants or antipsychotics.

TABLE 13-11. Treatments for Conditions Associated with Multiple Sclerosis

Symptom	Drugs
Spasticity, gait difficulty	Baclofen, diazepam, dantrolene
Overactive bladder	Oxybutynin, tolterodine, desmopressin
Overactive bowel	Dicyclomine
Constipation	Fiber, fluids
Depression	Antidepressants
Paresthesias	Tricyclic antidepressants, carbamazepine

●●● OPIOIDS

Endogenous Opioid System and Pain Management

Opioid analgesics are used primarily to treat severe pain, although they may also be exploited to treat cough (hydrocodone, dextromethorphan) or diarrhea (diphenoxylate) and occasionally are used for anesthetic purposes. Specifically, opi*ates* are plant alkaloids derived from the opium poppy. Opi*oids* are chemically related compounds. These compounds, like many drugs, work by binding to receptors for natural neurotransmitters within the body. In this case, it appears that the endogenous opioids (endorphins, dynorphins, and enkephalins) are peptides found in regions of the nervous system involved in transmitting, organizing, and perceiving pain. The opioid receptors are categorized into three families: mu (μ), kappa (κ), and delta (δ). The major player for pain management is the μ receptor, with κ also playing a significant role in spinal transmission of pain.

The opioid receptors work through inhibitory G-protein signaling (decreasing cAMP synthesis) that results in decreased firing of presynaptic neurons in the spinal cord or postsynaptic firing of neurons in the CNS. In the former case, this occurs through decreases in calcium influx, while the latter is mediated primarily through increases in sodium outflow and a resulting hyperpolarization of neurons. In each case, the pain signal is either blocked or diminished or is not *perceived* as noxious ("dulled").

Opioid Analgesics

Hydrocodone, Dextromethorphan, Diphenoxylate, Morphine, Hydromorphone, Meperidine, Methadone, Fentanyl, Oxycodone, Codeine, Nalbuphine, Butorphanol, and Pentazocine

Naloxone and Naltrexone (Antidotes)

The opioid analgesics are categorized as strong, moderate, or weak agonists (Table 13-12). The prototypical strong opioid agonists are morphine (a precursor of heroin), hydromorphone, meperidine, methadone, and fentanyl. This designation as "strong" reflects not only their analgesic characteristics but also their abuse liability and their ability to cause respiratory depression. These drugs are used to treat moderate-to-severe pain. Because of abuse potential, most opioid agonists are classified as controlled substances by the U.S. Drug Enforcement Administration (DEA). Morphine is the prototypical compound to which other opioids/opiates are compared.

Methadone has a very long half-life, which causes the drug to accumulate. This prolonged duration of activity is ideal for using methadone to wean heroin addicts from the illicit substance, since withdrawal symptoms occur later and are

TABLE 13-12. Opioid Analgesic Drugs

Drug	Mechanism of Action	Indication	Side Effects/Comment
Morphine	Strong opiate; μ-agonist	Analgesic	Poorly bioavailable Side effects shared by most opioid drugs: respiratory depression, nausea, vomiting, dizziness, confusion, constipation, abuse potential
Meperidine	Strong opiate; μ-agonist	Analgesic	Treatment for postoperative shivering
Methadone	Strong opiate; μ-agonist	Analgesic, heroin recovery	Used in maintenance therapy for recovering opiate addicts because it has a long $t_{1/2}$
Fentanyl	Strong opiate; μ-agonist	Analgesic	100 times more potent than morphine
Oxycodone	Moderate μ-agonist	Analgesic	Excellent bioavailability; significant abuse liability
Codeine	Moderate μ-agonist	Cough suppressant, analgesic	Frequently combined with aspirin or acetaminophen
Pentazocine	κ-agonist and partial μ-agonist	Analgesic	Lower abuse potential than others
Buprenorphine	Partial μ-agonist and weak κ-agonist	Analgesia and treatment for opiate addiction	Partial agonist with weak analgesic activity; alleviates symptoms of opiate withdrawal

less severe with methadone compared with heroin. This is an example of using a drug with *cross-tolerance* but more favorable pharmacokinetics (longer half-life). There is concern that methadone may cause cardiac arrhythmias (including torsades de pointes) by delaying myocardial repolarization.

At the opposite end of the spectrum, meperidine has a short duration of action, necessitating frequent dosing. Because of its short half-life, meperidine is often used during labor, since its short duration of activity produces less respiratory depression in infants. One of the metabolites of meperidine metabolism may accumulate in patients with renal failure, causing seizures, dysphoria, and agitation. An additional short-acting opioid is fentanyl, which is often used as a surgical anesthetic adjunct. Fentanyl may also be used for pain relief for regional (intrathecal) anesthesia. Unique dose forms of fentanyl include long-acting transdermal patches and short-acting lollipops. Note, however, that these alternative fentanyl dose forms could be deadly to an opioid-naïve child.

Moderate opioid agents include codeine and hydrocodone. These drugs are usually the first to be tried when NSAIDs are insufficient to control pain. Another moderately effective therapeutic is oxycodone, although this drug has a high potential for abuse. The abuse potential relates to the relatively high doses in which it is packaged and the discovery that alternative routes of administration (intranasal ["snorting"] or intravenous) produce a rapid "high."

Weak opioid analgesics include nalbuphine, butorphanol, and pentazocine. These drugs have mixed effects, with full agonist activity at κ receptors and partial agonist activity at μ receptors. Recall that a partial agonist competes with the endogenous opioid (with a smaller effect) leading to an overall antagonist effect. These pharmacologic actions permit pain relief with minimal risk of respiratory depression and less likelihood for abuse.

Side effects following opioid administration are significant. In addition to respiratory depression (the predominant cause of death in overdose victims), there is miosis (a defining characteristic), cough suppression (an indication for the moderate μ agonists codeine and hydrocodone), emesis, constipation due to slowed gastrointestinal motility (diphenoxylate is prescribed as an antidiarrheal), urinary retention and reduced uterine tone (prolongs labor) due to effects on smooth muscles, and histamine release (specific to morphine). Additional adverse effects are included in Box 13-4.

In the event of opioid/opiate overdose, two antagonists at μ and κ receptors, naloxone and naltrexone, can be administered to reverse life-threatening respiratory depression or hypotension. Of course, administration of these drugs will also precipitate withdrawal symptoms in patients who are physically dependent on opioids/opiates (Table 13-13).

New classes of nonopiate analgesics have also been developed. These other analgesics include tramadol and ziconotide. Tramadol binds weakly to μ receptors but also inhibits reuptake of norepinephrine and serotonin. Thus, this drug may modulate the emotional aspects of pain. Tramadol lowers the seizure threshold and may cause seizures in patients who are predisposed. Ziconotide is the first in a new class of nonopiate pain relievers. The drug blocks N-type Ca^{++}

Box 13-4. ADVERSE EFFECTS OF OPIOID ANALGESICS

- Miosis
- Respiratory depression
- Cough suppression
- Emesis
- Elevated intracranial pressure
- Postural hypotension
- Constipation
- Urinary retention
- Itching, urticaria

TABLE 13-13. Opioid Withdrawal Signs and Symptoms

Symptoms	Signs
Regular Withdrawal	
Anxiety	Diarrhea
Dysphoric mood	Fever
Increased pain sensitivity	Increased blood pressure
Insomnia	Piloerection ("goose bumps")
Irritability	Pupillary dilation
Muscle aches	Sweating
Nausea, cramps	Tachycardia
Opioid craving	Vomiting
Restlessness	Yawning
Protracted Withdrawal (Relapse Liability)	
Anxiety	Cyclic change in weight, pupil
Drug craving	size, respiratory center
Insomnia	sensitivity

Note that a symptom is reported by the patient while a sign is something you measure or observe.

CLINICAL MEDICINE

Characteristics of Addiction and Abuse

Potent opioid full agonists are the most effective analgesics, but they are accompanied by strong abuse liability. This is because opioid agonists can produce euphoria. With chronic use, however, the body develops tolerance and dependence, requiring more drug to produce the "high," and the body simultaneously depends on the drug to maintain homeostasis. This is a dangerous behavioral combination that leads to the unique physical and psychological dependence that underlies addiction. These characteristics render the strong opioid agonists (along with nicotine and alcohol) the most addictive drugs. Unfortunately, because of this, some patients suffer because physicians are reluctant to prescribe opioids for pain. The fear of addiction is largely unfounded in patients with legitimate pain. Proper administration of opioids to alleviate pain has a low risk of addiction, although physical dependence will occur. The medication must be slowly tapered in these patients following therapeutic treatment of the pain.

channels, preventing the release of neurotransmitters that are involved with pain transmission. Ziconotide is administered only intrathecally and may cause psychosis, cognitive impairment, hallucinations, or changes in mood or consciousness.

Management of Migraine Headache Pain

Sumatriptan, Rizatriptan, Zolmitriptan, Frovatriptan, Naratriptan, and Almotriptan

Note: These drugs end in "-triptan."

Certainly any of the analgesics (NSAIDs, opioids/opiates) can be used to treat headaches, including migraines. The underlying etiology of migraine headaches is thought to involve dilation of cerebral and cranial arteries mediated at least in part by release of substance P, prostaglandins, leukotrienes, and bradykinins—all of which propagate pain responses. The "triptans" have found a unique niche in pharmacotherapy as a result of their ability to block neurogenic inflammation. Triptans are drugs that act as selective agonists at serotonin 1B and 1D receptor subtypes. Overall, triptans prevent release of vasoactive substances, block inflammation, and constrict arteries.

Sumatriptan is the prototypical agent to which the others are compared. Differences among agents primarily are either pharmacokinetic (oral rizatriptan and zolmitriptan nasal spray are fast-acting; frovatriptan has the longest duration of activity) or relate to adverse effects (naratriptan and almotriptan are usually the best tolerated).

Owing to vasoconstrictive effects, triptans are contraindicated in patients with ischemic heart disease, a history of myocardial infarction, uncontrolled hypertension, arrhythmias, asthma, or pregnancy. The drugs are commonly associated with chest tightness or pressure; sensations of warmth, tingling, or burning; hypertension; tachycardia; and a bad taste in the mouth.

●●● SEDATIVE-HYPNOTIC AND ANXIOLYTIC AGENTS

GABA Receptor Modulators

The sedative-hypnotic and anxiolytic agents generally are barbiturates and benzodiazepines, which are both GABA receptor modulators. *Sedation* refers to a calming effect that decreases excitement and moderates hyperexcitability. *Hypnosis*, in the pharmacologic sense, refers to drowsiness and the promotion and maintenance of sleep. *Anxiety* disorders are a large family of clinical problems that were previously known as psychoneuroses. These include various phobias, social anxiety disorder, generalized anxiety disorder, obsessive-compulsive disorder, and posttraumatic stress disorder. Just as agents that activate or potentiate GABA (the most common inhibitory neurotransmitter in the brain) are effective in calming the overactivity of epilepsy, they also are effective as anxiolytics and sedative-hypnotics. Barbiturates and benzodiazepines are useful in the treatment of panic attacks and generalized anxiety, various phobias, insomnia, and as discussed above, epilepsy and spasticity. Furthermore, they are used adjunctively for general anesthesia (Table 13-14).

Benzodiazepines

Diazepam, Alprazolam, Clonazepam, Lorazepam, Temazepam, Triazolam, and Flumazenil (Antidote)

Note: Most of these drugs end in "-olam" or "-epam."

The GABA$_A$ receptor is a pentameric ligand-gated chloride channel (see Fig. 13-2). (In contrast, the GABA$_B$ receptor is a

TABLE 13-14. Sedative-Hypnotic/Anxiolytic Drugs

Drug	Mechanism of Action	Indication	Side Effects/Comment
Diazepam	Benzodiazepine	Anxiety disorders, status epilepticus, anesthetic premedication, muscle relaxant	Relatively safe drugs Produce cognitive impairment, increased reaction time, lightheadedness, nausea, vomiting
Alprazolam	Benzodiazepine	Anxiety disorders, phobias	See diazepam
Midazolam	Benzodiazepine	Anesthesia adjuvant	See diazepam
Triazolam	Benzodiazepine	Insomnia	See diazepam
Zolpidem	Non–benzodiazepine agonist at the GABA receptor	Insomnia	Dizziness, confusion
Phenobarbital	Barbiturate	Seizure disorders, status epilepticus, sedation	Induction of P-450 metabolic enzymes; respiratory depression, drowsiness, vertigo, nausea, vomiting, diarrhea
Secobarbital	Barbiturate	Insomnia, sedation, seizure disorders (acute)	Induction of P-450 metabolic enzymes; respiratory depression, drowsiness, vertigo, nausea, vomiting, diarrhea
Ethanol	Unknown but thought to interact with GABA receptor	Used as an intoxicant and for its sedative-hypnotic effects	Dysphoria, sedation, vomiting, coma, respiratory depression

7TM-GPCR with a completely different pharmacologic profile.) The prototypical benzodiazepine for anxiolysis is diazepam, which acts by binding to $GABA_A$ receptors to enhance the actions of GABA; in other words, it acts as an allosteric modulator of GABA receptors. Specifically, benzodiazepines increase the *frequency* of chloride channel opening. Clinically useful benzodiazepine anxiolytics include alprazolam, clonazepam, and lorazepam. Benzodiazepines may be used primarily for their hypnotic effects to facilitate sleep in patients with insomnia. Examples include temazepam and triazolam.

Benzodiazepines differ from each other pharmacokinetically, primarily with respect to their onset of activity and their duration of action. Diazepam acts very quickly and has a long half-life. This prolonged duration of action can cause "hangover" effects. Benzodiazepines are classified as controlled substances by the DEA because of their potential for abuse. Benzodiazepines cannot be discontinued abruptly or withdrawal symptoms will occur (Box 13-5). Following long-term use of benzodiazepines, it is wise to switch patients to diazepam, a benzodiazepine with a long half-life.

Adverse effects associated with benzodiazepines are primarily related to CNS depression (drowsiness, dizziness, incoordination), although respiratory depression is a concern if other CNS depressants are used simultaneously. In cases of benzodiazepine overdose, the $GABA_A$ receptor antagonist flumazenil can be administered. Compared with barbiturates, benzodiazepines have a superior safety profile, with CNS depression reaching a plateau prior to achieving a comatose state (Fig. 13-8).

Nonbenzodiazepine GABA-A Receptor Modulators

Zolpidem, Zaleplon, and Eszopiclone

Several nonbenzodiazepine compounds also interact with the $GABA_A$ receptors but have not been associated with tolerance. These drugs include zolpidem, zaleplon, and eszopiclone. Zaleplon's claim to fame is that it has a quick

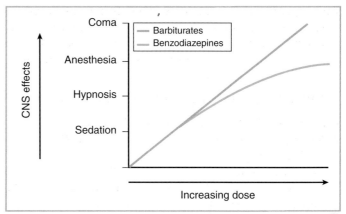

Figure 13-8. Relative safety of benzodiazepines compared with barbiturates.

onset of action and its actions are terminated in 4 hours. This short duration of action makes zaleplon ideal for patients who wake up in the middle of the night and cannot fall back to sleep, because as long as there are at least 4 hours until the patient must awaken, no "hangover effects" will be experienced.

Barbiturates

Phenobarbital and Secobarbital

While the benzodiazepines act by enhancing the action of GABA (serving to increase the frequency of chloride channel opening), the barbiturates also bind to the $GABA_A$ receptor, at a distinct site, and enhance GABA activity by facilitating the *duration* of time that the receptor chloride channel remains open. Phenobarbital and secobarbital are prototypical barbiturates. Because of their abuse liability and potential for overdose, the barbiturates are not so widely prescribed as the benzodiazepines. They do serve as a valuable tool in the treatment of seizure disorders, as described above.

Other Anxiolytics

Buspirone

Finally, buspirone, a partial agonist at serotonin 1A receptors ($5HT_{1A}$) is an effective treatment for generalized anxiety. Unlike benzodiazepines and barbiturates, however, it takes several weeks for maximal effects to be seen.

Alcohol

Ethanol is noteworthy because there is growing evidence that it exerts its sedative-hypnotic effects by binding to the $GABA_A$ receptor. Therefore, in many respects, it resembles the benzodiazepines and is synergistic with (and potentiates) both the pharmacologic and toxicologic effects of the benzodiazepines and barbiturates. For this reason, it can be viewed, in many cases, as a *natural* form of self-medication (i.e., calms the nerves). As we see below, however, this is a simplistic and dangerous view of this abused drug.

Box 13-5. SYMPTOMS OF BENZODIAZEPINE WITHDRAWAL

Following moderate drug usage

Anxiety, agitation
Increased sensitivity to light and sound
Paresthesias, strange sensations
Muscle cramps
Myoclonic jerks
Sleep disturbance
Dizziness

Following high-dose or long-term usage

Seizures
Delirium

●●● ABUSED RECREATIONAL DRUGS

Abused Drugs as False Messengers

Drugs of abuse (e.g., alcohol, nicotine, heroin, cannabinoids, and cocaine) are generally natural products that serve as false messengers at endogenous receptor systems. They basically bind to receptor systems and mimic natural neurotransmitters but generally with much greater potency (Table 13-15).

Alcohol

As discussed in the preceding section, ethanol (ethyl alcohol) exerts many of its effects on the $GABA_A$ receptor. It is not so simple a drug as the benzodiazepines, because of its other behavioral effects. At low doses, ethanol produces social disinhibition, feelings of pleasure, and even euphoria. At escalating doses, however, it interferes with motor control and produces dysphoria, sedation, vomiting, coma, and even death (through respiratory depression). The reinforcing nature of the drug and perhaps the seat of its abuse liability, is due to activation of the mesolimbic dopamine pathway. Like the opiates, following chronic use, ethanol produces behavioral and physiologic tolerance and physical dependence. Hence, withdrawal from severe alcohol dependence produces strong physiologic effects, including seizures (Box 13-6; see also Table 13-15). Such acute withdrawal effects are treated with benzodiazepines like diazepam. In fact, there is cross-tolerance between ethanol and the benzodiazepines. This means that, for certain physiologic effects, one will substitute for the other—not because they are structurally similar but because they interact with the same molecular target: the GABA-stimulated chloride channel. Chronic use of alcohol adversely impacts nearly every organ system in the body. Long-term alcohol abuse is treated with other pharmacologic agents that produce aversive effects by interfering with ethanol metabolism (disulfiram) or by modulating endogenous serotonin, opiate, or GABAergic systems (ondansetron, naltrexone, or acamprosate, respectively).

NEUROSCIENCE

Differentiating Between Tolerance, Dependence, and Addiction

Tolerance occurs when larger doses of drug are required to produce the same effect. Tolerance can occur for numerous reasons: innate tolerance is genetically determined, pharmacokinetic tolerance results from changes in drug metabolism, and pharmacodynamic tolerance is caused by adaptive changes in receptor density or second messenger characteristics. Cross-tolerance is sometimes used pharmacologically during detoxification to allow one drug to substitute for another.

Dependence can be either *physical* or *psychological*. Psychological dependence is manifested by cravings for a drug—probably the major cause of relapse. Physical dependence is virtually synonymous with *withdrawal*. Cessation of use of drugs that cause physical dependence will result in withdrawal symptoms. Importantly, tolerance and dependence are biological phenomena and *do not imply drug abuse*.

Abuse or *addiction* denotes an overwhelming compulsion and preoccupation with obtaining and using a drug. Not all drugs of abuse are associated with the same propensity to cause tolerance or dependence.

Cocaine and Psychomotor Stimulants

Cocaine and the psychomotor stimulants (amphetamine and methamphetamine) work directly through antagonizing dopamine reuptake and storage in the CNS. Cocaine blocks dopamine reuptake (and to lesser extent, norepinephrine and serotonin) through antagonism of reuptake transporter pumps. As a result, cocaine enhances dopamine activity within the nigrostriatal track (activating motor behavior). Simultaneously, cocaine acts directly on the mesolimbic dopamine pathway to serve as a behavioral reinforcer. Through other pathways, it produces euphoria. Interestingly, in keeping with the dopamine theory of affective disorders,

---

TABLE 13-15. Tolerance and Dependence Potential of Commonly Abused Drugs

	Dynamic Tolerance	Physical Dependence	Psychological Dependence	Withdrawal Syndrome
THC	+	—	+	—
Morphine	++++	++++	++++	++++
Ethanol	++	++++	+++	++++
Barbiturates	++	++++	+++	++++
Amphetamines	++++	+	+++	+
Cocaine	+	+	+++	+
LSD	+++	—	++	—
PCP	++	—	+	—
Nicotine	++	++	++	++
Caffeine	++	+	+	+

++++, pronounced effect; +++, moderate effect; ++, low effect; +, slight effect; —, no effect.

ANATOMY

Mesolimbic Dopamine Pathway

In nearly every case, administration of abused substances activates the mesolimbic dopamine pathway. This pathway (considered to be a ventral extension of the nigrostriatal tract) originates in the ventral tegmental area (VTA; A10 nucleus) and projects to the nucleus accumbens. The mesolimbic pathway appears to serve as the reinforcement circuit for the brain. That is, things that are generally good for the health and welfare of the individual and species (eating, drinking, sex) elicit its activity, which drives the behavior to be repeated. Abused substances—whether or not they have a dopaminergic mechanism—also activate the mesolimbic pathway. The difference is that they do so to a much greater extent. This may account for why there is such a strong drive to abuse many illicit drugs.

Box 13-6. SIGNS AND SYMPTOMS OF ETHANOL WITHDRAWAL

Alcohol craving
Tremor, irritability
Nausea
Sleep disturbance
Tachycardia
Hypertension
Sweating
Perceptual distortion
Seizures (12 to 48 hours after last drink)
Delirium tremens (rare in uncomplicated withdrawal)
    Severe agitation
    Confusion
    Visual hallucinations
    Fever, profuse sweating
    Tachycardia
    Nausea, diarrhea
    Dilated pupils

---

high doses of cocaine can produce manic behavior and acute psychoses. The drugs within the amphetamine family (amphetamine, methamphetamine, and methylenedioxymethamphetamine [MDMA]) have similar mechanisms of action and act by releasing intracellular pools of dopamine and reversing the dopamine transporter to pump neurotransmitter into the synapse. MDMA is important because it has 5HT (serotonin) activities and causes hallucinogenic effects as well. These compounds, in addition to their addictive liability, have significant, even fatal, side effects because of their potent peripheral sympathomimetic activities (see Chapter 6).

It is also noteworthy that stimulants such as amphetamine and methylphenidate, although certainly drugs of abuse, are widely used to treat behavioral disorders like attention-deficit disorder (ADD) and narcolepsy in both children and adults.

However, the newer nonstimulant atomoxetine, a drug that selectively inhibits reuptake of norepinephrine, is also enjoying widespread use for ADD behavioral conditions, since it is not associated with a potential for abuse. It has, however, been associated with hepatotoxicity.

Cannabinoids

Cannabis is the most widely used illicit drug in the United States. Smoking the cannabis plant volatilizes many plant alkaloids including the active ingredient, Δ-9-tetrahydrocannabinol (Δ9-THC). This compound interacts, with high affinity, at an endogenous receptor of unknown function—the cannabinoid receptor (for which there are central and peripheral nervous system forms). The natural ligand for these receptors is thought to be a derivative of arachidonic acid, anandamide. Use of cannabis produces a "high" that is distinct from that of alcohol, stimulants, or opiates. It is accompanied by impairment of short-term cognitive function, memory, reaction time, and perception (especially of time). Clinically, Δ9-THC is used as the prescription drug dronabinol to manage chemotherapy-associated nausea and vomiting and in AIDS-related anorexia.

Nicotine

Nicotine dependence contributes to the foremost preventable cause of death today—smoking. Besides the fact that the drug—a stimulant (a direct agonist at nicotinic acetylcholine receptors)—is reinforcing, its pattern of administration probably contributes significantly to its addictive nature. Each "puff" produces a small reinforcing effect, repeated many times over the course of a day. Combined with the fact that it is associated with pleasurable social activities, nicotine's pharmacology and the psychosocial behaviors associated with its use combine to create, for some individuals, the ultimate physical and psychological dependence. Withdrawal from nicotine, although unpleasant, is not life-threatening (Box 13-7). Nicotine is readily absorbed across membranes (skin, lung epithelium, oral membranes), and there are a variety of approaches to treating nicotine dependence including nicotine gums, lozenges, inhalers, and transdermal patches. Additionally, the antidepressant bupropion appears to reduce nicotine craving.

Box 13-7. SYMPTOMS OF NICOTINE WITHDRAWAL

- Irritability
- Anxiety
- Dysphoric or depressed mood
- Difficulty concentrating
- Restlessness
- Decreased heart rate
- Increased appetite or weight gain

COMPLEMENTARY AND ALTERNATIVE MEDICINE

St. John's Wort

Some patients use St. John's wort to treat depression. The product appears to be more effective than placebo and in some clinical studies was as effective as tricyclic antidepressants or SSRIs for treating mild to moderate depression. St. John's wort may inhibit serotonin reuptake, which would explain its antidepressant activity.

Typically, St. John's wort is well tolerated. The biggest concerns with this natural product are related to drug-drug interactions. St. John's wort induces hepatic microsomal CYP P-450 enzymes, altering the metabolism of many drugs and possibly rendering them ineffective. Additionally, St. John's wort decreases the effectiveness of oral anticoagulants. This supplement should never be used with other medications that alter serotonergic neurotransmission (i.e., triptans, prescription antidepressants, opioids, MAOIs) because of the risk of serotonin syndrome.

Melatonin

Melatonin is often used by people who have difficulty sleeping, especially if their insomnia is related to jet lag or shift-work. Melatonin is synthesized endogenously in the pineal gland. Its primary role seems to be regulation of circadian rhythm, endocrine secretions, and sleep patterns. Light inhibits melatonin secretion; dark stimulates its secretion.

Patients should not drive or operate heavy machinery for 4 to 5 hours after using melatonin. Although usually well tolerated, supplements have been reported to cause transient drowsiness, headache, dizziness, depression, and mild anxiety. Melatonin may increase the risk of bleeding in patients taking oral anticoagulants. Additionally, sedation may be exacerbated by concomitant use of other CNS depressants (e.g., alcohol, benzodiazepines, antihistamines). Although speculative, melatonin may increase blood glucose in patients with diabetes, exacerbate seizure disorders in susceptible individuals, and worsen hypertension in some patients.

Kava

Kava, a popular social drink in Pacific Island countries, is sometimes used as a supplement to treat anxiety disorders. Although a variety of pharmacologic effects have been noted with kava, including anxiolytic, sedative, anticonvulsant, local anesthetic, spasmolytic, anti-inflammatory, and analgesic activities, the mechanisms for these effects are unknown and do not appear to be mediated via known pathways.

When used orally, kava can cause gastrointestinal disturbances, headache, dizziness, drowsiness, miosis, and extrapyramidal effects. Hepatotoxicity is also a concern with kava. Kava may inhibit hepatic P-450 enzymes, and it exacerbates CNS sedation when used with other CNS depressants. Owing to the hepatic toxicity, the U.S. FDA is in the process of banning kava in the United States, and several other countries have already done so.

TOP FIVE LIST

1. Anesthetics, antiepileptics, and sedative hypnotic drugs generally work by modulating ion channels (primarily GABA-stimulated Cl^- channels, but also Na^+ and Ca^{++} channels).
2. Antidepressants work by blocking biogenic amine reuptake (inhibiting norepinephrine and/or serotonin transporters).
3. Antipsychotic agents are antagonists of dopamine (or serotonin) receptors.
4. Neurodegenerative diseases are targeted by agents that treat symptoms (increasing dopamine activity for Parkinson's disease; increasing acetylcholine activity for Alzheimer's disease); however, there are currently no cures.
5. The opioids stimulate (and simulate) natural analgesic systems in the CNS (endorphins and enkephalins).

Case Studies

CASE STUDY 1

A 54-year-old homeless male, who admits to smoking cigarettes all his adult life, is admitted to the hospital with evidence of tuberculosis. This gentleman weighs 65 kg, and he tells you that he was diagnosed with CHF and asthma "many years ago." For the past 15 years, he has been obtaining theophylline samples from a physician who volunteers at the local homeless shelter, so you decide to continue the drug while he is hospitalized. In the hospital, the patient has been receiving 100 mg theophylline every 12 hours. However, you realize that theophylline is metabolized by P-450 microsomal enzymes, and you've placed the patient on several medications that alter the metabolism of theophylline, including ciprofloxacin, which is known to increase theophylline levels, and rifampin, which is known to induce the P-450 enzymes, thus reducing theophylline levels. You decide that it is best to obtain laboratory data to determine what the patient's plasma levels of theophylline are because of these potential drug interactions. The laboratory report indicates that the patient's plasma concentration of theophylline is 3.6 mg/L (target range is 5–15 mg/L).

1. Knowing that the published value of volume of distribution (Vd) for theophylline is 0.48 L/kg, calculate this man's Vd for theophylline.

2. Knowing that the published $t_{1/2}$ for theophylline in a smoker is 4.5 hours, what is the rate at which theophylline is cleared in this patient?

3. What loading dose should this patient be given to quickly increase his theophylline plasma level to 10 mg/L?

CASE STUDY 2

A 68-year-old patient is transferred to your practice. She is concerned because she has been taking the same medication for 60 years for her asthma, but it doesn't seem to be working very well lately. She says that she has taken the same dose of theophylline all her life—ever since she was 8 years old—and she wanted her previous doctor to increase the dose, but he wouldn't. She is certain that the reason her asthma has been under poor control for the past few months is because her doctor refuses to prescribe more. (In actuality, her previous doctor had suggested discontinuing the theophylline entirely and switching her to a long-acting corticosteroid/β_2-agonist combination, since theophylline requires careful monitoring, has numerous drug interactions, and severe toxicities, but she refused because she had heard that steroids are "bad for you.")

"Theophylline has worked for my entire life. When it stopped working recently, my doctor refused to increase the dose. Why would a drug I've taken my whole life suddenly stop working?"

You review her medications and find that she is also currently taking cimetidine for gastroesophageal reflux and rifampin for a severe staphylococcal bone infection. You check her serum theophylline levels and find that they are 4.0 mg/L (target range is 5–15 mg/L).

1. What are some of the considerations for dosing a drug with a narrow therapeutic index (e.g., theophylline) throughout the lifespan of a patient.

2. Are there any pharmacokinetic interactions between rifampin and theophylline that could impact this woman's theophylline plasma levels?

3. Are there any pharmacokinetic interactions between cimetidine and theophylline that could impact this woman's theophylline plasma levels?

CASE STUDY 3

A 16-year-old female comes to the ER with severe abdominal cramps. She is sweaty and appears feverish. Upon workup, she becomes nauseated and vomits pill fragments. She reports that she ingested "a hundred pills, but I don't remember the type." Upon examination, her temperature is 101.2° F, her blood pressure is 128/72, her pulse is 120 beats per minute, and her respiration is 34 breaths per minute.

1. What is your initial management strategy for this patient after addressing the ABCs (*a*irway, *b*reathing, *c*irculation)?

2. What over-the-counter (OTC) medicine could be responsible for the initial symptoms?

3. Initial arterial blood gas levels are drawn (pH 7.64; pCO_2 16 mm Hg; pO_2 98 mm Hg). What are potential mechanisms underlying this alkalosis?

4. Repeat labs are performed 2 hours after the patient receives 2 liters of normal saline. The results are now pH 7.27, pCO_2 16 mm Hg, pO_2 103 mm Hg. What are potential mechanisms leading to the secondary acidosis?

5. The patient's condition continues to worsen. What are your next courses of treatments?

CASE STUDY 4

A 33-year-old female is brought to the emergency room by her husband one Saturday morning. She complains of such a severe headache that she cannot open her eyes. Her oral temperature is 104.1° F. Her husband mentions, "my wife has a rash on the back of her head."

According to the woman's husband, she was previously in good health. On the previous day, the woman rose early in the morning to complete her exercise routine and remarked to her husband about what a great workout she had. However, as the day progressed, she noted a "large painful lump" on the back of her head. By evening, she noticed additional lumps and was concerned because the lumps were beginning to spread down the back of her head and neck. She also began experiencing diarrhea that evening. Although the woman had been seen by her family doctor "after hours" the previous evening, no definitive diagnosis had been made, and the woman was sent home. Throughout the night, the woman experienced severe diarrhea and vomiting.

Almost as soon as the patient arrived in the emergency department, she began complaining of an irregular heartbeat. An ECG revealed premature ventricular contractions; the woman denied a prior history of cardiovascular problems. Upon examination of the patient's head, the "rash" on the back of her head appeared to be spreading down her neck and across her face. At the ER, an astute attending physician correctly diagnosed the woman as having erysipelas. The patient has no history of drug allergies.

1. What is erysipelas, and which microorganisms are the most likely culprits?

2. What is the most likely cause of the patient's cardiac arrhythmias?

3. A scab is identified on the patient's scalp, and both group A streptococci and staphylococci are isolated and cultured. Blood cultures are negative, which is common with erysipelas (blood cultures are positive in only 5% of cases). Discuss an antimicrobial that is appropriate for this patient.

4. After 5 days of receiving an intravenous antibiotic, her fever finally subsided and she was discharged with a prescription for 10 additional days of therapy with oral dicloxacillin. Additionally, at the time of discharge, a first-year resident informed the patient that the laboratory had just called with results of a stool culture that had been conducted during admission, since the patient's abdominal pain and diarrhea had worsened while she was hospitalized. *Clostridium difficile* toxins were identified in the patient's stool culture. What is the source of this gastrointestinal microorganism, and how is this secondary infection treated?

CASE STUDY 5

A 70-year-old man with a history of long-standing hypertension and recently diagnosed type 2 diabetes mellitus comes to the oncology clinic. He has just found out the gastric pain that he attributed to a "flare-up" of his peptic ulcer disease is actually giant large-cell lymphoma, an aggressive neoplasm. As the director of the oncology clinic, you tell the patient that he will be receiving 6 to 8 cycles of a chemotherapeutic regimen known as CHOP, followed by consolidative radiation therapy to his stomach and lymph nodes. The patient asks for additional information about the CHOP regimen, and you explain that this is a combination of four different drugs: cyclophosphamide, doxorubicin, vincristine, and prednisone.

1. When explaining the long-term complications of doxorubicin to the patient, what do you warn him about and what can be done to prevent or minimize this?

2. When explaining long-term complications associated with vincristine, of what do you warn the patient?

3. What long-term complications are associated with cyclophosphamide, and how can they be prevented?

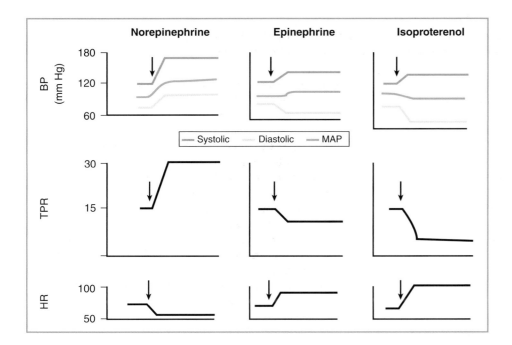

CASE STUDY 6

A clinical study is conducted in which a healthy volunteer is administered norepinephrine, epinephrine, and isoproterenol. Blood pressure (BP), total peripheral resistance (TPR), and heart rate (HR) are monitored during drug infusions. The results of this study are depicted in the accompanying figure.

1. **Explain the widely disparate results for these three adrenergic agonists.**

CASE STUDY 7

A 75-year-old male complains of "stomach pain" and massive rectal bleeding when passing stools. He is also gingerly holding his left shoulder. Upon questioning, he tells you that last week, he slipped on the ice and fell while shoveling snow. He was prescribed celecoxib by his family doctor for persistent shoulder pain and swelling. When the pain failed to resolve after a few days, this man scheduled a second appointment with his family physician. This time, his regular doctor was out of town, so he was seen instead by another partner in the practice, who prescribed ibuprofen. The pain has persisted for several weeks and during this time, he has been taking both celecoxib and ibuprofen regularly. In the middle of the night, the man was brought to the emergency room when he filled the toilet bowl with bloody stools twice. He was feeling faint and had nearly passed out before his wife was able to summon an ambulance. His past medical history includes hypertension and peptic ulcer disease. The hypertension is controlled with medication, and there have

been no ulcers in more than a decade. The following are the patient's pertinent laboratory values from his complete blood count (CBC), with normal values shown in parentheses:
Hemoglobin = 11.9 g/dL (13.8–17.2 g/dL)
Hematocrit = 34% (40.7% to 50.3%)
Mean corpuscular volume = 75.9 μm^3 (80.0–97.6 μm^3)
Mean corpuscular hemoglobin = 24.0 pg/cell
  (26.7–33/7 pg/cell)
Mean corpuscular hemoglobin concentration
  = 30.0 g/dL (32.7–35.5 g/dL)

1. **You suspect that because of his massive gastrointestinal bleeding, the patient is iron-deficient. What other tests might you wish to order to confirm your diagnosis?**

2. **What do you suppose contributed to patient's loss of iron?**

3. **Ultimately, surgical intervention was needed to halt the severe gastrointestinal bleeding, and the patient was discharged home with a prescription for iron supplements. What might you tell the patient and note in his chart regarding this iron therapy?**

CASE STUDY 8

A 45-year-old man enters a clinic for the first time. He tells the doctor, "I feel fine, but the nurse at work took my blood pressure. It was 150/100 mm Hg and 160/102 mm Hg on two different days. She says I need a check-up."

Despite a thorough examination to determine an identifiable cause for his hypertension, none was found, and the patient was given a diagnosis of stage 2 essential hypertension. The patient was instructed on lifestyle changes including (a) smoking cessation, (b) regular exercise, (c) alcohol limitations—no more than two beers per day, and (d) a low-fat, low-cholesterol, low-salt diet.

The patient was motivated to initiate these lifestyle modifications, so the physician prescribed only hydrochlorothiazide initially and scheduled a follow-up examination for 2 months later. The patient returned 2 weeks later with a painful, swollen, red big toe joint. His potassium level was 3.2 mEq/L (normal: 3.5 to 5.0 mEq/L) and uric acid was 11.9 mg/dL (normal: 3 to 8 mg/dL).

1. Account for the patient's painful toe and his abnormal laboratory values.

2. The patient's pharmacologic therapy was changed to atenolol. Although the patient's blood pressure had lowered to 132/94 with atenolol, his heart rate was only 50 beats per minute. The patient complained of easy fatigability and a reduction in exercise tolerance. Explain how atenolol causes these adverse effects.

3. Because the patient complained of other adverse effects associated with the β-blocker (e.g., reduced libido, sleep disturbances), it was decided that instead of lowering the dose, a drug from a different class would be tried. Atenolol was gradually tapered over a period of 1 week. Why was the dose of atenolol tapered slowly?

4. The patient was started on lisinopril. How does lisinopril work, and what adverse effects might the patient experience?

CASE STUDY 9

A 60-year-white male weighing 170 pounds is brought to the emergency room by his wife because his "ankles are swollen." You view the patient's extremities and note that he has stage 4 pitting edema in his ankles. The patient tells you that he has a history of poorly controlled hypertension. Before prescribing any medications, you ask the laboratory to check his Na$^+$, K$^+$, and serum creatinine. Pertinent laboratory values are:

K+: 3.5 [3.3–4.9 mmol/L]
Na+: 140 mmol/L [135–145 mmol/L]
Creatinine: 2.5 mg/dL [0.5–1.7 mg/dL]

1. What is this patient's creatinine clearance?

2. What is the best choice of medication to reduce this patient's edema on an outpatient basis?

3. At your suggestion, the patient follows up with the internal medicine department. In addition to having hypertension, he also finds out that he has type 2 diabetes. The internist gives the patient an additional prescription. Unfortunately, you see the patient again in the emergency room 2 weeks after his appointment with internal medicine. This time, he is complaining of an irregular heartbeat. An electrocardiogram (ECG) reveals that the patient has a prolonged PR interval and QRS duration, atrioventricular conduction delays, and a loss of P waves. Laboratory work reveals that his potassium level is elevated at 5.7 mEq/L. Which class of medication did the internist most likely prescribe for the patient's hypertension?

CASE STUDY 10

An 8-year-old boy with asthma has recently developed a nonproductive cough. His asthma has been well controlled over the last 3 years, since he started allergy desensitization immunotherapy (allergy shots). He is presently taking cromolyn (four puffs per day) as well as albuterol (two puffs) when needed or before exercise. He demonstrates good inhaler technique and uses a spacer. During your workup, you discover that the family has just "adopted" a puppy and the boy's asthma symptoms have been flaring up. His peak flow rates have been falling, and he has been having more nocturnal symptoms.

1. What is your plan to minimize and manage the child's asthma symptoms, given that the puppy remains in the household?

2. What adverse effects are especially of concern in a young child using inhaled corticosteroids?

CASE STUDY 11

A 49-year-old male has been given a diagnosis of hyperreactive airway disease and asthma. After a bout with influenza, he developed a recurrent cough that interferes with his job and active lifestyle. The cough and associated tight chest are unresponsive to over-the-counter cold and flu medications. The patient is somewhat surprised when you start working him up for GERD. He states that his stomach is fine and he has never had heartburn.

1. **What is the connection between asthma and GERD?**

2. **What agents can be given to the patient to treat his GERD symptoms?**

CASE STUDY 12

A. A 41-year-old woman is admitted for severe chest pains. She appears as a thin, flushed, nervous woman. Her complaints include nervousness, palpitations, weight loss despite strong appetite, and unexplained bruising. She states she is being treated for deep vein thrombosis with warfarin 5 mg/d. Physical examination reveals a BP of 190/95 mm Hg, pulse of 125 beats/min, and temperature of 102.6° F. Your exam also reveals droopy eyes, decreased visual acuity, an enlarged thyroid, atrial fibrillation, pitting edema, and tremor.

What is your initial diagnosis, and how would you treat the patient?

B. A 37-year-old female wants to breast-feed her first child. She requests information on contraception choices before leaving the hospital. She has a strong family history of cardiovascular disease and is presently a two-pack per day smoker. She previously had a conventional IUD device that was removed because of severe bleeding. She also states that spermicidal foams and condoms cause her itching and burning.

What type of contraception would you recommend to the patient?

Case Study Answers

CASE STUDY 1

1. Using the published value for Vd and the patient's weight, we calculate the patient's specific Vd:

$$Vd = (0.48 \text{ L/kg})(65 \text{ kg}) = 31.2 \text{ L}$$

2. Smokers are known to metabolize theophylline more rapidly than nonsmokers, and there is a "published" half-life that is used when dosing theophylline in a patient who is a cigarette smoker. Using the published $t_{1/2}$ value (4.5 hours) and the patient's estimated Vd (which we calculated in the previous question), we can now calculate the clearance for this patient:

$$Cl = \frac{0.693 \text{ (Vd)}}{t_{1/2}} = \frac{0.693 \text{ (31.2 L)}}{4.5 \text{ hr}} = 4.8 \text{ L/hr or } 80 \text{ mL/min}$$

3. Since the patient's plasma levels of theophylline are lower than the target values, we must give him a loading dose to quickly boost his theophylline values back into the target range. The following equation allows us to do this:

$$\text{Loading dose} = \frac{\text{(Vd)(Cp desired } - \text{ Cp initial)}}{F}$$

$$\text{Loading dose} = \frac{31.2 \text{ L (10 mg/L } - 3.6 \text{ mg/L)}}{1}$$

$$= 200 \text{ mg theophylline}$$

CASE STUDY 2

1. It is not uncommon for children to require higher theophylline dosages than adults do, so it is not entirely surprising that this woman has taken the same theophylline dose since she was a small child. There probably are two pharmacokinetic reasons for this. One has to do with volume of distribution, the other with hepatic metabolism. Recall that when clinicians dose theophylline, they are aiming for theophylline levels between 5 and 15 mg/L in the serum. Theophylline's volume of distribution is relatively restricted; it does not distribute into fatty tissue. In childhood, a larger percentage of the body is made up of water versus adipose tissue. This water, in essence, "dilutes" theophylline, so even though a child weighs less than an adult, there is more total body water in a child in which the theophylline is diluted. Children are routinely given larger mg/kg doses of theophylline than adults are.

  Secondly, during early childhood, the metabolic capacity of the liver reaches its peak level. After approximately 9 years of age, the liver's metabolic capacity begins a slow decline. Therefore, children hepatically metabolize theophylline faster than adults do, often necessitating larger doses than for adults.

  Although she weighs more now than she did as a child, her body composition is composed of less water (and more fat) and her hepatic metabolic capability declined with age (even in the absence of overt hepatic disease); therefore, she may actually require less drug on a mg/kg basis than she did as a child to maintain theophylline levels within the 5 to 15 mg/L target range. In spite of these factors (favoring effectiveness), the drug is currently ineffective. Something else is going on.

2. Rifampin is a potent inducer of P-450 hepatic enzymes. Since theophylline is metabolized by these same enzymes, rifampin could decrease theophylline levels, rendering theophylline less effective. This probably is what has occurred and probably is the reason this woman is having more breathing difficulties recently.

3. Cimetidine is a potent inhibitor of P-450 hepatic enzymes. Since theophylline is metabolized by these same enzymes, cimetidine could increase theophylline levels, leading to theophylline-related toxicities.

CASE STUDY 3

1. After the ABCs are addressed (airway, breathing circulation), the D component (decontamination) of toxicology management should be initiated. Orogastric lavage should be initiated, followed by ingestion of activated charcoal. Activated charcoal binds the toxic substance, preventing absorption. The patient is usually put into a left side (left lateral; decubitus), head down (Trendelenburg) position, to protect the airway from emesis and to limit transit of gastric contents into the small intestine.

2. Aspirin (salicylate) poisoning is consistent with the patient's initial symptoms. Salicylates directly stimulate the respiratory center in the medulla to cause hyperpnea and tachypnea. This rapid deep breathing leads to an initial respiratory alkalosis. The elevation in body temperature is consistent with salicylate uncoupling of oxidative phosphorylation. Salicylates are gastric irritants and will trigger vomiting and cramps.

3. Salicylates directly stimulate the respiratory center in the medulla to cause hyperpnea and tachypnea. This rapid deep breathing leads to an initial respiratory alkalosis. The increased respiration rate results in increased CO_2 removal at the lung, which decreases H ion concentration in plasma. Remember that $CO_2 + H_2O = H_2CO_3 = H^+ + HCO_3^-$.

4. Compensation for the initial respiratory alkalosis is achieved by increased renal excretion of HCO_3^-, accompanied by a decrease in renal bicarbonate reabsorption. This mechanism explains the low bicarbonate levels in the plasma of the first blood sample. By uncoupling oxidative phosphorylation, plasma CO_2 levels increase faster than CO_2 can be removed by enhanced respiration (now driven by acidosis), furthering exacerbating acidosis. In addition, derangement of carbohydrate metabolism leads to accumulation of lactic acid and pyruvate, and impaired renal function leads to accumulation of sulfuric and phosphoric acids. As metabolic acidosis worsens and urine acidifies, excretion of weak acid salicylate metabolites will decrease.

5. To reduce the metabolic acidosis, an intravenous bolus of sodium bicarbonate or addition of sodium bicarbonate to D5W (5% dextrose in water) should be initiated. Additional, oral activated charcoal can be administered. To correct for low K^+ plasma levels (increased excretion of K^+ is an indirect result of diminished reabsorption of bicarbonate), intravenous potassium can be delivered. In extreme cases, hemodialysis can be started to remove salicylate metabolites. In the case of salicylate-induced seizures, phenobarbital may be administered.

2. Since the patient has no prior history of cardiovascular disease but has a high fever and has been having episodes of diarrhea and vomiting for more than 12 hours, her cardiac arrhythmias are probably related to electrolyte disturbances, especially hypokalemia.

3. Although it is possible that streptococci or staphylococci isolated from a scab on the patient's scalp are simply normal flora, you cannot rule out the possibility that either one (or both) of these microorganisms might be the cause of her current infection. Most of the penicillins will provide adequate coverage against streptococcal organisms; however, whenever staphylococci are isolated, it must be assumed that the organisms make β-lactamases. Therefore, a penicillinase-resistant penicillin is the most appropriate drug of choice for this patient. Since the patient was quite ill by the time she came to the emergency room, it is appropriate to admit her and initiate intravenous nafcillin.

4. *Clostridium difficile* may be part of a patient's normal gastrointestinal flora, but this bacterium often overgrows under opportune conditions, such as during or immediately following antibacterial therapy. Alternatively, the organism may have been acquired at the hospital, since many institutions report difficulties controlling the spread of this bacterium from patient to patient, probably as a result of poor hand-washing techniques on the part of the staff. Typically, metronidazole is the first-choice antibiotic used to treat *C. difficile* infections; however, patients should be warned that strict avoidance of alcohol is imperative. Vancomycin is the only other antibiotic reliably used to treat infections caused by *C. difficile*. Although most patients initially respond to treatment with metronidazole or vancomycin, as many as 3% to 5% of patients will continually relapse. Use of probiotics may be considered, since this type of therapy addresses the real issue underlying *C. difficile* diarrhea, which is not the mere presence of the microorganism in the gastrointestinal tract but rather an absence of "healthy" bacteria that can keep clostridial growth in check. Probiotic therapies replace some of the missing "healthy" bacterial species and have even been used successfully in patients who were refractory to treatment with metronidazole and vancomycin.

CASE STUDY 4

1. Erysipelas is an infection of subcutaneous tissues. Patients often have a fever and dermatologic findings. Muscle and joint pains, nausea, headache, and skin discomfort often are noted as well. A defect in the skin barrier permits the infection to occur, e.g., trauma, abrasion, skin ulcer, insect bite, eczema, or psoriatic lesions. Group A streptococci are the most common organisms responsible for erysipelas, followed by groups G, C, and B streptococci or staphylococci.

CASE STUDY 5

1. Doxorubicin is associated with cardiotoxicity that may be life-threatening. The likelihood of cardiotoxicity and its severity is related to the cumulative dose received. Because of the patient's history of hypertension, he is already at risk of cardiotoxicity. Other risk factors include preexisting cardiac disease, prior thoracic radiation therapy, and very young or very old age. A technitium-99 based Multiple Gated Acquisition scan (MUGA scan) should be obtained prior to initiating therapy to evaluate

ejection fraction. Doxorubicin therapy is often discontinued if left ventricular ejection fraction falls <45%, since additional therapy could lead to irreversible heart failure.

2. Vincristine is associated with dose-limiting neurotoxicity, especially peripheral neuropathy. Those with existing neurologic diseases and the elderly are most susceptible. Typically, neurotoxicity is a cumulative effect that occurs only after several treatments. As a result, patients should be given a neurologic assessment at baseline and prior to each treatment. If the patient has a history of long-standing diabetes mellitus with accompanying peripheral neuropathies, vincristine could aggravate them.

3. Cyclophosphamide is associated with secondary myeloproliferative and lymphoproliferative malignancies, bladder fibrosis and bladder cancer, and sterility. Bladder problems may be prevented by maintaining adequate hydration and administering mesna therapy.
(Mesna stands for sodium 2-mercaptoethane sulfonate, an agent that reacts with acrolein and other urotoxic metabolites of cyclophosphamide or ifosfamide to form stable, nonurotoxic compounds. Mesna does not have any antitumor activity, nor does it appear to interfere with the antitumor activity of antineoplastic drugs.)

However, under conditions of fight-or-flight, cardiac output must increase, and increased perfusion of skeletal muscles also is necessary. This is accomplished through mechanisms that produce the physiologic tracings shown for epinephrine. Epinephrine stimulates α- and β-receptors. When epinephrine stimulates β_2-receptors in the vasculature, the typical α effect is overridden, leading to vasodilation and accompanying decrease in TPR (thereby increasing blood flow to the muscle). Therefore, diastolic pressure falls. Simultaneously stimulation of β_1-receptors within the heart produces a dramatic increase in heart rate and contractility. There is a corresponding increase in systolic pressure with a modest change or no change in mean arterial pressure.

The effect of epinephrine is most dramatically illustrated by comparison with infusion of isoproterenol, a β-selective agonist. Here, there is a dramatic drop in TPR because the β_2 response is unopposed by any α_1 effect. Additionally, systolic pressure rises because of the increased blood pressure that results from stimulation of mycoardial β_1-receptors. The foregoing discussion is of great importance because of the tendency to lump all adrenergic agonists into one large class of stimulatory agents. Based on their roles in the integrated physiology of the autonomic nervous system, there is tremendous diversity in pharmacologic responses to these agents.

CASE STUDY 6

In this clinical study, intravenous infusion of norepinephrine produces a rise in both systolic and diastolic blood pressure. Stimulation of α-receptors, accompanying vasoconstriction, and the increase in total peripheral resistance (TPR) (see the middle tracing) are responsible for the rise in blood pressure.

However, when administering adrenergic agents, don't forget about the baroreceptors. Because of reflex actions of baroreceptors, heart rate actually declines. Therefore, despite the fact that norepinephrine also stimulates β-receptors on the heart, because of the reflex activity of baroreceptors there may actually be a decline in pulse rate as sympathetic outflow is blocked and vagal (parasympathetic) tone temporarily predominates.

A common misconception is to consider epinephrine and norepinephrine as having the same pharmacologic actions. Compare the results of norepinephrine infusion with the results of epinephrine infusion. Following infusion of epinephrine, there is a rise in systolic pressure with a *fall* in diastolic pressure. This is counterintuitive and arises specifically because of stimulation of β_2-receptors in the vasculature.

Under normal conditions, the body is under the control of sympathetic norepinephrine-releasing nerves. These nerves "talk" directly to α_1-receptors and lead to vasoconstriction and increased TPR. This is the minute-to-minute regulation of blood pressure that prevents postural hypotension.

CASE STUDY 7

1. Perhaps the best indicators of iron deficiency anemia are a decrease in serum ferritin level and an elevated total iron-binding capacity (TIBC). Additionally, a peripheral blood smear might be performed, which would be expected to reveal hypochromic microcytic red blood cells if your suspicion is correct.

2. The patient has a history of peptic ulcer disease. Despite that history, two different physicians prescribed nonsteroidal anti-inflammatories for him, and the second doctor failed to tell the patient to stop taking the celecoxib when the ibuprofen was recommended. Although celecoxib is COX-2 specific, gastrointestinal bleeding may still occur, even when it is used alone, and this patient was taking celecoxib concomitantly with ibuprofen. Use of the NSAIDs caused the gastrointestinal bleeding, which in turn caused the iron deficiency.

3. Iron may cause constipation, but this can be prevented with a stool softener. Iron may also cause stools to darken in color. Iron therapy will most likely be continued for 3 to 6 months to ensure saturation of all iron stores. Serum ferritin will be the best predictor to monitor iron stores after correction of hemoglobin and hematocrit.

CASE STUDY 8

1. Hydrochlorothiazide, a first-line antihypertensive drug for most patients, may cause hyperuricemia and hypokalemia. In this patient, hyperuricemia precipitated an acute gout attack, thus the reason for the painful, swollen, red toe.

   Patients need to have potassium levels monitored with both thiazide and loop diuretics. Unless a sufficient amount of K^+ is obtained from dietary sources (e.g., bananas, orange juice), a potassium supplement is often necessary.

2. Atenolol is a β_1-selective antagonist; that is, the drug prevents norepinephrine from interacting with β_1-receptors. When β_1-receptors in the myocardium are blocked, both resting heart rate and exercise-induced heart rates are slowed.
   β-Blockers can precipitate AV blockade, too.

3. During therapy with β-blockers, there is up-regulation of β-receptors. Rapid discontinuation of β-blockers can promote a hyperadrenergic state, leading to tachycardia.

4. Lisinopril is an angiotensin-converting enzyme (ACE) inhibitor. ACE inhibitors prevent conversion of angiotensin I to angiotensin II. Since angiotensin II is a potent vasoconstrictor in the arteries and veins, lisinopril will lower total peripheral resistance by acting in a balanced fashion throughout the vasculature. Additionally, since angiotensin II stimulates aldosterone release, this drug will prevent Na^+ and fluid retention that is mediated by the renin-angiotensin-aldosterone system.

   ACE inhibitors may cause hyperkalemia, and up to 40% of patients may experience a dry cough, thought to result from bradykinin accumulation. Angioedema of lips and tongue may also occur. In the event of a persistent cough, the patient can be switched to an angiotensin receptor blocker.

CASE STUDY 9

1. Creatinine clearance is calculated according to the following formula:

   $$\text{CrCl (mL/min)} = \frac{[(140 - \text{age})(\text{body weight in kg})]}{(\text{Serum creatinine})(72)}$$

   1 pound = 2.2 kg, so the patient weighs 77 kg. We know the patient's age and we know his serum creatinine measurement, so we can calculate creatinine clearance.

   For this patient,

   $$\text{CrCl (mL/min)} = \frac{[(140 - 60)(77 \text{ kg})]}{(2.5)(72)} = 34 \text{ mL/min}$$

2. Because of their action in the loop of Henle (the region of the nephron with the greatest potential for sodium reabsorption), loop diuretics like furosemide are the best choices for reducing this patient's fluid overload. Spironolactone is rarely used in men because of its antiandrogenic side effects. Thiazides cannot eliminate large amounts of fluid. Additionally, given the patient's declining kidney function, furosemide is a superior choice to hydrochlorothiazide, since most thiazides are ineffective at low glomerular filtration rates. Mannitol is used only intravenously, so it is not appropriate for outpatient management of edema. A potassium supplement is often prescribed along with furosemide to counteract the loss of K^+ associated with the use of loop diuretics.

3. The patient's electrocardiogram findings are consistent with hyperkalemia. Angiotensin-converting enzyme (ACE) inhibitors such as enalapril, as well as angiotensin receptor blockers (ARBs) elevate serum potassium levels by interfering with the downstream actions of aldosterone in the kidneys. Since the patient was already taking potassium supplements, the addition of an ACE inhibitor or an ARB caused his potassium levels to rise to dangerously high levels, despite the loop diuretic that he was taking.

   Periodic monitoring of potassium levels is imperative when combining medications such as diuretics, potassium supplements, ACE inhibitors, or ARBs, which can alter potassium levels. Additionally, patients should be cautioned about eating certain foods that contain large amounts of K^+ such as bananas, orange juice, and potassium-containing "salt" substitutes while taking prescription potassium supplements or potassium-retaining medications.

CASE STUDY 10

1. The boy should be reassessed for allergy to dog dander. (A common misconception is that allergies to dogs are caused by dog hair. They are not. Pet allergies are caused by pet dander.) The puppy should be barred from the second floor, where the child's room is located (trigger avoidance). Carpeting in the child's bedroom should be replaced with wood or rubberized flooring to minimize accumulation of pet dander in the bedroom. The house should be dusted and vacuumed regularly with a vacuum that has a high-quality filtration system (preferably one that is vented outdoors). Electrostatic filters can also be placed over air vents in the house. Regular bathing of the puppy may help.

   If additional pharmacotherapy is needed, cromolyn can be discontinued and replaced with inhaled corticosteroids. In addition, montelukast, a leukotriene receptor antagonist, might be added to the treatment regimen. If necessary, a long-acting β_2-agonist may also be added. In essence, stepwise therapy might be instituted until the child's symptoms are brought under control.

2. Corticosteroids cause linear growth suppression. This is seen even with inhaled corticosteroids. There is an average height difference of 1 cm per year between children treated with inhaled corticosteroids and controls. However, the risks of not adequately controlling asthma are more dangerous than the growth suppression.

   As for all patients using inhaled corticosteroids, the child should rinse his mouth with water after using the inhaled corticosteroid to prevent thrush (an oral fungal infection).

CASE STUDY 11

1. Airway constriction occurs in response to refluxed gastric acids. Results from some studies suggest that as many as 63% of children with asthma may have GERD.

2. A proton pump inhibitor, such as omeprazole, may be added to the patient's other medications, which include nasal and orally inhaled glucocorticoids as well as a leukotriene receptor antagonist.

CASE STUDY 12

A. You suspect that the patient is experiencing life-threatening thyrotoxicosis (thyroid storm). As you are ordering thyroid tests to confirm your diagnosis, you aggressively manage cardiac events and fever with β-blockers and aspirin. To stabilize the patient before thyroid surgery, you use a combination of thionamide and iodide to suppress the overactive thyroid gland.

B. You might suggest a progestin-only "mini-pill" during the period of time that she is breast-feeding. Estrogen-containing formulations may suppress lactation. However, you will caution her that this type of contraception requires a commitment to take the pill at the same time each day to achieve maximal efficacy. Another option would be medroxyprogesterone injection every 3 months. However, you must warn her of the possibility of bone loss, a recently identified complication of depot medroxyprogesterone. After she finishes breast-feeding her child, you may switch her to a low-dose estrogen/progestin formulation. You might counsel her that smoking and estrogen contraception places her at high risk for thromboembolic events.

Index